FIRST AID FOR THE

WARDS

FOR THE CLINICAL YEARS

INSIDER | **2nd Edition** | **ADVICE**

TAO LE, MD
University of California, San Francisco, Class of 1996
Johns Hopkins University, Fellow in Allergy and Clinical Immunology

VIKAS BHUSHAN, MD
University of California, San Francisco, Class of 1991

CHIRAG AMIN, MD
University of Miami, Class of 1996

NADER POURATIAN, PhD
Student Editor
Geffen School of Medicine, Class of 2003

JESSICA NORD, MD
Student Editor
Geffen School of Medicine, Class of 2002

McGraw-Hill
Medical Publishing Division

New York   Chicago   San Francisco   Lisbon   London   Madrid
Mexico City   Milan   New Delhi   San Juan   Seoul
Singapore   Sydney   Toronto

*The **McGraw·Hill** Companies*

First Aid for the Wards, Second Edition

Information from the following title was adapted and incorporated with permission: Segen JC, *Current Med Talk*, Appleton & Lange, 1995.

1 2 3 4 5 6 7 8 9 0   CUS/CUS   0 9 8 7 6 5 4 3 2

ISBN 0-8385-2578-4

Notice

Medicine is an ever-changing science. As new research and clinical experience broaden our knowledge, changes in treatment and drug therapy are required. The authors and the publisher of this work have checked with sources believed to be reliable in their efforts to provide information that is complete and generally in accord with the standards accepted at the time of publication. However, in view of the possibility of human error or changes in medical sciences, neither the authors nor the publisher nor any other party who has been involved in the preparation or publication of this work warrants that the information contained herein is in every respect accurate or complete, and they disclaim all responsibility for any errors or omissions or for the results obtained from use of the information contained in this work. Readers are encouraged to confirm the information contained herein with other sources. For example and in particular, readers are advised to check the product information sheet included in the package of each drug they plan to administer to be certain that the information contained in this work is accurate and that changes have not been made in the recommended dose or in the contraindications for administration. This recommendation is of particular importance in connection with new or infrequently used drugs.

This book was set in Goudy by Rainbow Graphics.
The editor was Catherine A. Johnson.
The production supervisor was Lisa Mendez.
Project management was provided by Rainbow Graphics.
The interior designer was Elizabeth Sanders.
The index was prepared by Oneida Indexing.
Von Hoffmann Graphics was printer and binder.

This book is printed on acid-free paper.

To all our contributors, who took time to share their experience, advice,
and humor for the benefit of students
&
To our families, friends, and loved ones, who endured and assisted in the task
of assembling this guide.

Contributing Authors

JENNIFER LAFEMINA
Geffen School of Medicine, Class of 2003

ZACHARY V. EDMONDS
Geffen School of Medicine and Anderson
School of Management, Class of 2003

JEANNINE RAHIMIAN, MD, MBA
Geffen School of Medicine
Resident in Obstetrics & Gynecology

Faculty Reviewers

LLOYD BROWN, MD
Associate Director, Pediatric Residency
    Training Program
Cedars-Sinai Medical Center
Associate Professor of Pediatrics
Geffen School of Medicine

BARRY H. GUZE, MD
Professor Psychiatry and Biobehavioral Sciences
UCLA Neuropsychiatric Hospital

SIMERJOT K. JASSAL, MD
Chief Resident, Department of Medicine
Geffen School of Medicine

MARTHA LOVE, MD
Chief Resident Psychiatry and Biobehavioral
    Sciences
UCLA Neuropsychiatric Hospital

PEGGY B. MILES, MD
Director, Faculty Services
Director, Internal Medicine Clinics
Cedars-Sinai Medical Center

PERRIN PLENINGER, MD
Associate Professor of Neurology
Geffen School of Medicine

RITA OREGON, MD
Assistant Clinical Professor
Department of Obstetrics and Gynecology
Olive View Hospital

SRINATH SANDA, MD
Staff Physician
Departments of Internal Medicine and Pediatrics
Cedars-Sinai Medical Center
Assistant Clinical Professor of Medicine
Geffen School of Medicine

CHRISTIAN DE VIRGILIO, MD
General Surgery Residency Program Director
Harbor-UCLA Medical Center
Associate Professor of Surgery
Geffen School of Medicine

Contents

Chapter 7: Psychiatry 369

Preface

The change from the passive and controlled environment of the classroom to the fast-paced and active world of the wards can be stressful, confusing, and downright frightening at times. The purpose of *First Aid for the Wards* is to help ease the transition wards students must make as they begin their clerkship rotations. This book is a student-to-student guide that draws on the advice and experiences of medical students who were successful on the wards. It is our hope to familiarize you with life on the wards and to pass on some of the "secrets of success" that we picked up along the way in our training. The facts and wisdom contained within this book are an amalgam of information we, the authors, wished we had known at the beginning of our third year of medical school. *First Aid for the Wards* has a number of unique features that make it an indispensable guide for MD, DO, and DPM students:

- Insider advice from students on how to succeed on your clinical rotations.
- Sample H&P notes, daily progress notes, procedure notes, post-op notes, labor and delivery notes, and admission orders.
- Specific advice on how to give both concise and detailed oral patient presentations.
- Descriptions of typical daily responsibilities and interactions on each core rotation, including medicine, pediatrics, obstetrics and gynecology, neurology, psychiatry, and surgery.
- Key wards lingo with definitions courtesy of Dr. Joseph Segen and *Current Med Talk*.
- High-yield topics outlining the signs and symptoms, differential diagnosis, workup, and treatment of the important and commonly encountered diseases of each rotation.
- Student- and peer-reviewed evaluations of more than 160 commonly used handbooks, reference books, texts, and electronic resources, specifically addressing their usefulness to medical students on the wards.

First Aid for the Wards is meant to be a survival guide rather than a comprehensive source of information. It should supplement information and advice provided by other students, house staff, and faculty. It is designed not to replace reference texts as a source of information but rather to provide some essential background information for each core ward rotation. Although the material has been reviewed by medical faculty and students, errors and omissions are inevitable. We urge readers to suggest improvements and identify inaccuracies. We invite students and faculty to continue sharing their thoughts and ideas to help us improve *First Aid for the Wards* (see How to Contribute, page xxi).

Baltimore   Tao Le
Los Angeles   Vikas Bhushan
Los Angeles   Chirag Amin
Los Angeles   Nader Pouratian
Los Angeles   Jessica Nord

Acknowledgments

This collaborative project would not have been possible without the thoughtful comments, insights, and advice of the many medical students and faculty whom we gratefully acknowledge for their support in the development of *First Aid for the Wards*.

Special thanks to Andrea Fellows, our tireless editor, Selina Bush, our developmental editor, the section editors, contributors, and faculty reviewers for bringing the book together under constant pressure. For enthusiasm, support, and commitment for this project, thanks to our acquisitions editor, Catherine Johnson. For copyediting support, we thank Bridget Mooney. For speedy typesetting of all those last-minute changes, we thank the staff at Rainbow Graphics.

For helping to review the books in this edition, we thank Maria Rumsey, Rosanna Gray-Swain, Christian Ramers, Jennifer Moranda, Matthew J. Elias, Alexander C. Tsai, Jane Bang, Rahul Tendulkar, Erica Goorevich, Donna Mazloomdoost, Kiran Beyer, Ginger Bohl, Nirav Shah, Wes Crisp, Daniel Perry, Andrew Tang, Tracy Mueller, Michael Huang, George Dittrick, Robin L. Epp, Devi Nampiaparampil, Melissa MacCoy-Zale, Justine Yun, Thomas Carroll, Brooke E. Hohn, Liezl Irisari, Justin B. Rufener, David Lee, Jennifer R. Chan, Gretchen Kluesner, Andrew C. Eppstein, Edward Piepmeier, Amitpal Johal, Sandeep M. Chadha, Jose A. T. Suros, Matthew Sunderlin, Alicia Rogers, David Vadnais, Mila Felder, Tony Recker, Melanie J. Donnelly, Bismruta Misra, Barry McKenzie, Lily Limsuvanrot, Lemi Luu, James Kong, Chris Carlson, David Lloyd, Borislava Burt, Claire Najim, Parmi Suchdev, Lin Jin, Matthew Hurford, Parka Oldenburg, Sabah Igbal, Michael Baldovsky, Stephanie Hemm, Julianna Whiteman, Michele Brown, Geneen Gin, Sandra Taylor, Shelby Clarke, Sean Frederick, Kishore Vellody, Sara Myers, Laurent Dreyfuss, Stephen Moses, Stephanie Fong, Deborah Lloyd, Joan Cavin, Nandish Thukral, Ellen Amador, Kristin Egan, Jason Morgan, Amish Patel, Kari Hultgren, J Anspach, Carrie Bassett, Fernando Fleischman, Nathan Radcliffe, and Jeremy Graff.

Thanks to Geffen School of Medicine, Harvard Medical School, UC San Francisco School of Medicine, and the University of Washington School of Medicine for sharing their curriculum materials.

We apologize if we have forgotten anyone. Please e-mail us for the next edition.

How to Contribute

First Aid for the Wards is a work in progress—a collaborative project that was refined through the many contributions and changes received from students and faculty. The authors and McGraw-Hill intend to update *First Aid for the Wards* so that the book grows both in quality and in scope while continuing to serve as a timely guidebook to survival and success on the wards. We invite you to participate in this process by passing on your own insights.

Please send us:

- Tips for survival and success on the wards.
- New topics, diagrams, and tables that you feel should be included in the next edition.
- Mnemonics or algorithms you have used on the wards.
- Personal ratings and comments on books that you have used while on the hospital wards, including books that were not reviewed in this edition.
- Your medical school's handbook to the clerkships.
- Corrections and clarifications.

For each entry incorporated into the next edition, you will receive a **$10 Amazon.com gift certificate**, as well as a personal acknowledgment in the next edition. Significant contributions will be compensated at the discretion of the publisher.

The preferred way to submit suggestions and contributions is via electronic mail. Please include name, address, school affiliation, phone number, and e-mail address (if different from address of origin). If there are multiple entries, please consolidate into a single e-mail or file attachment. Please send submissions to:

firstaidteam@yahoo.com

You can also use the contribution forms on the following pages. Feel free to photocopy these forms or attach additional pages as needed. Please send your contributions and corrections, neatly written or typed, to:

Attn: Contributions
First Aid for the Wards
1015 Gayley Ave., #1113
Los Angeles, CA 90024

Note to Contributors

All entries become properties of the authors and are subject to review and edits. Please verify all data and spelling carefully. In the event that similar or duplicate entries are received, only the first entry received will be used. Include a reference to a standard textbook to facilitate verification of the fact. Please follow the style, punctuation, and format of this edition if possible.

Contribution Form I

For entries, facts, corrections, diagrams, etc.

Contributor Name:_____

School/Affiliation:_____

Address:_____

_____

Telephone:_____

E-mail:_____

Topic:

Signs & Symptoms:

Workup:

Treatment:

Notes, Diagrams, Tables, or Mnemonics:

Reference:

Please seal with tape only.
No staples or paper clips.

- (fold here) -

BUSINESS REPLY MAIL
FIRST-CLASS MAIL PERMIT NO. 74036 LOS ANGELES CA

POSTAGE WILL BE PAID BY ADDRESSEE

FIRST AID FOR THE WARDS
1015 GAYLEY AVE. #1113
LOS ANGELES CA 90024-8980

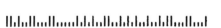

- (fold here) -

Contribution Form II

For book reviews

Contributor Name:_____

School/Affiliation:_____

Address: _____

_____

Telephone:_____

E-mail:_____

We welcome additional comments on books rated in this edition, as well as reviews of texts not included in this edition. Please fill out each review entry as completely as possible. Please do not leave "Comments" blank. Rate all books using the letter grading (A^+ to C^-), taking into consideration the other books on that subject.

Title/Author: _____

Publisher/Series: _____   ISBN Number: _____

Rating: _____   Comments: _____

_____

_____

Title/Author: _____

Publisher/Series: _____   ISBN Number: _____

Rating: _____   Comments: _____

_____

_____

Title/Author: _____

Publisher/Series: _____   ISBN Number: _____

Rating: _____   Comments: _____

_____

_____

Title/Author: _____

Publisher/Series: _____   ISBN Number: _____

Rating: _____   Comments: _____

_____

_____

Title/Author: _____

Publisher/Series: _____   ISBN Number: _____

Rating: _____   Comments: _____

_____

You will receive personal acknowledgment and a $10 gift certificate for each entry that is used in future editions of First Aid for the Wards

Please seal with tape only.
No staples or paper clips.

--------------------------------- (fold here) ---------------------------------

**NO POSTAGE
NECESSARY
IF MAILED
IN THE
UNITED STATES**

BUSINESS REPLY MAIL
FIRST-CLASS MAIL PERMIT NO. 74036 LOS ANGELES CA

POSTAGE WILL BE PAID BY ADDRESSEE

**FIRST AID FOR THE WARDS
1015 GAYLEY AVE. #1113
LOS ANGELES CA 90024-8980**

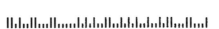

--------------------------------- (fold here) ---------------------------------

User Survey

Contributor Name:_____

School/Affiliation:_____

Address:_____

_____

Telephone:_____

E-mail:_____

What student-to-student advice would you give to a student about to begin his or her clerkships?

Is there any advice in this book that you believe should be altered or amended? How can it be improved?

Have you experienced any "difficult situations" on the wards that were not covered in this edition or that you feel should be handled differently? Do you have any advice to others on how to deal with similar situations?

What would you change about the high-yield topics? Were the entries too superficial, too detailed, or just right?

How else would you improve *First Aid for the Wards*? Any other comments or suggestions? What did you like most about the book?

Please seal with tape only.
No staples or paper clips.

-- (fold here) --

NO POSTAGE
NECESSARY
IF MAILED
IN THE
UNITED STATES

BUSINESS REPLY MAIL
FIRST-CLASS MAIL PERMIT NO. 74036 LOS ANGELES CA

POSTAGE WILL BE PAID BY ADDRESSEE

FIRST AID FOR THE WARDS
1015 GAYLEY AVE. #1113
LOS ANGELES CA 90024-8980

-- (fold here) --

Guide for Wards Success

INTRODUCTION

For the past two years, you have been learning medicine in classrooms, labs, the library, and the floor of your bedroom. During this period, you may have spent some time on the hospital wards, observing, taking histories, and practicing physical exams. Up to this point, however, your presence on the wards has largely been superfluous. All that is about to change. You are finally about to practice medicine. You will now be an integral part of an organized team and will be given real responsibilities. And yes, you will have your own patients.

So relax.

The transition from the controlled environment of the classroom to the dynamic and often chaotic wards will be one of the most exhilarating periods in your training. The purpose of this book is to make your transition to the wards as smooth and stress free as possible by familiarizing you with the inner workings of each service and the common pitfalls that many students encounter. Some common mistakes that students make when coming to the wards include:

- Not understanding the responsibilities and expectations for the rotation.
- Not seeking timely feedback.
- Not using appropriate pocket references and clinical texts.
- Not knowing what to study on the wards.
- Inefficient organization and execution of daily work.
- Insufficient preparation for oral presentations for attending rounds.
- Not streamlining personal and family responsibilities.
- Scheduling key rotations too early or too late.

In this section, we will offer advice to help you avoid these pitfalls and be more productive in your clinical rotations. It is important, however, to first understand the wards experience itself.

THE TEAM

To succeed on the wards, you should understand how your team works and how you fit in. Your goal should be to function as a productive team member, to care for your patients, and, of course, to learn. Winning friends and allies on the team can help ensure that you get the best teaching and support possible and that you always get the benefit of the doubt. For example, if you help the intern with daily patient care, also known as SCUT WORK, he or she may prep you for the inevitable PIMP questions that the attending or resident may ask. On the other hand, making the intern or resident look bad in front of the attending will compromise your team's trust in you.

SCUT WORK: Menial, non-patient-care-related activities that are often passed to medical students (externs) or interns, although they are actually the responsibility of other health-care workers; the array of "scut" details is vast and includes obtaining supplies; performing ward paperwork; going to the pharmacy, laboratory, and emergency room with specimens or paperwork; acting as an orderly; cleaning the nurses' station; going for pizza; and so on. Scut duties are often cited as a subtle form of "medical student abuse."

PIMPING: A practice in which persons in power ask esoteric questions of junior colleagues, usually with the sole purpose of publicly demeaning them, which most often occurs on ward rounds with a chief of service in a university hospital. The interrogating "pimper" is theoretically interested in correct answers; the "pimpee," usually a medical student, is interested in self-esteem, although correct answers to the questions gain neither recognition nor relief from this form of harassment. Pimping serves to establish a "pecking order" among the medical staff. DISADVANTAGE: It suppresses spontaneous or intellectual questions or pursuits, creates an antagonistic atmosphere, and perpetuates medical student abuse (JAMA 1989; 262:2541–2; 263:1632c).

A medical team typically consists of the following members:

Attending

As the head of the team, the attending is usually involved in the most critical treatment decisions affecting your patients, such as whether a patient needs chemotherapy versus radiotherapy for that tumor. The logistics (e.g., scheduling, fine-tuning of treatment) are typically left to the resident and intern. On certain surgical services, the chief resident acts as the head of the team and reports to several "attending" surgeons. The attending is legally and morally responsible for the actions of each member of the team. Thus, the attending is ultimately responsible for educating and evaluating the resident, intern, and medical students.

You will have far less contact with the attending than with the other members of your team. Because the attending sees you mostly during attending rounds, buffed oral presentations are usually the key to making a good impression on him or her. The attending will also see your admit note and will often ask you questions at the patient's bedside. Therefore, knowing the patient inside out will keep you from falling on your face. You should also have a basic understanding of the patient's problem and the rationale behind the treatment plan.

Resident

The resident (PGY-2 and up) is a house officer who has gone through internship. As such, he or she works closely with the attending to devise and manage the treatment plan for your patient. The resident is also responsible for teaching you and the intern via didactics or informal pimping. Do not be afraid of pimp questions. No one expects you to be able to answer all of them. Junior medical students often report to interns, whereas subinterns usually report directly to the resident.

The resident monitors and sometimes supervises your daily activities. You can make a strong impression by making concise work-round presentations, demonstrating a strong fund of knowledge regarding your patient's illness and how it affects your treatment plan, maintaining an awareness of all events pertaining to your patient (e.g., the latest CXR results), showing hustle and effort in scut work, and providing occasional review articles that address treatment issues affecting your patients. The best articles you can find are often "review articles" from respected journals in the field. If the team has a conference scheduled, find out the topic ahead of time and copy articles for the team.

Intern

Intern rules: Eat when you can, sleep when you can, leave when you can.

The intern (PGY-1) provides the "muscle" that gets the practical aspects of wards work done for the team and is responsible for executing the treatment plan under the direct supervision of the resident. Any patient care that does not get done falls in the lap of the poor intern. Because interns are usually the most overworked members of the team, they do little didactic teaching, but they are excellent sources of information on how to get tasks done quickly and efficiently. While you are a physician-in-training, they are teachers-in-training. The junior clerk often reports directly to the intern.

Interns can be your best friends; keep them informed.

Inasmuch as they were recently students, interns are your most natural allies. Although interns are not usually involved in your formal evaluations, they will let the resident know how you're doing. Keeping your intern up to date on patients will earn points. Lightening the scut burden will allow your intern to finish earlier and spend more time working in the OR or reading about patients' problems. It should also give the intern more time to go through the patients with you. So volunteering for "thankless" duties will not only win the intern's gratitude but also get you more one-on-one teaching in return. In contrast, neglecting scut work will force the intern to do it all to the detriment of your education.

Subintern

The subintern is a fourth-year student who has the same responsibilities as the intern. Although subinterns have no responsibility for evaluating or teaching you and usually do not cover your patients, they can often be a valuable source of clinical pearls and practical information about the wards and applying for residency. Often, however, subinterns are overwhelmed by the amount of responsibility heaped upon them, so don't take it personally if they run past you in a frenzy down the hallway.

Nurse

A good rapport with the nursing staff is one of the keys to a successful and enjoyable rotation. Ward nurses carry out the written physician orders and attend to the daily needs of the patient. Nurses are experienced in patient care and know a great deal about what is going on with patients. Accordingly, they can often give you the "scoop" on your patient when you preround in the morning.

Nurses can make or break your rotation.

Learn the names of the nurses who are caring for your patients and treat them as your equals. (Do not walk around barking orders rudely, or you will quickly find out how critical it is to get along with the nurses, especially when you are trying to sleep on call.) Respect the nurses' opinions, but also double-check with your resident or intern. If something goes wrong, you will often be held responsible.

Never leave a mess for the nurse to clean up, and make sure you exchange relevant clinical information. If nurses like you, they may feed you extra information on your patient, clue you in on important treatment issues, and take the time to teach you important scut skills, such as placing Foley catheters or inserting IV lines. Be friendly yet assertive when asking for help.

Never leave a mess.

NURSE PRACTITIONER: A nurse certified to diagnose illness and physical conditions and perform therapeutic and corrective measures within a designated specialty area of practice. NPs may write orders for routine laboratory and clinical tests and prescribe routine drugs (i.e., not controlled substances), devices, and immunizing agents as specified in his or her privileges in a particular health care environment or hospital; all such orders must be countersigned by an attending physician.

PHYSICIAN ASSISTANT: An individual who is qualified to perform a wide variety of medically related tasks under a physician's supervision, including taking a patient's history and performing physical examinations and autopsies. EDUCATION: Two postgraduate years beyond college or university, training as a physician assistant, surgeon assistant, or pathologist assistant. Physician assistants may then subspecialize for a one- to two-year period in various fields, including neonatology, pediatrics, emergency medicine, and occupational medicine.

CURRENT *Med Talk*

Ward Clerk

The ward clerk deals with many administrative issues affecting your patient. Specifically, he or she takes written orders off the charts, schedules procedures and lab tests, requests consults, and does discharge work on your patient. If a patient has gone somewhere for a diagnostic study, the ward clerk often knows where that patient is and when he or she will return (the only thing worse than not being able to find your patient's chart is not being able to find your patient).

Pharmacist

Sometimes staff pharmacists, residents, and/or students round with the team. Do not hesitate to hit them up for valuable information regarding toxicity, drug interactions, dosing in different disease states, and efficacy. Pharmacists are especially helpful on the medicine wards, where pharmaceuticals make up a large part of the internist's armamentarium.

Other Hospital Staff

Other members of the hospital staff include PHYSICIAN ASSISTANTS, NURSE PRACTITIONERS, nutritional services, physical therapists, social workers, respiratory therapists, IV/blood draw (phlebotomy) teams, radiologic technicians, and laboratory technicians. All are important members of the hospital staff who are responsible for key aspects of your patient's care. Learning from their experience will thus make you a better ward clerk. For example, if you want to learn the finer points of IVs, you might want to tag along with the IV team on a day when you have extra time. Similarly, social workers are integral team members, often providing patient counseling, psychosocial assessment, and housing and transportation arrangements. Being on the wards is often the student's first exposure to the ubiquitous hospital "THREE-PIECE SUITS."

CURRENT *Med Talk*

> "THREE-PIECE SUITS": A colloquial and nonspecific term for any businessperson, which in the health care industry includes "medicrats" (MD/MPHs, i.e., physicians with a master's degree in public health, hospital administrators), pharmaceutical representatives ("detail men"), and financial officers ("bean counters") who function in a medical center's bureaucracy.

A DAY ON THE WARDS

A Typical Medicine Day

The typical medicine day also applies to pediatrics, neurology, and psychiatry. Please refer to the chapters that follow for specific advice and information on each rotation.

Prerounds: 7:00–8:00 AM. As your patient's primary caretaker, you note and evaluate any event affecting your patient that occurred since you left the hospital the previous day (see Table 1.1). Much of this information can be obtained by asking the overnight (cross-covering) house officer or the patient's nurse and by reviewing the chart. You can also discuss your plan prior to rounds with the intern who is following your patient. Note that interns are usually rushed in the morning, as they generally carry more patients. You should allow 15 to 20 minutes per patient at the beginning, until you become more efficient.

Work rounds: 8:00–9:30 AM. During work rounds, you round with the team (minus the attending) and give a very brief (less than 30-second) presentation on your patient to the resident in "SOAP" format. During this time, you also discuss your patient's problem and develop a plan with a to-do list for the day. Make sure to write down these chores immediately, as they may quickly be forgotten as you move on to the next patient. Have the chart available to write orders, and have them signed by the resident as you discuss the patient. Most of the pimping you get is restricted to your patient's care—another reason to know your patient inside out.

> **SOAP**
> **S**ubjective
> **O**bjective
> **A**ssessment
> **P**lan

Work time, aka "Hour of Power": 9:30–11:00 AM. This is when you and the intern crank on the scut. Speed and efficiency during this critical period will determine what time you and the intern go home. Understand that studies and consults scheduled later in the day are often not accomplished until the next day. Typical tasks include:

- Placing orders in the chart
- Scheduling studies (e.g., CT scans)
- Requesting consults
- Procedures (e.g., paracentesis)
- Drawing blood for key labs
- Discharge paperwork
- Progress notes

Attending rounds: 11:00 AM–noon. During attending rounds, you meet with the entire medical team and the attending physician to discuss all newly admitted patients and to follow up on current patients. On postcall days, you

---

TABLE 1.1. Preround Checklist.

❏ Review the events since last night by checking the charts for new notes, talking to the cross-covering intern, and touching base with the nurse.

❏ Subjective status: Ask the patient how he or she feels.

❏ Objective status: Vital signs/brief physical exam focused on findings that are relevant to current problems.

❏ Check new labs, culture results, study results, and radiographs.

❏ Your plan for the patient for today (break it down by problem).

---

formally present your patient—a four- to six-minute ordeal—to the attending. As shallow as it may seem, acing the formal presentation is key to scoring points with the attending, since this may be the only chance you get to demonstrate your strengths face to face. Attendings depend on a smooth presentation in their efforts to understand a patient's story and to formulate a diagnostic and therapeutic approach. A choppy or poorly organized presentation is painful to listen to and makes it difficult to concentrate on the patient's problems. Try not to read your presentation from your notes, as this makes it more difficult to follow.

During attending rounds, you will receive didactic teaching related to the patient's problems. It can be very helpful to read up on these topics beforehand. Do not hesitate to volunteer to organize a presentation on a disease or some aspect of its management; this gives you another chance to shine by demonstrating your sincere interest. Preparing brief handouts on your patient's disease (describing the clinical presentation, differential diagnosis, diagnostic findings and labs, complications, treatment, and prognosis) will make you a stellar student in the eyes of your team.

Radiology rounds are often part of attending rounds and occur with variable frequency. You may be asked to provide the radiologist with a 10- to 30-second bullet presentation prior to reviewing the films on each patient.

Noon conference: Noon–1:00 PM. If your service offers a noon conference, don't miss it. First, there is often free food, courtesy of the service or a pharmaceutical representative. Second, noon conferences typically cover bread-and-butter topics that are geared toward house staff and medical students.

Afternoon work: 1:00 PM–? In the afternoon, you plow through the rest of your to-do list and write your progress notes. During this time you will also check the results of any consults, studies, and labs that came back in the afternoon and will adjust your treatment plan with the intern accordingly. On some days there will be additional conferences, some of which may be oriented toward medical students. If the service was light and you were a total stud(ette) during the Hour of Power, you may find yourself ready to go home by 4 PM.

A good sign-out is the mark of a good student.

Signing out: When the day is over and you have completed your daily chores, you have one critical responsibility left. "Signing out" involves a transfer of information to someone who will be responsible for your patients while you are home watching *ER*. Depending on your team, this may involve no more than an update of pending tests and your patient's condition to the resident or intern who is covering your patient. Alternatively, you may need to sign out to the cross-covering intern on call, who will be covering your patient overnight—in which case you will need to give a brief description of your patient, current problems, medications and allergies, and any responsibilities you may be passing on to the cross-covering intern (e.g., "Please check the patient's wound site at 10 PM"). You should also document the patient's code status (full code vs. Do Not Resuscitate [DNR]), whether IV access is absolutely necessary (must it be restarted if it happens to fall out?), and whether you want blood cultures if the patient spikes a fever overnight.

A Typical Surgery Day

The surgery day starts earlier and ends later than a typical medicine day. Many of the same activities occur, but often at a quicker pace to make time for the OR. Differences are noted below.

Prerounds: 5:00–6:00 AM. This is just like medicine prerounds—but, in addition, you will be checking wounds and drains on postop patients. You may also be expected to write brief progress notes before work rounds.

Work rounds: 6:00–7:30 AM. If progress notes are not written during prerounds, they will be done here. Some services actually write notes during afternoon rounds or even twice a day. Otherwise, surgery work rounds are similar to medicine work rounds.

Preoperative preparation: 7:30–8:00 AM. During this period, you and a house officer work with the anesthesiologist to prepare the patient for the operation. This usually includes positioning the patient, placing a urinary catheter, and prepping the operative area.

Surgery: 8:00 AM–5:00 PM. This is where you have the most exposure to the attending. Depending on the needs and preferences of the team, your role may range from simple observation to retraction, suctioning, and tying and cutting sutures. The operating theater is often a place for rampant pimping, so bone up on your reading the night before the case. Alternatively, keep a pimp answer book in your locker for easy review. Know your anatomy.

Pimp questions often fly fast and furious in the OR.

Floor work: 8:00 AM–5:00 PM. If you are not in the OR during this period, you are doing the daily scut work on your patients with a resident. This may include wound checks, pulling staples, pulling chest tubes, and getting consults. Often, you and another medical student will switch off between the OR and the surgical floors. Convey your relative desire to be in the OR and your case preferences to the chief.

"Afternoon" rounds: 5:00–7:30 PM. Sometimes more aptly called "evening" rounds, these rounds allow the team to review the day's events and plan the next day. Afternoon rounds usually start soon after the last surgery of the day has been completed. These presentations are generally more casual and abbreviated than the morning presentations.

Postrounds work: 7:30 PM–? Sometimes afternoon rounds generate a short list of tasks that the team must accomplish before going home.

This is just a sample schedule; times may vary depending on your institution, the number of patients on the service, and the number and length of operative cases. On clinic days, the morning schedule is usually similar, as rounds must be completed before the start of clinic. The evening schedule may be lighter depending on whether there is clinic scheduled in the afternoon and how many patients need to be worked up or admitted for surgery the next day.

As a third-year student, you will work with the team to admit one to three patients on a call night. This has the potential to be a scary experience, but it need not be if you follow a few simple rules. In general, the admissions process follows a loose sequence of events. Your resident receives the ER call. You both throttle to the ER to conduct a history and physical exam (H&P) on the patient, formulate an assessment and plan, write the appropriate admission orders, and then move the patient up to the floors (or the units). Generally, your resident decides which case(s) you will work up and admit—although you could try to request the *type* of case assigned to you (e.g., cardiac, infectious).

The "Call"

Patients are usually admitted through the emergency department. Others are admitted from a clinic or transferred from an outside hospital or other medical and surgical services. The resident is usually given a one-line description of the patient's complaint, such as "33-year-old African-American female with abdominal pain" or "67-year-old Caucasian complaining of chest pain and dizziness." Immediately generate a differential diagnosis (e.g., skin, musculoskeletal, pulmonary, cardiac, and gastrointestinal) and use this to guide your initial approach to the patient's workup. Classic mnemonics such as "MINT CANDY" will help you develop and organize a consistent differential diagnosis. You will then ask questions, look for physical signs, and review old records for information that will help you "tease out" a likely diagnosis.

Reviewing Objective Data

The patient will usually have some preliminary testing done in the ER, so review the evaluation sheet to see what the ER doctors were thinking. Do a quick chart review, paying close attention to the latest discharge summaries, past hospitalizations, and problem lists. Of course, you may have time for only some of the above if your patient is unstable or in critical condition.

The Chart Review

Many of your patients have previously been admitted to the hospital. If this is the case, the past medical records should be in the ER when you arrive. If there is no old chart, ask the clerk if one exists and whether it has been ordered to the ER; a focused chart review before you see your patient can give you a good idea of his or her previous health status and health issues. Concentrate on the discharge summaries from each admission, since they are typed, concise, and provide a summary of the hospital course as well as a list of the patient's problems and discharge medications. Medical student admission notes are useful in that they often contain more detailed information on the

---

Quick framework for a differential diagnosis—

MINT CANDY
Metabolic
Infectious
Neoplastic
Trauma
Collagen vascular disease
Allergies
'N'ything else
Drugs
Youth (congenital)

social history and physical exam. You should also look for studies such as an ECG, recent echocardiograms, and past blood work so that you can compare them to current values. Knowing the patient's baseline will give both you and your team a better understanding of how sick the patient currently is (e.g., has the patient's chronic anemia worsened significantly? Are there new ECG changes?).

Focus on past discharge summaries and medical student admission notes.

Interviewing the Patient

At this point, you may have modified your differential diagnosis on the basis of your chart review. Keep a mental note of these potential diagnoses as you begin the patient interview. Sometimes the H&P may be conducted as a team, with the medical student leading the history taking while the residents take notes. At other times you will evaluate the patient alone and then present the patient to the team before they conduct their own H&Ps. Remember, your H&P skills will be judged by your residents and almost always count toward your final clerkship evaluation. So be organized, and try to prepare a mental outline of your questions before you see the patient.

If possible, avoid the "SHOTGUN APPROACH" to asking questions. This involves showering the patient with a barrage of nonfocused questions in the hopes of stumbling on a fact that might lead you closer to a diagnosis. Instead, ask about pertinent positives and negatives in the history. Admittedly, experience helps in developing a focused and directed H&P, and there is nothing wrong with being overly thorough. However, you will look sharper if you can conduct an interview that focuses on the pertinent issues; you can ask about nonurgent issues after your patient has been admitted to the floor.

Remember to begin your interview with open-ended questions (e.g., "What brought you to the hospital?"), which will give the patient some degree of control over the interview process. Then gradually move toward more structured questions (e.g., "Was your pain dull or sharp?") if the interview loses focus or if the patient wanders off the subject. Above all, don't get discouraged if the interview does not go smoothly. The medical interview is an art form that can be mastered only through repeated practice.

The Physical Exam

You should also conduct the physical exam as thoroughly as possible and in the same sequence every time. As a third-year student, you will need to develop solid physical exam skills. Each patient provides you with excellent practice, so time allowing, don't skimp on any part of the exam, including the rectal exam. You will soon enough be forced to do limited problem-oriented exams. Ask for supervision and feedback from a resident so that you can fine-tune your examination skills.

Two reasons not to do a rectal exam:
(1) you don't have a finger, or
(2) the patient doesn't have a rectum.

"SHOTGUN APPROACH": A diagnostic method or technique in which every conceivable parameter is measured in order to detect all possible clinical or laboratory nosologies, however remote the possibility that a rare disease is present. An often-criticized result of practicing "defensive medicine," increasing the cost of health care without improving patient management.

SUTTON'S LAW: A guideline evoked to temper the enthusiasm of externs and other novices in clinical medicine who want to "work up" an acute abdomen for porphyria, metastatic medulloblastoma, or other esoterica while ignoring a particular disease's most common causes. The "law" is attributed to the noted bank robber Willie Sutton, who, when asked why he robbed banks, reportedly replied, "That's where the money is." To apply Sutton's law, then, is to search for the most likely cause of a symptom (i.e., to "go where the money is").

Putting It All Together

After conducting the H&P and reviewing the medical records, labs, and studies, you will present the case to your resident(s) and formulate your assessment and plan. Give a short, three- to five-minute presentation similar in format to a full oral presentation, and present your most likely diagnoses. Include other, less likely considerations as well, as this shows depth and thoroughness in your evaluation of the case. Of course, if you can surreptitiously and quickly consult any pocketbooks about your leading diagnoses, you will be better prepared for the impending onslaught of pimp questions.

"Show me the money."

Sometimes you will be unsure of the diagnosis. Don't fret; your thought process and reasoning ability are more important at this stage than hitting the exact diagnosis. Do, however, support your current diagnoses with both subjective and objective data; rank your differential diagnoses in order of likelihood (remember SUTTON'S LAW); and present a thorough plan for each. This plan may include anything from more diagnostic studies to obtaining further consultation from other services.

Admission Orders—

ADC-VAANDIMSL
Admit to
Diagnosis
Condition
Vitals
Allergies
Activity
Nursing Orders
Diet
IV Fluids
Medicatons
Special Studies
Labs

KEY NOTES AND ORDERS

Admit Orders

Admission orders are written soon after the patient's acute problems and management plans have been discussed with your team and at least a working diagnosis has been rendered. Orders are written in a standard format; "ADC VAANDIMSL" is one of a few versions of the mnemonic for admission orders. Here is an example of orders for a patient admitted for pneumonia:

Sample Admit Order

6/10/02 12:02 PM

ADMIT TO: Ward, service, your name/intern's name, beeper number.

DIAGNOSIS: If there is no clear diagnosis, give the two or three most likely suspects (e.g., pulmonary embolism vs. CHF exacerbation) or the presenting complaint (e.g., chest pain), or what diagnoses you are trying to exclude (e.g., rule out MI).

CONDITION: Satisfactory, stable, fair, guarded, critical.

VITALS: Per routine, q4h, q1h, q shift.

ALLERGIES: Mention the specific reaction to the drug (e.g., rash); note NKDA if no allergies.

ACTIVITY: Ad lib, out of bed to bathroom (with assist), out of bed to chair, strict bed rest, ambulation with crutches.

NURSING ORDERS: Strict I/Os, oxygen, daily weights, telemetry, glucose checks, Foley cath, NG tube.

DIET: Regular, 1800 cal ADA, low sodium, soft mechanical, NPO.

IV FLUIDS: Hep lock, KVO, type of solution (D5, NS, D5 1/2 NS, etc.) and rate of infusion (e.g., D5 1/2 NS + 20 mEq/L KCl at 125 cc/hr).

MEDICATIONS: Don't forget antibiotics and prn medications.

SPECIAL STUDIES: ECG, CXR, CT, etc.

LABS: AM labs: CBC, electrolytes, BUN, Cr, glucose, etc.

CALL HOUSE OFFICER: Temp > 38.4, pulse > 120 or < 50, SBP < 90 or > 180, resp rate < 8 or > 30, O_2 sat < 90%.

ADA = American Diabetes Association

I/O = Intake/output

KVO = Keep vein open

NG = Nasogastric

NKDA = No known drug allergies

NPO = Nothing by mouth

NS = Normal saline

SBP = Systolic blood pressure

COMMON PRN MEDICATION ORDERS

"Prn" is the abbreviation for *pro re nata*—Latin for "as the need arises."
Acetaminophen (Tylenol) 650 mg PO q4h prn temp > 101.5°F
Bisacodyl (Dulcolax) 10 mg PO/PR qd prn constipation
Diphenhydramine (Benadryl) 25 mg PO qhs prn insomnia
Maalox 10–20 cc PO q1–2h prn dyspepsia
Lorazepam (Ativan) 1–2 mg IM/IV q6h prn anxiety/agitation
Promethazine (Phenergan) 25 mg PO/IM/IV q4h prn nausea

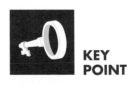

KEY POINT

Characterizing the Chief Complaint—

OPQRST

Onset
Progression
Provocation
Palliation
Quality
Region
Radiation
Symptoms
Severity
Time

Medical Student Admit Notes

Depending on the policies of your medical service, you may be given varying amounts of time to get the admit note into the chart. Use that time wisely to learn more about your patients' problems. Regardless of the time and circumstance, you should have the admit note in the chart before work rounds the next morning. The HPI and the assessment and plan are the two most challenging portions of the admit note to write. A well-written admit note is a testament to your thought processes and fund of knowledge.

HPI. Deciding which pieces of information belong in the HPI can be a difficult process at this stage of your career. Do not forget to characterize the chief complaint; for this purpose, use the mnemonic "OPQRST": Onset, Progression, Provocation, Palliation, Quality, Region, Radiation, associated Symptoms, Severity, Time course.

Also include the pertinent positives and negatives that support your diagnosis, and rule out the other main suspects. Present the information in chronological order. If information on the patient's past medical history (PMH), family history (FH), health-related behaviors, or social history (SH) is pertinent to the reason for admission, it should be included in the HPI.

By presenting the correct combination of pertinent positives and negatives as well as medical, social, and family history, the ideal HPI will lead the reader toward the most likely diagnosis and the differential diagnosis. The optimal HPI will also demonstrate the interviewer's reasoning and logic in assessing the patient's history.

Although you should include only pertinent positives and negatives in your history, as a medical student you should do a complete review of systems (ROS) with every patient you see. Especially early on, when your fund of knowledge may be limited, you should systematically ask about symptoms relating to all the major organ systems (constitutional, HEENT, cardiovascular, respiratory, GI, GU, neurologic, musculoskeletal, and endocrine), since you might not know ahead of time if a particular symptom is pertinent.

Other pieces of the history that are important include PMH, current medications (meds), allergies, FH, and SH.

Assessment and plan. In your assessment and plan, start off with a brief summary of the case. Give your presumed diagnosis at the end of the summary; then you can launch into a discussion of the case. Take the time to read up on your patient's diagnosis and management as well as his or her other important medical problems. Present your formulation of your patient's current health issues using a problem-list-based approach. Alternatively, you may use a systems-based approach if you have a more complicated patient (e.g., in the ICU). Each problem has an assessment and plan. In the assessment of the primary problem, the reader wants to know (1) why you think this is the diagnosis, and (2) why the other possible diagnoses are less likely to be correct. Other incidental problems get a brief one-line assessment. In the plan, outline your initial treatment plans (e.g., medications, procedures) and what additional workup needs to be done to further characterize the diagnosis or to clinch that diagnosis if it is still unclear at this point.

A few other pointers on the admit note are as follows:

- As you write the admit note, you'll come to realize that there are a few holes that need to be filled in. Try to identify all the gaps at once so that you don't keep shuttling between the patient and your note.
- Be prepared to use the most common abbreviations. Avoid obscure abbreviations that may not be recognizable or that may be mistaken for something else. Don't coin your own.
- The admit note (like all your progress notes) becomes part of the legal record. Thus, opinionated comments that are not relevant to the patient's care are faux pas. "Chart wars" are unprofessional and can create unwelcome medicolegal liability.
- Neat handwriting wins points. Messy handwriting can always be improved by slowing down. There is little point to writing an illegible note.

These tips should get you started. A more detailed discussion on admit notes can be found in any of a number of texts on medical history and physical examination.

Progress Notes

A PROGRESS NOTE is a daily written record of all events pertaining to a patient. An example is provided on p. 19. On medical-type services (including pediatrics, psychiatry, and neurology), progress notes are typically written in the afternoon. On surgical-type services (including OB/GYN), progress notes are written before work rounds in the morning. Make sure your intern or resident reviews and cosigns your notes. Most students write progress notes in the SOAP format described below.

- **Subjective.** This component includes the patient's own observations concerning changes in symptoms, any significant events in the last day, and any physical complaints.
- **Objective.** This includes vital signs; a focused, brief physical exam; and any laboratory and study results.
- **Assessment and plan.** This is your impression of the objective and subjective information and what the appropriate diagnostic and treatment regimen will be. Your plan should be concise and laid out so that someone else reading your note can easily understand the team's plan for your patient.

A&O × 4 = Alert and oriented to person, place, time, and situation

abx = Antibiotics

A/P = Assessment and plan

BRBPR = Bright red blood per rectum

c̄ = With

CC = Chief complaint

C/C/E = Clubbing/cyanosis/edema

CN = Cranial nerve

CTAB = Clear to auscultation bilaterally

D/C = Diarrhea/constipation

DOE = Dyspnea on exertion

DTRs = Deep tendon reflexes

EOMI = Extraocular movements intact

F/C/S = Fevers/chills/sweats

HA = Headache

h/o = History of

HSM = Hepatosplenomegaly

ID = Identification

M/R/G = Murmurs/rubs/gallops

MAE = Moves all extremities

MS = Muscloskeletal

MVI = Multivitamin infusion

NABS = Normal active bowel sounds

Sample Admit Note

MS3 Admission H&P
Time and Date: 6/10/02, 1:30 PM

ID/CC: 42-year-old Caucasian woman, former IV drug user, HIV+ c̄ CD4 count of 250, complains of 3 days of painful neck rash and diffuse itching.

HPI: Patient has been HIV+ × 3 years, no opportunistic infections. She complains of sudden-onset painful neck rash 2 days prior to admit. Noted vesicle formation on L neck and deltoid c̄ pruritus, as well as severe burning/stinging pain. Used warm compresses for symptomatic relief. She felt "drained" and stayed in bed × 2 days, denies any F/C/S, no N/V, no abdominal pain, no diarrhea. No arthralgias/myalgias, no cough, no SOB, no HA. She denies any vesicles on face, no ear pain, no eye pain or visual changes. She is unaware of any childhood history of chickenpox, denies any chemical or plant contacts or contact with others with similar symptoms. Denies any recent changes in medication.

PMH:

---

1. HIV+ × 3 years. Last CD4: 250, 3 months ago. Denies any OIs.

---

2. Pneumonia 3–4 × in past 3 years. Hospitalized but cannot relate dates, durations, or diagnoses. Recalls having a chest CT in past and has never had to take prophylactic abx. Chart currently unavailable for review.

---

3. Cellulitis of extremities several times in the past. Patient unable to recall details or dates.

---

4. Hepatitis C Ab+.

MEDS: Indinavir 800 mg PO qid.

Zidovudine 300 mg PO bid.

ddC 0.75 mg PO tid.

ALL: NKDA.

FH: Noncontributory.

SH: Patient is homeless. Moved from Chicago to San Francisco 4 years ago. She is unmarried and has 4 children, no family on the West Coast. She is intermittently followed by the HIV clinic at San Francisco General Hospital. + tobacco: 1 ppd × 20 years; + EtOH 1 pint vodka per day, no h/o withdrawal; + h/o IV drug use, none × 6 years.

ROS: Constitutional: no fatigue/weakness, no N/V, no F/C, no night sweats, no recent weight change.

HEENT: Denies headaches, visual changes, blurry vision, hearing changes, tinnitus, vertigo, rhinorrhea, nasal congestion, epistaxis, sore throat.

NECK: As noted above. No stiffness or masses.

CV: No chest pains, no palpitations, no DOE, no orthopnea.

RESP: No SOB, no cough, no wheezing.

GI: No recent change in appetite, no dysphagia, no jaundice, no abdominal pain, no D/C, no melena, no BRBPR.

GU: No sexual dysfunction, no dysuria, no hematuria, no polyuria, no stones, no nocturia, no frequency, no hesitancy; no genital sores, rashes, or discomfort.

NEURO: No seizures, no paresthesias, no numbness, no motor weakness, no difficulties with gait.

EXTREMITIES/MS: No edema, no joint stiffness, no change in ROM.

ENDOCRINE: No heat/cold intolerance, no excessive sweating, no polyuria, no polydipsia.

PSYCHIATRIC: No depression, no change in sleep pattern, no change in motivation.

PE: GEN: Somnolent, arousable to alertness, in mild distress due to pain and pruritus.

VS: T 37.1 BP 111/80 HR 112 RR 18, 99% O_2 sat on 2L NC.

SKIN/HAIR/NAILS: Vesicular rash c̄ erythematous base, clustered, on L lateral and posterior neck and L deltoid, anteriorly to clavicle, stops at midline anterior and posterior.

HEENT: NC/AT, PERRL 4 → 3, EOMI, mild conjunctival injection bilat, TMs clear without vesicles, O/P is dry with poor dentition, no vesicles or open lesions, no thrush.

NECK: 1 posterior SCM node 1 × 1 cm, supple neck.

BREAST: Deferred at this time per patient request.

LUNGS: CTAB, no rales, no wheezes.

CV: Tachycardic, reg rhythm, normal S1/S2, no M/R/G. Good distal pulses.

ABD: Soft, NT, NABS, ND, no HSM.

GU: Deferred at this time per patient request.

EXT: No C/C/E. Cool and dry. Numerous old needle-track scars.

NEURO: A&O × 4. CN II–XII intact. MAE, DTRs 2+ & symmetric, sensation intact. Normal and symmetric strength, tone, and bulk throughout

LABS:

8.2 \ 13.3 / 297   142 | 105 | 8 / 92   T. Bili 0.7; AST 38; ALT 20; Alk Phos 77
/ 40.0 \\   4.0 | 29 | 0.8 \\   PT/INR/PTT: 12.4/1.2/32.2

Ca 8.3; Mg 2.3; Phos 3.9   Albumin 3.6; amylase 82

CXR: Increased interstitial markings, o/w negative.

A/P: 42-year-old woman c̄ HIV, presenting with likely herpes zoster in L C3/C4 dermatomal distribution.

1. **Herpes zoster:** The differential in this case is rather narrow given the history and presentation. A contact dermatitis is unlikely, although a possibility. Given the specific dermatome distribution, which stops at the midline, reactivation is far more likely than a primary varicella infection. The patient's HIV status places her at risk for zoster dissemination. Admit for involvement of 2 contiguous dermatomes and monitor for signs of dissemination.

NC = Nasal cannula

NC/AT = Normocephalic/atraumatic

ND = Nondistended

BP = Blood Pressure

NT = Nontender

N/V = Nausea/vomiting

OI = Opportunistic infection

O/P = Oropharynx

o/w = Otherwise

PE = Physical Exam

PERRL 4 → 3 = Pupils equal, round, responsive to light from 4 mm to 3 mm

ppd = Pack per day

ROM = Range of motion

RR = Respiratory Rate

SCM = Sternocleidomastoid

SOB = Shortness of breath

TM = Tympanic membrane

VS = Vital Signs

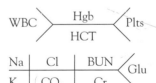

- Acyclovir 500 mg IV q 8 hours

- Benadryl 25–50 mg PO q 6 hours prn pruritus

- TyCo#3 1–2 tabs PO q 4 hours prn pain

- Isolation protocol to protect other immunocompromised patients on floor

2. **HIV:** CD4 > 200, no h/o opportunistic infections.

- Continue current medications as noted above

- Will arrange follow-up appointment with HIV clinic

3. **EtOH:** Monitor for signs of EtOH withdrawal.

- Thiamine 100 mg IV

- Folate 1 mg IV

- MVI 1 amp IV

- Ativan 1–2 mg IV q1–2h prn agitation

4. **Code status:** Patient is Full Code.

5. **Disposition:** Patient is homeless. Will consult social worker for discharge planning.

Procedure Notes

An intern will usually cosign everything you do — orders, notes, etc.

Before performing any procedure, you must obtain informed consent from the patient and document it in the chart. In addition, a procedure note must be written and placed in the chart for any invasive procedure performed on a patient, including a lumbar puncture, thoracocentesis, paracentesis, and central line placement. The note itself should be concise and should document the date and time, indications, consent, preparation of the patient, anesthesia used (if any), details of the procedure, yield, any studies sent, and any complications.

Writing Daily Orders

Make it clear to your team that you want to write orders for your patients (they will be cosigned). This will accomplish at least two critical goals. First, you will receive valuable practice in prescription writing and drug dosing. Second, you will automatically stay current with your patient's treatment regimens. Things to keep in mind when writing prescriptions are as follows:

- Make sure your prescription has all of the following essential information:
  - Time and date
  - Generic drug name
  - Dose
  - Route of delivery (PO, IV, IM, SQ)
  - Frequency
  - Signature; include your printed name, title (e.g., MS-III), and beeper number

BR = Bathroom

BS = Bowel Sounds

c/w = Compared with

nl = Normal

RA = Room air

RRR = Regular rate and rhythm

Sample Progress Note

Date and Time: 6/11/02, 10:00 AM

Hospital Day #2: Medicine Service

S: No events overnight. Patient "feels OK," reports continued pruritus, although significantly improved c/w yesterday. Good sleep last night, good pain control. No other complaints. Has not noticed any progression of rash.

O: VS: T 36.6 BP 110/65 HR 90 RR 18, 97% O_2 sat on RA.

I/O: 950 cc/BR.

SKIN: No change in distribution or size of vesicles on L neck/shoulder, although some have crusted over. No new vesicles on body.

HEENT: PERRL, EOMI, no conjunctival injection, TMs clear, no vesicles, O/P moist and clear.

LUNGS: CTAB, no rales, no wheezes.

CV: RRR, nl S1/S2, no M/R/G.

ABD: Soft, NT, +BS.

LABS:

$$\frac{7.9}{} \diagdown \frac{12.8}{37.2} \diagup 260 \qquad \frac{134 \mid 103 \mid 8}{3.6 \mid 25 \mid 0.8} \diagdown 90$$

A/P: 42-year-old woman with herpes zoster, afebrile and comfortable, doing well.

1. **Herpes zoster:** No evidence of dissemination or spread to other dermatomes. Good pain control, tolerating IV acyclovir well.

   - Atarax prn pruritus.

   - Continue IV acyclovir, TyCo#3.

2. **HIV**

   - Continue AZT, indinavir, and ddC.

   - Plan to speak with HIV clinic today to arrange follow-up care.

3. **EtOH:** No sign of alcohol withdrawal at this time. Continue to monitor.

4. **Dispo:** Social worker to speak with patient this afternoon re housing and $.

Sample Procedure Note

Procedure: Diagnostic lumbar puncture.

Indication: Suspected meningitis.

Consent: Patient gave informed consent.

Complications: None.

Patient was placed in left-lateral decubitus position with spine flexed, and the L4–5 interspace identified. Under sterile conditions the area was prepared with Betadine, anesthetized with 1% lidocaine 5 cc, spinal needle introduced into L4–5 interspace without difficulty. Opening pressure 130 mm, 8 cc clear, nonturbid spinal fluid collected, sent for protein, glucose, Gram stain, cell count, culture. Patient tolerated the procedure well.

- Write legibly; do not use abbreviations.
- Have the prescription cosigned immediately by a house officer. Your signature alone is not sufficient.
- If it's an important order, also pass the order verbally to the nurse or the ward clerk.
- Just because a written order exists does not mean it was executed. Check nursing records frequently to be sure orders were properly carried out. Check the IV bag label to see if the correct IV meds are being given.

Writing Prescriptions

Before you discharge a patient from the hospital or when you see a patient in an outpatient setting, you may need to write a prescription. Clearly, as a medical student, you cannot sign the prescription. You can, however, gain valuable practice by asking your residents or attending if you can fill in the prescription. Remember that whoever cosigns your prescription is liable for any errors you may make, so be sure to fill in the appropriate medications, dosages, route of administration, schedule, quantity, and number of refills. If you're not sure why a patient is being discharged on a particular medication, don't be afraid to ask. This will show that you are interested and are trying to understand the rationale behind the care of the patient.

Sample Prescription
Name: John Smith
Hospital ID: 222-22-255
Rx: Keflex 500 mg
Disp: #40
Sig: Take one tab PO qid × 7 days
Refills: None
Generic OK

THE ORAL PRESENTATION

During your clerkships, no skill is more important to master than the delivery of a focused, fluent, and concise oral presentation. You will be called upon to present patients under varied circumstances and time constraints for the rest of your professional life, so getting a good handle on this skill early is critical to success on the wards. Indeed, it is the primary basis upon which you will be judged during attending rounds.

Practice, practice, practice your presentations!

When done effectively, oral presentations should approach an art form that will leave your audience with a solid comprehension of your patient's health care issues. When done poorly, however, such presentations will leave your audience confused and groping for further clarification. The ability to amass voluminous amounts of information is easily acquired, but organizing that information, synthesizing it, and using it to tell a succinct story can be challenging. Above all, the story must make sense to you before you can tell it to anyone else. So don't expect to get away with just reporting snippets of data that you've culled from old charts and don't fully understand.

The Formal Presentation

Classically, the formal oral presentation is given in seven minutes or less. Although it follows the same format as a written report, it is not simply a regurgitation. A great presentation requires style as much as substance; your delivery must be succinct and smooth. No time should be wasted on superfluous information; such matters can be covered later in your admit note. Ideally, your presentation should be formulated so that your audience can anticipate your assessment and plan; that is, each piece of information should clue the listener into your thinking process and your most likely diagnosis.

More emphasis should be given to the patient's *current* state (CC, HPI, PE, labs, A/P) than to past events (PMH, FH, SH). Furthermore, body language, eye contact, posture, and the like all contribute to a polished presentation.

The following are the categories of information that you should be prepared to furnish during an oral presentation.

Identification/chief complaint. Ideally, this introductory portion of the oral presentation should be a one-line bullet presentation that includes identifying information and chief complaint (e.g., "Mr. Veza is a 71-year-old diabetic Filipino male with long-standing hypertension who is admitted for a two-day history of dyspnea, bilateral pedal edema, and chest pain").

History of present illness. The HPI is the cornerstone of the medical presentation. The HPI you present will be very similar to the written HPI in that you will be providing pertinent positives and negatives that will move the audience toward your diagnosis. When done well, the HPI will have the feel of a story.

Past medical history. Do not repeat information that was already mentioned in the HPI. If any information is relevant to the patient's chief complaint, it should be included in the HPI. Omit any extraneous information from your oral presentation (e.g., childhood chickenpox in an elderly man with an acute MI).

Allergies/medications. You need not present the dosage for each medication, but make sure you've written it down just in case you're asked.

Social history. Include at least a brief social history; it is always relevant. Remember that you are presenting another human being, not a disease.

Health-related behaviors. Again, this may be short or even nonexistent if the information is included in the HPI. This category usually includes tobacco, alcohol, and illicit drug use as well as a sexual history.

Family history. This section includes both positive and negative findings and should be very short, as any relevant information should have been mentioned in the HPI.

Review of systems. This section is often omitted entirely; anything directly relevant should have been mentioned in the HPI.

A well-done presentation is like a riveting story.

Physical exam/labs/other tests. Depending on your attending's preferences, you may present just the highlights or give a very thorough report of the physical findings. Ask your attending in advance what he or she prefers. Most will want just pertinent positives and negatives reported. Others, however, may want a more formal approach detailing each physical finding and lab/other test values. In general, unless otherwise specified, present *all* the physical findings and lab/other test values; you will never be faulted for being too thorough. Always use simple declarative sentences when you present a physical finding (e.g., "There were no murmurs, rubs, or gallops on cardiac exam" instead of "Cardiac exam was unremarkable").

Assessment and plan. By the time you reach the assessment and plan, you should have successfully "set the dinner table" so that your audience will be waiting hungrily in anticipation of their meal. Indeed, this section is the meat of the presentation. As in your admit note, you may give a short summary of the case, including only pertinent positives and negatives, as a preface to your assessment and plan; this is particularly useful in complicated cases with multifactorial diseases. Presumably, you will have read as much as possible about each of your patient's preexisting illnesses and potential diagnoses. Know in advance how to differentiate each potential diagnosis and what each workup entails. Also know both the acute and long-term management of each diagnosis entertained, and incorporate this knowledge accordingly into your assessment and plan.

Again, you can present the assessment and plan in the form of a problem or according to organ system; doing so makes it less likely that you will miss anything important. March through each problem on the list, give your assessment, and outline a plan succinctly. Finally, if you really want to impress your team, pose a question for discussion relating to, for example, the acute management of a problem. Of course, you should offer to give a short presentation on that topic based on a literature review!

The "Bullet" Presentation

The one-minute "bullet" presentation is an extremely concise synopsis of the case presentation. You may give bullet presentations during work rounds and to consultants or other health care providers who are unfamiliar with your patient. Ideally, the history, physical exam, laboratory findings, and assessment-and-plan sections are each summarized into one sentence. You have time to include only the most pertinent positive and negative findings, usually encompassing anywhere from 15 to 20 facts about the case. Practice this skill with each patient you write up and present. Initially, you may try writing down the most important information from each of the write-up sections and then develop a cohesive one-minute presentation. With practice, you will soon be able to filter the vast amount of information from memory.

Procedures

Procedures are done for a variety of reasons. Some are diagnostic, while others are therapeutic and potentially lifesaving—but all are vital to the care of your patient (see Table 1.2). You can learn procedures by doing them under supervision or by carefully observing while they are being performed. Reading about a procedure in a manual beforehand maximizes your learning (see the book reviews at the end of Chapter 2). At the same time, a procedure is not just technique; you should also understand its indications, contraindications, and potential complications. A few tips about procedures are as follows:

- Before performing any significant procedure, obtain informed consent from the patient. To do so, you must explain the procedure, its indications, its risks and benefits, any alternative options, and the risks and benefits of not having the procedure. Be sure to document the patient's consent or place a signed consent form in the chart. Some hospitals allow students to consent patients for simple procedures and operations; others do not.
- Have everything you need ready at the bedside (think through what you will require in advance).
- Gather enough materials for multiple tries (expect to miss the first IV or venipuncture).
- Position the patient and yourself for comfort (e.g., raise the bed so you don't have to bend over; ensure that you have adequate lighting).
- Always remember universal precautions.
- Prepare for a potential mess by having gauze and disposable drop cloths positioned as necessary.
- Clean up after yourself. Discard all of your sharps in the proper receptacle.
- Write a procedure note for any invasive procedure, including lumbar puncture, thoracocentesis, paracentesis, and central line placement, and place it in the chart.

Communicating with Patients and Family Members

As your patient's primary care provider, you should be the main communication link between the team and the patient and family. So here are some tips that will help you become the "Great Communicator":

- Respect the privacy and wishes of the patient. Never discuss patients in the elevator, the cafeteria, or other public places.
- Be as honest and direct as possible. Update family members regarding the progress of their loved ones. If it were your grandmother in the hospital, you would want the doctor to keep you informed.
- Immediately inform the patient of any upcoming studies and events.

TABLE 1.2. Common Procedures for a Junior Student.

Basic	Advanced
Arterial blood gas	Arthrocentesis
Blood culture	Chest tube insertion
ECG	Central line placement
IV placement	Lumbar puncture
Nasogastric tube placement	Obstetrical delivery
Surgical knots	Paracentesis
Suturing	Thoracocentesis
Urine (Foley) catheterization	Wound dressing changes
Venipuncture	

- At the beginning, break bad news with a resident or an attending at your side. They have more experience in helping patients and families deal with the emotional repercussions of an illness. They can also help you deal with any possible backlash.
- Choose a quiet time to talk (i.e., when nursing and ancillary staff are not around) and a private location.
- Keep technical jargon to a minimum, and explain any medical terminology you use.
- Always finish with "Do you have any questions?"
- Never fudge an answer. If you are unsure, tell the family that you will consult your team and get back to them promptly.
- Beware of becoming less understanding and empathic toward patients as the year progresses. Studies have shown that a decrease in empathy correlates with high Medical College Admission Test (MCAT) scores!

Consults

Your team will often have a diagnostic or treatment question that requires the expertise of a specialist. Obtaining a consult involves filling out a consult request form as well as making a courtesy call to tell the consultant about the patient. Consultants dread receiving a request from a junior clerk who gives a rambling presentation and does not know why the request is being made. You can make the consultant's day much more pleasant (as well as impress him or her) by giving a concise, one-minute bullet presentation that includes patient identification, a pertinent present medical history, a pertinent past medical history, medications, allergies, physical exam, key lab results, and study results. This brief presentation should be followed by a clear question for the consultant.

Always have a clear question to ask a consultant.

Before calling the consultant, review the patient and the consult request with your resident or intern. If you don't understand the reason for the consult, you may end up bouncing between an irritated consultant and an impatient resident. If you are professional in your interactions with consultants, they will be more likely to convey the recommendations directly to you rather than bypassing you in favor of the intern or resident.

Checking Labs and Studies

During a typical ward day, labs and study results should be checked during pre-rounds, in the afternoon, and whenever stat labs or important studies are expected back. Anything pertinent should be reported to your intern or resident. If a patient is unstable, make sure you check more frequently to see if the labs are back. Whenever possible, look at the blood smear or CXR yourself instead of reading the report.

Reading Up on Your Patient's Problems

Aside from one-on-one teaching and conferences, you will be expected to learn through independent reading. In this context, it is critical to understand the rationale behind the treatment plan for your patients, so knowledge of the pathophysiology of their condition is necessary. Your first priority is therefore to read about your patients' problems. Next, read about other patients being carried by the team with active and interesting problems. Knowing about other patients' problems keeps you involved in patient discussions during rounds. Depending on what you want to learn and when you can learn it, you will be using multiple sources of information:

Pocketbooks and handbooks. When you have five minutes before attending rounds, you can quickly read a pocket resource to get the "big picture" about a disease. A classic example is the *Washington Manual of Medical Therapeutics*.

Compact reference books. These books are generally meant to be read cover to cover during the course of a rotation. Whether that actually happens is anybody's guess. These texts cover diseases in moderate detail and are ideal for reading up on interesting patients.

Textbooks. These tomes comprehensively cover diseases in great detail. *Harrison's Textbook of Medicine* is an example. You should read about your own patients' problems in a clinical reference.

Journal articles. Sometimes even *Harrison's* can't tell you all you need to know about a patient's disease. If this is the case, you should search MEDLINE to find a review or a study that answers your burning questions. Journal articles discuss the latest treatment regimens and contain information that is two to four years more recent than that in a reference book. For diseases in which our understanding is constantly evolving, such as HIV, a literature search may be mandatory. If you find a helpful paper, it is highly appropriate to photocopy that paper for your team. The truly enthusiastic student may also present the findings as well as a critique of the paper, perhaps in a one-page handout. A quick and helpful shortcut is to print several article titles along with abstracts for your resident or attending. Let them choose which ones to photocopy.

Being a "Dispenser"

Sometimes the student serves as a mobile supply cart for the attending and house staff. This may sound demeaning, but simple things such as having extra gloves, 3 × 5 index cards, tongue blades, or pens will save time on rounds and make your team members' lives a little easier. So keep your pockets stocked. Attendings will often borrow your stethoscope and penlight. Make sure you get your pen back if borrowed (attendings are especially notorious for disappearing with them) or bring extras every day.

TIPS FOR WARDS SURVIVAL

Efficient Time and Patient Management

Getting out at a reasonable hour ultimately depends on your ability to work closely with your team and efficiently execute your duties, although complicated patients will certainly make your days longer. Some people will swear that they have a "black cloud," meaning that for some unknown reason they are swamped with more work and more admissions than others. Believe it or not, studies have been done to determine whether "black clouds" really exist. In fact, people with "black clouds" do not have more work. Instead, they just function differently, perhaps working inefficiently or creating more work for themselves. You should therefore appreciate the fact that learning to be efficient will be the key to maintaining your own sanity and getting a good evaluation. Here are some tips to help you take better care of your patients without depriving you of sunlight (unless you're on surgery).

Commit all tasks to a to-do list. Write down each task immediately. You will be bombarded with multiple responsibilities, so it is inevitable that you will forget something. You should thus try to add even the "smallest" tasks to your to-do list. When it comes to your patient's care, there is no such thing as a small task. Check off your chores as they are accomplished, and roll over any unfinished ones to the next day's to-do list.

Prioritize your tasks. You will have time to get things done in the morning and the afternoon. In medicine, if key tasks aren't done during the Hour of Power, you won't have a chance to work on them until the early afternoon. Think about what you need to do first to ensure that your patient does not stay any longer than necessary. For example, consults and studies must be requested in the morning or they will not get done that day (see Table 1.3). If you plan to discharge a patient, take care of the paperwork and placement issues early.

TABLE 1.3. Example of Prioritized Tasks.

Do Now	Do Next
Request consults	Progress notes
Schedule studies	Check routine labs
Do discharge paperwork	Follow-up consults
Check stat or crucial labs	Follow-up studies

Organize tasks by location whenever possible. Always think about what tasks can be done while you are in a particular location. If you find yourself in the radiology department for the purpose of looking at Patient A's CXR, for example, you should also take care of any other radiology-related tasks you might have, such as looking at Patient B's head CT and Patient C's abdominal films. If Patient B is on a different floor from your other patients, take care of tasks related to him while you're there, such as requesting that cardiology consult and scheduling the patient for a CXR.

Learn to maximize the hospital information system. A good hospital information system (HIS) can be your friend. Some systems can handle custom patient lists, print labs and problem lists, and can even perform literature searches.

Keep scut essentials on board. Supply carts are always in the third place you look. If you find a mother lode of supplies, load up on the suture removal kits, blood-draw supplies, and other essentials you need to get through your scut without seeking a supply cart every time you go to a different floor. Also, carry a beeper. Ideally, your medical school or hospital will provide you with a permanent beeper for your third and fourth years. If they do not, many students advise that you get your own. The easier you are to reach, the more you will stay involved with patient care. In addition, there is nothing worse than hanging around waiting for an admission without a pager, when you could be in the library or call room.

Organizational Aids ("Peripheral Brains")

Another key to being an efficient ward clerk is to have and use the right organizational aids. The pros and cons of the most popular organizational aids are discussed below. Regardless of the type of aid you choose, however, you should remember to come prepared on day one; don't wait until halfway through your first rotation to start your system. If a given system doesn't work for you, you can always change it—but you need to be organized from the very start.

Clipboard. Many students start out with a clipboard as their preferred mode of organization. The clipboard gives you lots of surface area to organize patient information and tasks. It also gives you the ability to hold additional items such as progress notes, journal articles, and lab requests. However, a clipboard is easy to lose. Throughout the day you will find yourself putting your clipboard down to do a physical exam or pull sutures. A clipboard can also get overstuffed with miscellaneous papers. Most fashion-conscious students thus discard their clipboards when they come to feel comfortable with note cards.

Binders. Three-ring binders can be extremely helpful, particularly on medicine services, where much patient information is accumulated. Tabs can help you locate patient information quickly without shuffling through papers or cards.

Data sheets. Many people prefer 8½ × 11 sheets that can be folded in half and put in the pocket. You can carry separate sheets for the patient's H&P and lab data. Shop around for a format you like (ask your residents or fellow medical students) or make your own.

Note cards. Most house staff and senior students use note cards to organize their patients, scut lists, and clinical cheat sheets. Note cards are compact and slide easily into your pocket. Because of space considerations, note cards also force you to organize your thoughts and record only important information. In addition, they are much less obtrusive when you are presenting. However, note cards may force you to use abbreviations and tiny print to the point where they are barely legible. Here are some pointers regarding note cards:

True fear is misplacing your patient cards before a presentation.

- Blank note cards can often be found at the nurses' station.
- A ring binder or clip allows you to keep your cards together. You will need to punch holes in the cards. An alternative is to maintain a small pocket spiral-bound notebook.
- Use a high-quality, fine-point pen (e.g., Pilot fine ballpoint) to minimize "microglyphics." Do not use felt-tip pens, as they may run if the card gets wet.
- Consider using a different color card for the patient's admission history and physical.
- Create an "if found" card with your name and pager number. Losing your cards is like having an unscheduled lobectomy. You have not known true fear until you have misplaced your patient cards.
- Create a card with key phone numbers on it (team pagers, lab, x-ray, nursing stations of each ward, etc.). This is key. It will save you time and will often help members of your team.

Personal digital assistants. Also known as electronic organizers, these handheld computers are increasingly common on the wards with students, residents, and attendings alike. Some medical schools already require their medical students to own PDAs. They are useful for their ability to hold personal addresses, phone numbers, and appointments. You can also record as a document file the clinical pearls you pick up during conferences and on the wards. Perhaps more significantly, medical software is now available for the PDA. Resources range from medical calculators to full-text reference books. Most PDAs also have infrared ports so that information can be exchanged between PDAs.

Beware: Keep track of your PDA at all times. It can grow legs!

Some of the more current and useful resources are discussed within the Top-Rated Books and Software section. Palm, Handspring, Sony, Casio, and Compaq all offer PDAs, each with unique characteristics and specifications. The choice of a PDA should depend on personal preference, memory capacity, price range, and other features. Remember that those PDAs operating on the Palm operating system cannot interface with those running on a Windows CE operating system. One should choose a PDA with at least 8 megabytes of memory and should inquire about the expandability of a PDA, especially with respect to memory.

Unlike note cards and clipboards, PDAs require a significant investment in both time and money. Also, since PDAs are a small but valuable piece of equipment, they are always at risk of being misplaced or stolen.

Surviving Call Nights

A travel alarm is essential for surviving call nights. Do not rely on the hospital operator to wake you up. Also make an "on-call" bag with a toothbrush, a hairbrush, a razor, and a change of clothes if you are working in a clinic the next day. Sleep whenever possible; eat whenever possible. Hang out in the residents' lounge to watch TV, and bring a review/mini-reference book to learn about your patients' problems when you have down time.

Evaluations

Third-year evaluations are crucial to a successful residency application.

Your third-year evaluations are critical, as they make up the majority of your dean's letter. Residency directors looking to recruit the best medical students examine third- and fourth-year evaluations first. Unfortunately, preclinical performance does not always predict clinical success. During the first two years, your fund of knowledge is everything; during the clinical years it is only one of many criteria by which you will be judged. As a result, doing well during the first two years provides little guarantee that you'll be successful on the wards.

Written evaluations. Written evaluations are usually subjective assessments written by the attending or the senior resident. They should include a compilation of comments and observations from evaluation forms filled out by all residents and attendings who worked with you during the rotation. Written evaluations are easily influenced by personal factors and can be dangerous, since they are often quoted verbatim in the dean's letter. A single interaction (both positive and negative) can easily be seen by an attending as representative of your performance during the entire rotation.

Students who ask for verbal feedback fare better on their written evaluations.

Maximizing your evaluations. It is critical to stay on top of your evaluations by getting feedback from your attendings and residents at an early stage, before potentially negative material ends up in your written evaluations. At least one study has shown that asking for verbal feedback before the resident or attending completes your written evaluation results in higher written evaluation marks. At the beginning of the rotation, you should thus ask both your attending and your resident what their expectations are. Then, two weeks into the rotation, meet with your attending and with your resident one on one to see if you are meeting their expectations and if there are any areas in which you can improve (e.g., notes, rounds, procedures, communication). Sit down with your attending and resident at the end to review your performance. Your persistence will not only provide invaluable feedback but also demonstrate initiative that will not go unnoticed.

Within weeks, the clerkship office should have written evaluations on file. Visit the office to review them; with any luck the results will be pleasant. However, if you believe your evaluation is an inaccurate representation of your performance, now is the time to bring it to the attention of the clerkship director or the dean of students. It may be too late to change them by the time dean's letters are written during the summer of your fourth year.

Do not allow evaluations to affect your self-perception. Evaluations can vary widely. However, do not ignore trends or patterns in your evaluations, as they more or less reflect the consensus perception of your performance.

Honors/Grades

Most schools have a grading system of one sort or another, such as "honors/pass/fail" or the traditional letter grading system, to gauge your clinical performance. Make sure you have a clear understanding of the criteria for achieving honors and "A's," as clerkship directors often fail to volunteer this information (sometimes intentionally). Note that objective standards (e.g., mini-boards exams) and subjective standards (e.g., Did the student fit in well with the team?) are often used together. Looking at an evaluation form can also tell you what specific skills and performance criteria will be used to judge you. Also keep in mind that getting honors is not necessarily everything. Although honors are certainly helpful for residency (icing on the cake), it is more important to perform consistently well on rotations, which will be reflected in your dean's letter.

Also remember that your final grade in a rotation does not completely rely on your performance on the wards. In most instances, a final examination will also be administered. Unfortunately, the final examination rarely correlates well with what you have learned or have been taught during your rotation. In fact, the final examination is sometimes specifically intended to evaluate a different competency domain than your rotation performance. Consequently, you must make time to study independently for the final examination as well. This is, of course, in addition to studying and learning about your patients—although if you're savvy, you may be able to coordinate the two!

Letters of Recommendation

If your attending wrote you a glowing evaluation or has given you very positive feedback, you may ask for a letter of recommendation while details of your valor are still fresh. Letters of recommendation are used when you apply for residency positions. If you ask for a letter early in the third year, have the attending update the letter when your career path becomes clearer.

DIFFICULT SITUATIONS

The junior clerk is faced with a host of new situations that may require social and political savvy. Unfortunately, however, the junior clerk is typically at the bottom of the totem pole and has little political leverage. Failure to handle these situations can lead to anything from simple embarrassment to patient endangerment.

Confidential counseling is available.

Do not hesitate to seek help if things become overwhelming. The wards can be a very stressful environment. Remember that getting help is not a sign of failure; rather, it is a testament to your ability to understand your limits. The three main areas of stress for medical students are academic pressures, social issues, and financial problems. Try to recognize your stressors. If necessary, seek help from your medical school, as this will not reflect negatively on your evaluations or dean's letter; schools are more concerned with your well-being than anything else. Most institutions will also have discreet counseling available at little or no cost. Remember that your fellow classmates are in the same situation and may be facing similar issues. So this is a time to reach out to others and talk about your feelings, concerns, and fears.

CURRENT *Med Talk*

UNIVERSAL PRECAUTIONS: A method of infection control in which all human blood, certain body fluids (to wit, amniotic fluid; CSF; pericardial, peritoneal, pleural, and synovial fluids; saliva in dental procedures; semen; vaginal secretions; and any fluid grossly contaminated with blood) as well as unfixed organs or tissues of human origin, HIV-containing cell or tissue cultures, and HBV-containing culture media or other solutions are treated as if known to be infected with HIV, HBV, and/or other blood-borne pathogens **(Federal Register Dec 6, 1991, p 64107, col 2)**; in the absence of knowledge of the nature of the fluid, it should be treated as if potentially infectious. UPs consist of the constellation of safeguards for handling materials, tissues, and fluids that may contain human pathogens; exposure to blood and body fluids is minimized by using isolation materials and removable and disposable barriers (latex and vinyl gloves, protective eyewear, masks and gowns, and "disposable sharps" containers). Body fluids that require universal precautions include blood (serum and plasma) and all body fluids containing visible blood as well as maternal milk, semen, vaginal secretions, and cerebrospinal, synovial, peritoneal, pleural, pericardial, and amniotic fluids.

Needlesticks

Being stuck by a needle or other sharp is probably the most feared incident any health care worker faces. As a medical student, you are at higher risk because of your inexperience with handling sharps as well as your limited knowledge of where things are in the hospital. Here are some useful tips:

- Always practice UNIVERSAL PRECAUTIONS. You won't always know a patient's HIV or HBV/HCV status. So wear gloves whenever handling any blood products or starting IV lines. Protect your eyes with a face shield or glasses to guard against splashes (e.g., a vomiting patient, arterial spray in surgery, or a trauma case in the ER). Wear a gown to protect other exposed areas (as well as your clothing) from contamination.
- Don't rush. Slow down and think about what you are doing. Be especially careful in the ER and in surgery, where needles and other sharps are being passed around you.
- Plan ahead. Have all of the necessary materials for the procedure you are about to perform at the bedside. Anticipate needing more than one needle for blood draws in case you miss (ditto for IVs). Find the sharps container ahead of time so you do not have to walk around the room with a needle in your hand.
- Dispose of contaminated sharps immediately (like a loaded gun) into the nearest sharps container. You are responsible for your own sharps. Never simply leave a needle on a table or a bed, as you may forget it is there or someone else may be stuck by it (you could easily forget about the needle if you suddenly leave the room for a Code Blue). If you absolutely have to put a contaminated sharp down, announce it ("sharp on the table") so that others are aware. If others are in the room when you are carrying a sharp to the disposal container, let them know you are carrying a sharp.
- Never recap, bend, or break any needles/sharps.
- Don't force a needle into a sharp container that is full.
- Get vaccinated against HBV!

Never recap, bend, or break a sharp.

Despite your best efforts, the unthinkable may still occur. If you are ever stuck by a contaminated sharp, try to remember the following:

- Don't panic. Take a deep breath. You cannot change what has already occurred, but your actions now are still very important.
- Make sure the patient is safe, and discard the sharp properly.
- Wash the involved area with soap and water or Betadine.
- Call the Needlestick Hotline as soon as possible and inform one of your team members. Report exactly what has happened and follow the appropriate protocol. The hotline will give you information and facilitate blood testing, counseling, and possible HIV prophylactic treatment.

Always report a needlestick.

Do not hesitate to speak with team members, fellow students, friends and family, or counselors about what has happened. A needlestick can be extremely traumatizing (in many ways, it can be like a brush with death). If you feel you need to leave early to go home, tell your resident.

CURRENT
Med Talk

MEDICAL STUDENT ABUSE: A widely extant practice in which medical students are psychologically "abused" by superiors (interns, residents, fellows, and attending physicians) in the form of badgering, belittling, and being forced to perform menial, degrading tasks; see pimping, scut work. Note: The opinion has been privately voiced by some health care workers that abuse is part of the medical student experience, which helps "harden" them for the realities of practicing medicine (**JAMA 1996; 275:414–6**).

Abusive or Inappropriate House Officers

House staff typically work long hours and lead hectic lifestyles. However, that does not give them an excuse to vent their frustrations on you (MEDICAL STUDENT ABUSE). If the situation does not resolve, you should bring it to the attention of the clerkship director, ombudsperson, or student dean. This is, of course, an awkward situation, since you are being evaluated by the house officer. Avoid bringing the issue to the attention of the attending, as doing so can further disrupt the dynamics of the team.

On the other hand, you may receive unwanted attention, such as being asked out for a drink by the resident. You may avoid an awkward situation by suggesting that perhaps the entire team go out for drinks. If the resident is insistent, you may have to be more direct. If this leads to a negative working relationship, you may have to bring it to the attention of the clerkship director or the student dean in order to resolve the situation as well as to protect yourself from any unfair evaluations.

Inappropriate Procedures

Be aggressive in volunteering for any procedures that may be appropriate to your skill level (residents love highly motivated students). However, do not allow yourself to be pushed into performing any procedure with which you are not comfortable; this is dangerous both for you and for the patient and is not an optimal learning situation. Good house officers will acknowledge your maturity if you say, "I'm not comfortable with this procedure. Can you walk me through it, or can I watch this one and perform the next one?"

Overly Competitive Classmates (aka "Gunners")

Learn to trust and depend on your classmates.

The desire to achieve recognition and high marks can cloud the better judgment of your classmates (and sometimes your own). When there is more than one student to a team, a sense of do-or-die competition may arise, leading to excessive "brown-nosing" or backstabbing behavior. This way of thinking must be curbed at the very start of any rotation. Your classmates are some of your most valuable resources, so make it clear that cooperation and support are key to learning and doing well on the rotation. Also remember that residents and attendings have all been junior students themselves and can thus spot brown-nosing and backstabbing behavior easily. So take the initiative; keep your classmates informed of scheduled events, share procedures, teach each other, and share information. Address backstabbing behavior immediately and firmly. As they say in psychiatry, set clear limits. If the pattern persists, bring it to the attention of your intern or resident. Always maintain the moral high ground; you'll sleep better at night.

Patient Death

Despite the best efforts you and your team might make, some of your patients will die under your care. The first patient death can be particularly disturbing, especially if you developed any personal attachments to the patient. You should thus consider discussing the patient's death with your team or other students if they are receptive. Good social and family support also helps. Seek confidential counseling if necessary. As you continue your clinical training, you will learn to deal more effectively with patient death. However, do not distance yourself so much from the patient that you lose the human perspective.

The first few patient deaths are often very disturbing to the student.

Sexual Harassment

The power structure of a medical team can lead to abuses of attending and house staff privileges. Female students are especially vulnerable to snide remarks and outright inappropriate behavior. However, confronting the offender immediately is an option you should exercise only if you feel that you can handle it. In any case, document the event(s) clearly and unambiguously. Record the exact circumstances and nature of the incident(s), and identify any witnesses. Then make an appointment to see your student dean as soon as possible, and review the school's written policies. Your dean should be able to confidentially evaluate the information and determine the best course of action. Your school may also have a sexual harassment prevention office or a dean or ombudsperson in charge of a sexual harassment protocol.

Sexual harassment is a highly charged issue, so you will want to have as many backers as possible before you confront an offender. If you decide that the degree of harassment is mild, you may elect to tolerate the situation or wait until the rotation is finished for the sake of preserving your evaluation and team dynamics. This is a personal decision. However, continue to document all offending incidents in the event that you do change your mind and decide to act. At the end of the rotation, consider using evaluation forms to state your case so that you can help prevent this behavior in the future.

Document harassment. Then see your student dean.

Difficult or Violent Patients

Not all patients are pleasant and enjoyable to work with. To the contrary, patients can sometimes be manipulative, hostile, verbally abusive, and even vio-

Personal safety is a priority with potentially violent patients.

lent. Often, however, such negative behavior is a physical manifestation of the patient's anger and frustration. So do not take anything personally. You need not like every patient you care for, but each deserves your best efforts and respect. You should also use common sense when dealing with difficult patients. Never hesitate to call on more experienced house staff to intervene when situations escalate. And never, ever retaliate against a patient. When dealing with agitated or potentially violent patients, keep the following in mind:

- Remember that your own safety must come first.
- Never let the patient get between you and the door.
- Keep the door open.
- Visit the patient only with a nurse or house officer.
- Assess restraint status.
- Rule out reversible causes of increased agitation and lability.

Difficult Family Members

Having a sick loved one in the hospital places considerable stress on family members and friends, and sometimes the anger, frustration, and sadness are redirected toward you. So again, do not take anything personally. When dealing with family members, find out who the chief decision maker is, especially if the patient is incapacitated or is not competent to make his or her own decisions. Do not, however, let family members push you into speculating about a treatment course. If you are unsure about anything, check with your team before giving the family a definitive answer. Again, know when to seek help from your team or a social worker in order to defuse highly charged or emotional situations.

"Narcolepsy"

Do whatever it takes to stay awake!

During your preclinical years, no one ever noticed if you fell asleep after lunch in a roomful of people. On the wards, however, everyone will notice when you doze off. Although occasionally falling asleep is understandable given your state of frequent exhaustion, constant snoozing will leave a bad impression. The best remedy is to get more sleep. Other students become believers in coffee; however, be aware that caffeine withdrawal is a real clinical syndrome! Another option is to remain standing during rounds and conferences. Although this may raise a few eyebrows, remember that it's your learning (and to some extent your evaluation) that is at stake. If you have to, consider taking a quick nap (30 minutes) during down time to reenergize yourself. Before you do this, however, make sure your resident or attending is not expecting you to do something at that time.

Personal Illness

Nobody can blame you for getting sick.

As students slip into the role of health care provider, they often come to believe that they are not allowed to get sick. In fact, it is a wonder that students do not get sick more often given the long work hours and relentless stress they face. When you get sick, however, your first priority has to be your own health. You cannot provide good patient care while sick, and you may transmit your illness to your patients. Do not dwell on your clinical responsibilities while you are ill; your team will likely get the job done just fine without your help. When sick, immediately page your resident or intern and let them know when you hope to return. If you are out for more than one day, try to keep track of events with your patients by speaking to your team once a day. This will help you slide back into the ward routine with minimal confusion. Use the down time to catch up on reading.

Time Off for Personal Obligations

When you need time off to attend to personal obligations such as a wedding, make arrangements with your resident as far in advance as possible, preferably at the beginning of the rotation. Arrange your call nights around the event if possible. If not, make up the call day elsewhere in the rotation. Try to limit major time off to once a rotation. Of course, there will be situations when you suddenly need time off, such as a family illness or a death. Again, give your team as much advance notice as possible, even if it is just one day. Everyone will understand. As with personal illness, try to keep track of your patients' events if possible. Otherwise, come in the evening before or very early in the morning of your next workday to review patient notes.

Strategies for Mental and Physical Health

Clinical clerkships are a very taxing time, but you must make a conscious effort to balance work and rest, as ignoring your body's needs will eventually compromise your clinical performance. Besides, how can you possibly tell your patients how to stay healthy if you do not care for yourself? (Actually, that is fairly easy, as most medical professionals do not practice what they preach.) Remember that your own health must come first, as you are no help to the team if you are ill. Most of the following advice is considered so basic that it is actually ignored.

Practice what you preach: stay healthy.

Streamline and/or delegate household chores when possible. Consider using an automatic bill payment service. Chip in for a bimonthly cleaning service. Schedule household chores while on an easier rotation in exchange for your roommate's doing them during the more time-consuming rotations. Make sure your roommate understands how difficult your schedule will be on the wards.

Stay grounded in friends and family. Your friends and family have been there for you during the preclinical years, but you'll need their support and companionship more than ever during the clerkships. Given the hours you may be keeping, it can become difficult to stay in touch at times, especially since many of your friends may be classmates who are equally overwhelmed. But make sure you make a solid attempt to return phone messages and remember birthdays, anniversaries, and the like.

Eat well. It is a well-known fact that hospital food and most lunches at noon conferences are considered risk factors for cardiovascular disease. You can still be picky without sacrificing speed. In addition, eat when you can. Being well fed is key to maintaining a high energy level. Load up with complex carbohydrates instead of fat and sugar snacks.

Exercise. "No kidding," you say—but this can be especially tough when you're exhausted from a long day on the wards. It's even worse if you view exercise as another chore. You must find an activity that you enjoy, whether it be walking or basketball. Exercising with a friend keeps you more committed and makes it more social. Consider joining a 24-hour gym so you can work out during the odd hours in which you are free. Another option is to have a treadmill or a bike at home so you can work out while watching TV or reading.

Find healthy ways to deal with stress. Unfortunately, alcohol and substance abuse is higher among medical students and medical graduates than in the general population. This abuse grows most rapidly between the second and fourth years of medical school. You should recognize that you are entering a significantly vulnerable group and be prepared to deal with the stress in ways other than using alcohol and drugs. Find a nonmedical activity, such as reading, running, or painting, that can help you escape the stress of medical school every once in a while. Put it on your schedule and make sure to do it for your health!

YOUR ADVANTAGES

Although you may think that starting on the wards is akin to getting tossed to the wolves, you are not going in empty-handed. Instead, you need to be aware of several advantages that you can maximize to work in your favor.

Enthusiasm

House staff may have a deeper fund of knowledge and more experience, but you can easily match or even surpass them when it comes to hustle, effort, getting there early, and staying late. Team members are often impressed by enthusiastic students, as are patients.

Time

The house staff's time is very precious. You, on the other hand, have plenty of time available. While the house officers have to do brief H&Ps, you have the opportunity and privilege to really learn about your patients. This often allows you to ferret out bits of information on H&Ps that can contribute to—or sometimes even drastically change—patient management. If your patients are frustrated at having to repeat their entire histories again, let them know that you will be able to give them more of your time than anyone else on the team.

Basic Science Knowledge

Not too long ago, you completed one of the most arduous tasks of medical school: passing the USMLE Step 1. Believe it or not, some of the minutiae that you memorized are still buried somewhere in your unconscious and will surface when you least expect it. By contrast, the interns and residents are years away from their basic science classes, so don't be surprised when you show them a thing or two on rounds in front of the attending (of course, don't make a habit of making your resident look dumb, or you may be less than happy with your evaluation). Discreetly feeding the tired intern or resident factoids for attending rounds helps them look good. This can build your reputation as a "team player."

"Low" Expectations

Remember that you are *not* expected to know the answer to every question, nor are you expected to know the set of orders written for a rule-out-MI protocol with your first patient. You will find to your surprise that residents are often impressed by your level of knowledge, even when you consider a question to be a relatively simple one. You are, however, expected to care about your patients and to make a sincere effort to be a contributing member of the team. As long as you show your resident that you are trying to be productive, regardless of how inefficient you are, your resident will be satisfied.

GETTING OFF TO A GOOD START

To further maximize your wards experience, here are some preparatory measures you can take in the months and weeks before your first rotation starts.

Scheduling Rotations

In the spring of your second year, you will go through the process of scheduling your third-year clerkships. Many schools have rotations prescheduled on tracks. Your only task is to choose a track, usually by lottery. Fortunately, there are only a few guidelines you need to know when scheduling your third-year clerkships.

Do not do your most likely specialty first. During the first few weeks of your clerkships, you won't even know where the bathroom is, let alone competently function as a clerk. It is therefore important to allow yourself a chance to get the general feel of the hospital wards and to understand your role, as well as to become comfortable presenting patients and writing notes. Your first rotation should be in a field that you are not likely to go into. For example, most students do not end up going into neurology; however, neurology (as opposed to psychiatry) has the look and feel of a medicine rotation. Make sure every member of your team knows that this is your first rotation; they will be more pleasant and forgiving.

Do not do your most likely specialty last. You will be scheduling your senior clerkships in the spring of your third year. If you're interested in pediatrics, you will want to have done your junior pediatrics before that crucial scheduling period so that you can decide if and when you will be taking any senior pediatrics rotations.

Avoid back-to-back tough rotations. This is a soft rule, especially if you've decided that you have no career interests in one of those specialties. However, you should be concerned about the possibility of burnout when "killer" rotations get scheduled together. Strategically place vacation time after especially difficult rotations to give yourself a chance to unwind.

Schedule an easy rotation before your most likely specialty rotation. Also a soft rule, this gives you time to relax and do some preemptive reading before you start that big rotation. Some students even recommend putting a little vacation time before a key rotation to do some heavy-duty reading.

Choosing Rotation Sites

Your rotations occur in a variety of hospital and clinical settings. Each type of setting has characteristics that will color your clinical experience. Consult senior students regarding the pros and cons of each site, including key attendings to seek out or avoid. The generalizations below don't always apply but should give you an idea of what to expect.

County. The county hospital is typically very busy yet understaffed. Chaos seems to be the baseline as interns and residents constantly battle high patient loads and constant fatigue. County hospitals usually serve the urban poor. In this "all hands on deck" state, you can expect to have more responsibility and more hands-on procedures but less guidance and didactic teaching. You can excel in this environment by being the perfect "SCUT MONKEY," taking care of all those little (but necessary) patient-care tasks. This helps get your team's census down before the next on-call onslaught. The discharge of county hospital patients tends to be more difficult and time-consuming owing to their social situations, so social workers will often become your best allies as you struggle to get your patients out of the hospital.

CURRENT *Med Talk*

"SCUT MONKEY": A highly colloquial and demeaning term that usually refers to a medical student who is relegated to the bottom rung of a team involved in patient management in a university-affiliated health care facility, and performs so-called scut work.

At the VA, know how to work the system.

VA. The VA system personifies the U.S. government in that things take twice as long to get done at twice the cost. Indeed, things sometimes don't get done at all without a little political back scratching and schmoozing. Therefore, being savvy with regard to the political hierarchy definitely helps. The VA population is also unique, consisting mostly of older men with a lot of time on their hands. This makes for an entertaining and forgiving patient population, like the former Marine martial-arts instructor who lets you stick him five times for a blood draw and then teaches you block-and-kill moves after rounds. Female students should be prepared, if necessary, to be a bit more cautious with these patients. Because the population is somewhat demographically restricted, you will also see the same diseases over and over again, including:

- CHF
- MI
- Chronic obstructive pulmonary disease (COPD)
- Lung cancer
- Diabetes
- Arrhythmias
- Gastrointestinal bleeding
- Peripheral vascular disease

Definitely read up on these diseases before you go to the VA. Often, patients remain in house owing to placement issues (where will the patient go after discharge) rather than medical issues. You may end up with a large yet inactive census if you neglect discharge planning.

Academic/university center. Ivory-tower medicine has its own unique approach toward treating patients. Medical and surgical services are top-heavy with consultants and fellows. As a result, residents and interns are often deprived of procedures, leaving even less for you to do. In addition, university hospitals are often tertiary and quaternary referral centers; thus, they get the patients that stump the community physicians. This is where you will see those "ZEBRA" cases, so be prepared to spend time with MEDLINE.

The high staff-to-patient ratio at academic centers also means that a lot of time is spent rounding and discussing the latest treatment for your patient's disease. You can stay ahead of the game by pulling current review papers in the literature for yourself and for the team. The quality of didactics is typically best in the academic center but can sometimes stray into the realm of cutting-edge research and basic science. Finally, a lot of the bigwigs at your school can be found in the academic center. Many students schedule key core and senior rotations there to rub elbows with the academic gods. Scoring an enthusiastic letter of recommendation from them can help make your residency application more impressive.

It should be noted, however, that this form of medicine is currently under siege. Rising managed-care competition plus dwindling Medicare and Medicaid reimbursements are forcing prestigious academic centers to forge new alliances and to scramble for managed-care contracts. Because academic centers have a concurrent and vital teaching mission, they are inherently more costly (IVORY-TOWER SYNDROME) and less efficient than HMOs. Many centers will adopt managed-care strategies to survive, but not all centers will be successful at balancing the bottom line and your education.

"ZEBRA": A somewhat hackneyed aphorism often quoted to wide-eyed medical students during their clinical rotations is *"When you hear hoofbeats, don't think of zebras"*; this variation of "Sutton's law" is designed to teach students a logical approach toward achieving a diagnosis, since common things occur commonly, and when one hears hoofbeats, one usually thinks of horses. (Note: In the Republic of South Africa, zebras are more abundant and the word *canary* is substituted.)

IVORY-TOWER SYNDROME: A highly colloquial ad hoc term for the blatant disregard that academic physicians have for economic realities when teaching medical students the practice of medicine; in the academic construct, information that is deemed extraneous to learning the foundations of medicine is regarded as unnecessary or unworthy of a medical student's time **(Am Med News 24 April 1995, p 15).**

Community hospital. Community hospitals are the antithesis of academic centers in that the focus here is on the patient's treatment and the bottom line. Patients thus tend to come in with bread-and-butter diagnoses, and the populations tend to be more skewed toward the middle class. Many of the physicians are, in addition, private community types—so if residents are present, they are sometimes relegated to "water-boy" status, carrying out orders rather than formulating treatment plans. In many cases, you will be working with a different private physician for each patient. Again, schmoozing is key to participating in a meaningful learning experience as well as to getting things done on your patients. Teaching is more relaxed and deals with the practical treatment approach. Nobody really cares if the long QT syndrome is linked to the Harvey ras (H-*ras*-1) oncogene on the short arm of chromosome 11 as long as you know what to do when a patient with a more common problem walks (or rolls) through the door.

Outpatient clinic. Reforms in medical education will lead to more time spent seeing patients in the outpatient clinic. Residents can blow through half a dozen patients in an afternoon; you'll be lucky if you manage to see three patients in the same amount of time. Keys to being a well-regarded outpatient clerk include obtaining a focused H&P guided by past clinic notes and studies and making a succinct presentation with pertinent positives and negatives that allow your resident or attending to clearly assess the problem. It is also crucial to learn the important things to ask and document as well as the nonessential information that is better left out, since time and efficiency are of the essence. Outpatient medicine is very different from inpatient care in that the patients are not "prisoners," so you cannot order all the tests at once and expect to get them back the same day. In this setting, you will also learn the frustration of patient noncompliance and missed appointments (think about that the next time you decide to blow off your dental appointment).

Before You Start on the Wards

Months before starting on the wards. A few months prior to your rotation, you should consider the following:

- Order an extra white coat or two from the AMA catalog. They have huge pockets both inside and out.
- Gather your medical supplies. Find a stethoscope that is light, yet one you can actually hear with. Test them out in the bookstore on your own heart, lungs, and belly; you're sure to get some strange looks, but doing so will help you decide whether you really need the Littmann Cardiology III.

Remember, too, that equipment is less pricey when ordered in bulk through medical schools—and you might even get a stethoscope for free if you can wrangle one from a pharmaceutical company. You may also want to buy a cheap stethoscope to have as an "extra" in case your good one walks off one day and you have no time to go to the bookstore to replace it.

One week before. You will feel less lost on the first day if you follow these general rotation-specific guidelines:

- If you're starting neuro, practice the neuro exam.
- If you're starting psych, practice or review the psych interview.
- If you're starting medicine, review normal values and the H&P.
- If you're starting surgery, review knots, sutures, and what goes in a preop, brief-op, postop, and progress note.
- Read the appropriate chapter in *First Aid for the Wards*.

The night before. On the night before your rotation starts, you should do the following:

- Get your white coat. Chances are that there is no safe place to leave anything in the hospital on your first day, so don't bring too much. Remember to bring your ID, your name tag, some money, extra pens, your stethoscope, *Pharmacopoeia* (for all rotations because it is tiny and will quickly translate all those brand names into generic names), your beeper (memorize the number so you can give it out), and a set of car or apartment keys.
- Set your alarm half an hour early, especially if you're not sure how to get either to the hospital or to your floor.
- Make sure you know where to go and when to get there. If in doubt, ask classmates who are on your team, or page a resident on the team.
- Recheck your alarm, especially the volume and the AM/PM settings.

The first day. On the first day of your wards experience:

- Eat a big breakfast.
- Arrive early.

- Make sure every member of your team knows this is your first rotation. That way, they are likely to be more tolerant toward you and to pay more attention to teaching you hospital basics, such as how to read a nursing chart, get labs or cultures off the computer, or page someone.
- Don't leave until the chief resident says to leave.
- If in doubt, ask when and where rounds will be the next day. Especially for surgery and medicine, bring an on-call bag with a toothbrush and toothpaste, underwear, socks, any medication you are on, and earplugs. Leave this gear in your car in case you are on call that first night.

Practical Information for All Clerkships

This chapter reviews some key high-yield skills and knowledge that you will need regardless of the rotation you are on. Topics include how to read a CXR, how to make sense of an ECG, how to manage your patients' fluids and electrolytes, and how to interpret acid-base problems. The final section lists key abbreviations with which you should be familiar and key formulas that you may need to solve clinical problems.

Be systematic in clinical problem solving.

You'll find that the most important thing you can do when learning the high-yield skills and knowledge presented in this chapter is to create a systematic approach. Whether you are solving an acid-base problem or interpreting a CXR, you will be far less likely to miss something essential if you are systematic. There are many different ways to approach each of these skills. Find one that you are comfortable with and stick to it. Your residents and attendings will be impressed!

READING KEY STUDIES

The Chest X-Ray

Many of your patients in the hospital and emergency room will have a CXR. Although a formal reading will be completed by a radiologist, it is important for you to learn the basics of interpretation.

There are many different ways to approach a CXR. Again, the key is to be systematic. When your attending asks for your impression of the study, you will earn points by walking through it step by step. One basic approach will be discussed below.

First, however, you should be familiar with a few common ways of making a chest film. Most of the studies you see will be one of the following:

- **Anteroposterior AP:** X-rays pass through the patient from front to back (anterior to posterior). Since the heart is farthest from the film, AP films often falsely enlarge heart size. They are less ideal films and are typically used when the patient cannot stand up (e.g., when portable films are obtained in an ICU patient).
- **Posteroanterior PA:** X-rays pass through the patient from back to front (posterior to anterior). These films yield a more accurate estimate of heart size.
- **Lateral:** Typically, the patient's left side is facing the film to avoid cardiac distortion. The lateral projection is named by the side closest to the film (e.g., left lateral). These films are used to pinpoint the location of abnormalities seen on AP/PA films, to assess AP diameter, and to check the posterior costophrenic angles for small (< 250-cc) effusions.

- **Decubitus:** Patients are lying on their sides (e.g., in a left decubitus film, the left side faces down). These films are used to evaluate the presence of free air or fluid (e.g., pleural effusion or pneumothorax).

When you set out to interpret a film, you should always begin by checking the patient's name and the date to ensure that you are looking at the correct film. No matter how stellar your interpretation may be, it won't count for much if you have the wrong patient.

Next, begin to assess the film systematically using the A-B-C-D sequence (see Table 2.1).

The ECG

Many books teach a detailed approach to the ECG (see Top-Rated Books). However, it is important to have a basic method for quickly scanning an ECG on the spot. There are many different methodologies for this, so again, pick one you like and stick with it. One basic approach is presented in Table 2.2.

Most studies you see will be 12-lead ECGs. Before you begin your reading, check the standardization mark. In a standard ECG set at 25 mm/sec, each small box represents 0.04 sec, and each large box (composed of five small boxes) represents 0.2 sec. See Figure 2.1 for identification of the elements of an ECG tracing.

Table 2.3 outlines the three degrees of atrioventricular (AV) block.

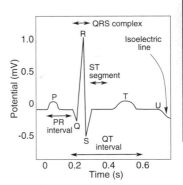

FIGURE 2.1. Sample ECG tracing

Be familiar with the fluid and electrolyte composition of different body compartments.

FLUIDS AND ELECTROLYTES

On the wards, you will be managing your patients' fluids and electrolytes from the outset. Although you aren't expected to be a pro on day one, it will help if you understand some key terms and concepts. You should become familiar with the basic fluid and electrolyte composition of the body, the types of fluids available, and the phases of fluid therapy. Keep in mind that the approach will differ somewhat from service to service and for adult and pediatric patients, but the basic principles remain the same.

Total Body Water

To order fluids, you will often need to estimate a patient's total body water (TBW). As a general rule, more body fat means less TBW. For calculations, use the following guidelines:

- 50% of lean body weight in adult females and the elderly
- 60% of lean body weight in young adult males
- 75–80% of lean body weight in infants

TABLE 2.1. The A-B-C-D Sequence.

Step	Process
Assessment	Assess the quality of the film using the mnemonic **PIER:** Position: Is this a supine AP film? PA? Lateral? Inspiration: Count the posterior ribs. You should see 10 to 11 ribs with a good inspiratory effort. Exposure: Well-exposed films have good lung detail and an outline of the spinal column. Overpenetration leads to a dark film with more spinal detail. Underpenetrated films are whiter with little spinal detail. Rotation: The space between the medial clavicle and the margin of the adjacent vertebrae should be roughly equal on each side. Also look for indwelling lines or objects (e.g., endotracheal tube, feeding tube, airway obstruction), which may reveal clues to the pathology in the film.
Bones and soft tissues	Scan the bones for symmetry, fractures, osteoporosis, or metastatic lesions. Evaluate the soft tissues for foreign bodies, edema, or subcutaneous air.
Cardiac	Evaluate heart size: the heart should be < 50% of the chest diameter on PA films and < 60% on AP films. Check for heart shape, calcifications, and prosthetic valves.
Diaphragms	Check diaphragms for position (the right is slightly higher than the left due to the liver) and shape (may be flat in asthma or COPD). Look below the diaphragms for free air.
Effusions	Pleural effusions may be large and obvious or small and subtle. Always check the costophrenic angles for sharpness (blunted angles may indicate small effusions). Check a lateral film for small posterior effusions.
Fields/fissures	Check lung fields for infiltrates (interstitial vs. alveolar), masses, consolidation, air bronchograms, pneumothoraces, and vascular markings. Vessels should taper and should be almost invisible at the lung periphery. Evaluate the major and minor fissures for thickening or fluid.
Great vessels	Check aortic size and shape and the outlines of pulmonary vessels. The aortic knob should be clearly seen.
Hilar/ mediastinal area	Evaluate the hila for lymphadenopathy, calcifications, and masses. The left hilum is normally higher than the right. Check for widening of the mediastinum (which may indicate aortic dissection) and tracheal deviation (which may indicate a mass effect or tension pneumothorax). In children, be careful not to mistake the thymus for a mass!
Impression	Always formulate a preliminary impression of the film. Even if it is incorrect, it will show that you have been thinking.

TABLE 2.2. ECG Interpretation.

Variable	Method of Assessment
Rate	Estimate the rate by counting the number of heavy black lines between consecutive R waves. Find an R wave on a heavy black line, and then start counting at the next heavy line: "300, 150, 100, 75, 60, 50 . . ." Rates over 100 are tachycardia; rates under 60 are bradycardia. Alternatively, use the formula 1500/RR number of small boxes between consecutive R waves. For bradycardia, you can count the number of cycles per 6-sec strip × 10.
Rhythm	Identify the basic rhythm and look for abnormal waves, irregularities, or pauses. Check the sinus rhythm: Is there a single P wave before each QRS complex? Is there a single QRS after each P wave? Do all of the P waves look alike? Are the P waves upright in lead II and inverted in lead aVR? Check for ectopic beats (premature atrial or ventricular contractions). Check the RR intervals for regularity of rhythm. An irregularly irregular rhythm suggests atrial fibrillation.
Intervals	Check the PR interval for AV block (> 0.20 sec). The classification of AV blocks is discussed in Table 2.3. Check the QRS for bundle branch block (> 0.12 sec). ■ Right bundle branch block (RBBB): RSR′ ("rabbit ears" pattern) in V_1 and V_2; wide S in I and V_6 ■ Left bundle branch block (LBBB): RR′ ("slurred" pattern) in I and V_6; wide S in V_1 Check the QT interval using the corrected interval: QTc = QT/RR. For a quick check, the QT interval should be less than half of the RR interval.
Axis	For a quick assessment of the axis, look at the QRS complex in leads I and II. If both are upright, the axis is normal. See Figure 2.2 for the diagnosis of axis deviation.
Hypertrophy	Right atrial hypertrophy (RAH): biphasic p in V_1, peaked first portion, > 2.5-mm height, or > 1 × 1 mm = "p pulmonale." Remember, right is height Left atrial hypertrophy (LAH): biphasic p in V_1, wide/negative terminal portion, > 0.8-mm duration = "p mitrale." Remember, left is length Right ventricular hypertrophy (RVH): R > S in V_1; S persists in V_5, V_6; right-axis deviation; widened QRS interval. Left ventricular hypertrophy (LVH): amplitude of S in V_1 + R in V_5 > 35 mm; left-axis deviation; wide QRS; inverted/asymmetric T wave.
Infarction	Look for Q waves (transmural infarct), inverted T waves, and ST elevation. Significant Q wave = 1 mm wide or > ⅓ amplitude of QRS. An inverted T wave may point to ischemia. ST depression may mean ischemia or subendocardial infarct (non-Q-wave MI).

TABLE 2.2. *(continued)* ECG Interpretation.

Variable	Method of Assessment
	Localize the infarct: • Inferior MI (dominant coronary, usually right): II, III, aVF • Lateral MI (left circumflex): I, aVL, V_5, V_6 • Anterior MI (left anterior descending): V_1–V_4 • Posterior MI (right coronary): large R and ST depression in V_1, V_2 • Septal MI: V_2, V_3
Electrolyte abnormalities	Hyperkalemia: peaked T waves → short PR interval → loss of P wave → wide QRS → sine wave. Hypokalemia: flat T wave → U wave → prominent U wave. Hypercalcemia: short QT interval. Hypocalcemia: prolonged QT interval. Excess quinidine (or very low potassium): torsades de pointes.

Fluid Compartments

The TBW is distributed between the intracellular (⅔) and extracellular (⅓) compartments. Extracellular fluid is further distributed between the interstitial (¾) and intravascular (¼) spaces. Fluid distribution can also be calculated as a percentage of body weight (BW):

- Intracellular water accounts for 40% of BW.
- Extracellular water accounts for 20% of BW.

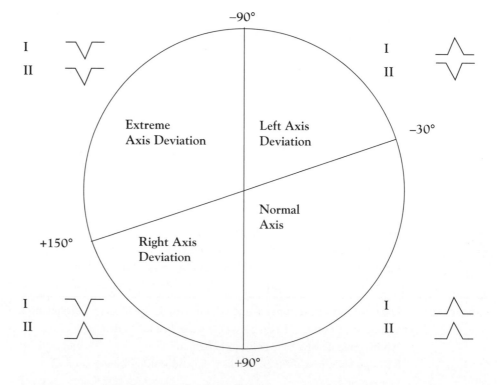

FIGURE 2.2. Quick Method of Axis Determination.

Degree	Characteristics
TABLE 2.3. Degrees of AV Block.	
First degree	Prolonged PR interval (> 0.2 sec) with normal tracing
Second degree 　Mobitz type I 　(Wenckebach) 　Mobitz type II	 Progressive lengthening of PR interval until a QRS is 　dropped Consistent ratio of conducted to dropped QRS complexes. 　Requires pacemaker.
Third degree	Complete dissociation between atrial and ventricular rates. Requires pacemaker.

- Interstitial water accounts for 15% of BW.
- Blood volume in adults accounts for 7% of BW.
- Blood volume in children accounts for 8% of BW.

IV Fluids

You will have different types of fluids to choose from in the hospital. Isotonic fluids include normal saline (NS) and lactated Ringer's (LR), which are frequently used for acute resuscitation. Note that resuscitation fluids do not contain dextrose, which can cause hyperglycemia and osmotic diuresis. On surgical services, LR is also typically a maintenance fluid of choice. The lactate is converted by the liver into HCO_3^- and then into CO_2 in the blood. As a result, this fluid should be avoided for maintenance in a patient with high CO_2 levels.

In general, maintenance fluids contain added dextrose and potassium. Dextrose prevents the breakdown of muscle for energy needs, provides fuel for the Krebs cycle, and prevents ketoacidosis. "D5" means 5% dextrose solution and "D5W" means dextrose in water. Potassium can be added after your patient proves that his or her kidneys work (i.e., there is urine output).

Don't add potassium until you know the kidneys work.

The components of common fluids are listed in Table 2.4. Values are in milliequivalents per liter. Normal plasma osmolarity ranges from 280 to 300.

Fluid and Electrolyte Therapy

The important elements of complete fluid therapy are acute resuscitation, provision of maintenance fluids, replacement of ongoing losses, and replacement of deficits. Some patients will present in an acutely dehydrated state and will require resuscitation and deficit replacement, while others may be admitted for an elective surgical procedure and will require only maintenance fluids.

Fluid resuscitation. If a patient is significantly volume depleted, the first goal is to rapidly replenish intravascular volume. It is important to realize that the ex-

Fluids	Na	Cl	K	HCO₃	Ca
Crystalloids					
NS	154	154			
D5 NS	154	154			
½ NS	77	77			
D5 ½ NS	77	77			
D5 ¼ NS	39	39			
D5W					
LR	130	109	4.00	28	3
3% NaCl	513	513			
Colloids					
Hespan	154	154			
Plasmanate	145	100	0.25		
25% albumin	130–160	130–160	1.00		

TABLE 2.4. Components of Common Fluids.

KEY POINT

THREE-FOR-ONE RULE

To replace 1 L of intravascular volume, you should give 3 L of isotonic solution. After one to two hours, 1 L of isotonic solution redistributes such that only 300 mL remains in the intravascular space. Thus, three to four times the estimated intravascular deficit should be replaced. Colloid solutions remain in the intravascular space for a longer period but are quite expensive and should be used sparingly in appropriate clinical situations (e.g., in edematous patients).

tent of clinical symptoms will depend not only on the volume lost but also on the rate of loss. Patients who have a gradual volume contraction may be well compensated, while patients with rapid volume loss may go into circulatory shock.

In adults, the standard resuscitation fluid is LR or NS. In a very dehydrated adult, a 1- to 2-L bolus may be given over 30 to 120 minutes. If the patient has a history of cardiac disease, a slower rate is recommended.

In children, you can ask parents about recent intake (bottle- or breast-feeding) and output (fewer than four to five wet diapers in 24 hours suggests dehydration). You should evaluate physical signs of dehydration, which are outlined in Table 2.5.

TABLE 2.5. Clinical Manifestations of Dehydration.

Symptoms/ Signs	Mild Dehydration	Moderate Dehydration	Severe Dehydration
Weight loss	5%	10%	15%
Pulse	Normal or slightly increased	Increased	Very increased
Blood pressure	Normal	Normal to orthostatic	Orthostatic to shock
Tears	Present	Decreased	Absent, sunken eyes
Mucous membranes	Normal	Dry	Parched
Mental status	Normal	Altered	Depressed
Anterior fontanelle (in children)	Normal	Normal to sunken	Sunken
Skin	Capillary refill < 2 sec	Delayed capillary refill 2–4 sec, decreased turgor	Very delayed capillary refill, > 4 sec, cool skin, acrocyanosis
Urine specific gravity	1.020	> 1.020, oliguria	Maximal, oliguria or anuria
Estimated fluid deficit	< 50 mL/kg	50–100 mL/kg	> 100 mL/kg

Mild to moderate dehydration in children may be treated with oral rehydration therapies (ORTs) such as Pedialyte or Ricelyte, which contain approximately 45–90 mEq/L sodium, 20 mEq/L potassium, 20 g/L glucose, and 30 mEq citrate or bicarbonate. IV fluid boluses with isotonic crystalloid (NS or LR) are used to rapidly expand intravascular volume within the following guidelines:

- 10 cc/kg bolus over one hour for mild dehydration.
- 20 cc/kg bolus over one hour for moderate dehydration.
- 30–50 cc/kg over one hour for severe dehydration or shock.
- Reassess urine output and clinical status and rebolus as necessary.

The second phase of fluid therapy involves provision of maintenance fluids, replacement of ongoing losses, and replacement of existing deficits.

Maintenance fluids. People in the hospital often order IV fluids on the basis of average fluid requirements. For example, an average order for an adult is D5 ½ NS + 20 KCl at 125 cc/hr. You can also calculate the exact water and electrolyte needs of a given patient, which will be more accurate if your patient differs from the standard 70-kg male. Maintenance fluid requirements are increased under certain conditions, including hyperventilation, sweating, fever, hyperthyroidism, renal disease, and GI losses.

KEY POINT

SAMPLE MAINTENANCE FLUID CALCULATION

Patient: A 24-kg child is admitted for elective surgery.

Maintenance fluids: $(100 \times 10) + (50 \times 10) + (20 \times 4) = 1580$ mL/day = 65.8 mL/hr

Maintenance electrolytes: Na = 3 mEq/100 mL $\times$ 1580 mL/day = 47.4 mEq/day

K = 2 mEq/100 mL $\times$ 1580 mL/day = 31.6 mEq/day

Answer: ¼ NS provides 34 mEq NaCl/L. If the child requires approximately 1.5 L/day, the child will receive 51 mEq of NaCl, which satisfies his requirement. The addition of 20 mEq KCl to each liter (after first void) will provide 30 mEq/day.

Appropriate fluid order: D5 ¼ NS + 20 mEq KCl to run at 65 mL/hr.

Water requirements are calculated using the following methods:

1. Holliday-Segar method (100/50/20 rule):

   - 100 mL/kg/day for the first 10 kg of weight.
   - Add 50 mL/kg for the next 10 kg.
   - Add 20 mL/kg for each kilogram over 20.
   - Sample calculation: A 70-kg adult would need $(100 \times 10) + (50 \times 10) + (20 \times 50) = 2500$ mL/day.

2. Hourly fluids (4/2/1 rule):

   - 4 mL/kg/hr for the first 10 kg.
   - Add 2 mL/kg for the next 10 kg.
   - Add 1 mL/kg for each kilogram over 20.
   - Sample calculation: A 70-kg adult would need $(4 \times 10) + (2 \times 10) + (1 \times 50) = 110$ mL/hr.
   - A shortcut is "40 plus the weight in kilograms." A 70-kg man would need $40 + 70 = 110$ mL/hr.

Electrolyte requirements for adults and children are shown in Table 2.6.

Replace ongoing losses. Evaluate the volume and composition of fluids lost through diarrhea, vomiting, chest tubes, or various other sources. Try to replace losses "cc for cc" with fluids of similar composition. The average composition of body fluids can be found in many pocket guides and textbooks.

Deficit therapy. Replacement of existing deficits will depend on the degree of dehydration (established by history and exam) and the type of dehydration (established by serum sodium, and generally classified as isonatremic, hyponatremic, or hypernatremic). A complete discussion of volume and electrolyte imbalances is beyond the scope of this book, but there are some basic facts that you should know.

TABLE 2.6. Electrolyte Requirements.

	Adults	**Children**
Na	80–120 mEq /day	3–5 mEq/kg/day or per 100 mL fluid
K	50–100 mEq/day	2–3 mEq/kg/day or per 100 mL fluid
Cl	80–120 mEq/day	3 mEq/kg/day or per 100 mL fluid
Glucose	100–200 g/day	100–200 mg/kg/hr

Deficit replacement generally takes place at a rate proportional to the rate of loss. In a patient with 2 L of acute blood loss, IV fluids should be given rapidly in the resuscitation phase. By contrast, in a patient with well-compensated chronic hypernatremic dehydration, replacement should be undertaken slowly to avoid rapid fluid shifts and potential complications.

1. **Isonatremic dehydration (Na 130–150 mEq/L):** This is the most common form of dehydration and involves a net loss of isotonic fluid. Begin treatment by estimating the fluid deficit based on the degree of dehydration (e.g., mild = approximately 5% BW). Some clinicians replace the entire deficit with isotonic solution; standard therapy is D5 ¼ NS in small children and D5 ½ NS in older children and adults. After urination, 10–20 mEq KCl can be added. Half of the deficit should be replaced over eight hours and the remainder over 16 hours.

2. **Hyponatremic dehydration (Na < 130):** There is a net loss of solute, so an additional sodium deficit must be replaced. The formula for calculating the sodium deficit is:

   Na deficit (mEq) = (desired Na − measured Na) × 0.6 × weight (kg)

   This sodium should be added to the patient's other fluid and electrolyte needs. Again, half of the deficit can be replaced over eight hours and the remainder over 16 hours. In chronic, severe hyponatremia however, the serum sodium should not be increased > 2 mEq/L/hr or 10–12 mEq/L/day because of the risk of central pontine myelinosis (CPM). In a symptomatic patient (e.g., one who has CNS symptoms), 3% NaCl may be given in an ICU setting to raise Na to > 120 mEq. The remainder of fluid replacement should proceed slowly. NS is the standard fluid and free water should generally be restricted.

3. **Hypernatremic dehydration (Na > 150):** There is a net loss of water relative to solute. This is typically due to decreased fluid intake in the presence of increased insensible losses (e.g., fever, burns) but may also be due to excess salt intake. Treatment involves replacement of the free water deficit, which is calculated using the following formula:

When in doubt, assume hyponatremia is chronic and do not replenish sodium rapidly.

$$\text{Water deficit (L)} = \text{TBW} \times (\text{actual Na} - \text{desired Na})/\text{desired Na}$$

Correction must be undertaken cautiously; if sodium is corrected too rapidly (> 0.5–1.0 mEq/L/hr), cerebral edema, seizures, and CNS injury may result. Sodium may be lowered by 10–15 mEq/L/day, not to exceed 25 mEq/L/24 hr or 5 mEq/L/hr. Thus, the replacement schedule is slower. In general, use D5 ½ NS, D5 ¼ NS, or D5W to correct half of the free water deficit over 24 hours. Then, follow serum sodium and correct the remainder of the deficit over 48 to 72 hours. Begin replacing potassium after the patient urinates, and remember to replace ongoing losses and provide maintenance fluids.

ACID-BASE CALCULATIONS

On almost every rotation you embark on, you will be asked to evaluate the acid-base status of a patient. You'll impress your residents and attendings if you can rapidly interpret your patient's acid-base status *and* provide a differential diagnosis for your patient's condition. There are several approaches to determining a patient's acid-base status, so you will probably encounter a different paradigm with each resident you meet and each new rotation you begin. The important thing is to be systematic and approach each case the same way. Presented below is one systematic approach to acid-base problems.

Two essential laboratory results are necessary for interpreting acid-base problems: an arterial blood gas (ABG) and an electrolyte panel. Using these studies, you will ask yourself four major questions:

1. **Does the patient have an acidemia (pH < 7 .36) or alkalemia (pH > 7.44)?** Normal pH is 7.40.

2. **Is the primary disturbance metabolic or respiratory?** In general, the quickest way to assess the primary disturbance is to look at the P_{CO_2} (normal P_{CO_2} is 40). If the P_{CO_2} has shifted in the *opposite* direction of pH (e.g., P_{CO_2} increases when pH decreases), then you know your primary disturbance is respiratory. Beware, however, of combined disturbances. See Table 2.7 for an algorithm to define the primary disturbance. Note that normal HCO_3^- is 24.

3. **Is compensation for the primary disturbance appropriate?** See Table 2.8.

4. **Is there an anion gap (AG) acidosis?** Regardless of whether you initially identified a metabolic acidosis, always check for an AG acidosis.

   a. Calculate the patient's AG.
   b. Calculate ΔAG. ΔAG = the calculated AG − the normal AG.

Compensatory mechanisms NEVER overcompensate or compensate completely.

TABLE 2.7. Method for Defining Primary Acid-Base Disturbance.

pH[a]	PCO_2	$[HCO_3^-]$	Primary Disturbance
< 7.36	↑	↑ or ↔	Respiratory acidosis
	↓ or ↔	↓	Metabolic acidosis
	↑	↓	Combined respiratory and metabolic acidosis
< 7.44	↓	↓ or ↔	Respiratory alkalosis
	↑ or ↔	↑	Metabolic alkalosis
	↓	↑	Combined respiratory and metabolic alkalosis

    c. Calculate ΔHCO_3^-. $\Delta HCO_3^- = [\Delta HCO_3^-]_{plasma} - [HCO_3^-]_{normal}$.
    d. Refer to Table 2.9 to determine if the patient has AG, non-anion-gap (NAG), or combined metabolic acidosis.

Some examples are as follows:

1. **Lab values:** pH = 7.11, PCO_2 = 16, HCO_3^- = 5, Na^+ = 140, K^+ = 4.0, $[Cl^-]$ = 115

    Step 1: Does the patient have an acidemia or alkalemia?

        pH = 7.11, so the patient is acidemic.

    Step 2: Is the primary disturbance metabolic or respiratory?

        PCO_2 = 16, which is lower than normal. PCO_2 has moved in the *same* direction as pH (i.e., down), so the primary disturbance is *not* respiratory, but metabolic. Consistent with a metabolic etiology, we see that $[HCO_3^-]$ = 5, which indicates that the major base, bicarbonate, is decreased. We conclude that this patient's primary disturbance is a metabolic acidosis.

    Step 3: Is the compensation for the primary disturbance appropriate?

        For a metabolic acidosis, we expect $PCO_2 = 1.5 * HCO_3^- + 8 \pm 2$. So in this case, we would expect $PCO_2 = 1.5 * 5 + 8 \pm 2 = 16 \pm 2$. We therefore conclude that the compensation is appropriate.

    Step 4: Is there an AG acidosis?

        First we calculate the AG, which is 20 (140 − 115 − 5). ΔAG therefore equals 8. ΔHCO_3^- = 19. Since ΔHCO_3^- is greater than ΔAG, we conclude that there is a combined AG and NAG metabolic acidosis.

    SOLUTION: Combined AG and NAG metabolic acidosis.

2. **Lab values:** pH = 7.67, PCO_2 = 30, HCO_3^- = 34, Na^+ = 140, K^+ = 3.0, Cl^- = 94

TABLE 2.8. Methods of Compensation for Primary Disturbance.

Primary Disturbance	Compensatory Mechanism	Calculating Appropriate Compensation	Compensation Is Inappropriate
Metabolic acidosis	P_{CO_2}	$P_{CO_2} = 1.5 * HCO_3^- + 8 \pm 2$ (Winter's equation) P_{CO_2} = last two digits of pH $P_{CO_2} \uparrow$ by 10 for every $HCO_3 \downarrow$ by 10	If actual P_{CO_2} is: Higher, there is also a respiratory acidosis Lower, there is also a respiratory alkalosis
Metabolic alkalosis	P_{CO_2}	$P_{CO_2} = 0.9 * HCO_3^- + 9$ $\Delta P_{CO_2} = 0.6 * HCO_3^-$ $P_{CO_2} \uparrow$ by 7 for every $HCO_3^- \uparrow$ by 10	If actual P_{CO_2} is: Higher, there is also a respiratory acidosis Lower, there is also a respiratory alkalosis
Respiratory acidosis	HCO_3^-	Acute: $HCO_3^- \uparrow$ by 1 for every $P_{CO_2} \uparrow$ by10 Chronic: $HCO_3^- \uparrow$ by 4 for every $P_{CO_2} \uparrow$ by10	If actual HCO_3^- is: Higher, there is also a metabolic alkalosis Lower, there is also a metabolic acidosis
Respiratory alkalosis	HCO_3^-	Acute: $HCO_3^- \downarrow$ by 2 for every $P_{CO_2} \downarrow$ by10 Chronic: $HCO_3^- \downarrow$ by 5 for every $P_{CO_2} \downarrow$ by 10	If actual HCO_3^- is: Higher, there is also a metabolic alkalosis Lower, there is also a metabolic acidosis

Step 1: Does the patient have an acidemia or an alkalemia?

pH = 7.67, so the patient is alkalemic.

Step 2: What is the primary disturbance?

$P_{CO_2} = 30$, which is lower than normal. P_{CO_2} has moved in the *opposite* direction from pH, so we can conclude that the primary disturbance is respiratory. We also check HCO_3^- to determine if there is a combined primary disturbance. $HCO_3^- = 34$, which indicates that the major base, bicarbonate, is increased. We therefore conclude that there is also a primary metabolic alkalosis.

Step 3: Is the compensation appropriate?

For a respiratory alkalosis, we expect HCO_3^- to decrease 2–5 mEq/L for every 10-mmHg decrease in P_{CO_2}. We would therefore expect HCO_3^- to be between 19 and 22. $HCO_3^- = 34$, which is higher than expected, so we once again confirm that there is a metabolic alkalosis in addition to the respiratory alkalosis.

TABLE 2.9. Determination of Acidosis Type.

ΔAG	ΔHCO_3^-	Type
0 ± 2	$> \Delta$AG	NAG acidosis
> 2	$= \Delta$AG	AG acidosis
> 2	$> \Delta$AG	Combined NAG and AG acidosis

Step 4: Is there an AG acidosis?

First, we calculate the AG, which is 12 (140–94–34). ΔAG therefore equals Ø and we can conclude that there is no underlying anion gap metabolic acidosis.

SOLUTION: Combined primary respiratory and metabolic alkalosis.

SLIDING-SCALE INSULIN

When patients are admitted to the hospital, you will often be asked to write a sliding scale insulin (SSI) in their admission orders. Scales differ significantly across institutions and may also be tailored to individual patients. Table 2.10 gives just one example of a scale you might see.

PATIENT EMERGENCIES

One of a student's worst nightmares is being all alone with a patient when something bad happens. In such a situation, the first rule is "Don't panic!" Immediately call for help (i.e., yell "Nurse, I've got a problem!").

Cardiopulmonary Arrest

Check for patient responsiveness first. In a loud voice, ask the patient, "Are you okay?" while you shake him or her. If the patient is unresponsive and does not pass the "eyeball test" (i.e., the patient looks very sick), do not hesitate to call a CODE BLUE. You will get all the help you ever wanted. Do not fear any embarrassment that would arise from calling an unnecessary code blue. Everyone will remember if you failed to call a necessary code.

In an emergency immediately call for help.

> CODE STATUS: The formally indicated (often through signed documents) status of a patient in a hospital with respect to his/her desire for resuscitative (i.e., CPR) efforts, should the need arise; unless the patient specifically requests that he/she *NOT* be resuscitated, i.e., DNR (do not resuscitate) status, CPR will be performed.
>
> CODE: *(noun)* A widely used (albeit highly colloquial) term for a cardiopulmonary arrest that is invariably accompanied by a frenzied fracas and frenetic fray. *(verb)* To suffer a cardiac arrest in a hospital environment.

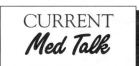

CURRENT *Med Talk*

Value[a]	SSI[b]
< 70	Give 1 amp dextrose and call house officer
71–150	Nothing
151–200	2 units
201–250	4 units
251–300	6 units
301–350	8 units
351–400	10 units
> 400	Give 12 units and call house officer

TABLE 2.10. Sliding-Scale Insulin Orders.

[a]Result of finger-stick blood glucose measurement.
[b]Regular human insulin administered subcutaneously.

KEY POINT

REGULAR INSULIN DOSING

Some patients need a regular insulin schedule. Type I diabetics generally require 0.4-0.6 unit/kg lean body weight. A typical dosing schedule is constructed in the following way:

⅔ total insulin in AM
  ⅓ regular
  ⅔ NPH
⅓ total insulin in PM
  ½ regular
  ½ NPH

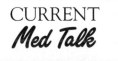

CURRENT *Med Talk*

CODE BLUE: A message announced over a hospital's public address system indicating that a cardiac arrest requiring medical attention is in progress; in a similar context, to be "coded" is to undergo CPR.

In a patient emergency:

1. Don't panic.

2. Get help.

3. Check ABCs.

4. Perform CPR if

necessary.

By the time you check ABCs (airway, breathing, and circulation), there should be hordes of physicians and other health care professionals who will take over. The patient's code status will be ascertained, and the resulting resuscitation will be driven by established advanced cardiac life support (ACLS) protocols. In a full-code situation, the medical student often does the chest compressions, places an IV, or helps defibrillate.

The basic sequence of a code blue is outlined as "A-B-C/D-E-F" (see below).

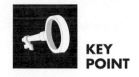

A-B-C/D-E-F SEQUENCE

Airway	Ensure airway patency (clear bronchotracheal tree)
Breathing	If patient is not breathing, begin intermittent positive pressure ventilation
Circulation	If patient does not have pulse, compress chest at 80–100 minute
Drugs/Fluids	Place IV line
ECG	Monitor cardiac rhythms
Fibrillation	Defibrillate

While the code is being activated, check **ABC**s:

- **Airway:** Determine if the patient is breathing. If not, adjust the patient's airway with a backward head tilt or a forward jaw thrust and reassess breathing.
- **Breathing:** If the patient is still not breathing, give two slow breaths. Then check the circulatory status of the patient.
- **Circulation:** Check the carotid pulses, one at a time, on both sides. Peripheral pulses are not reliable in these situations. If pulses are absent, initiate CPR. In adults and children, use the heel of your hand to compress the sternum one and one-half to two inches at the level of the nipples at a rate of 80 to 100 beats per minute (bpm). In infants, use the tips of the middle and ring fingers to compress the sternum one-half inch to one inch at a rate of at least 100 bpm. The ratio of compressions to breaths in adults is 15:2 and in children and infants 5:1. Check the ECG pattern, as this may alter further treatment. If no ECG is present, ask the nurse to call for one immediately.

If asystole is detected by ECG in more than one lead, continue CPR. In addition to chest compressions, transcutaneous pacing may be considered. The patient must be intubated. An IV is started immediately, and 1 mg of epinephrine and 1 mg of atropine (up to a maximum of 0.05 mg/kg) are pushed every three to five minutes.

If a ventricular fibrillation (VF) or ventricular tachycardia (VT) is detected with a ventricular rate greater than 150 bpm, cardioversion is necessary. While stable VT may be treated with medication, VF or unstable VT (i.e., low BP of no pulse) should immediately be treated with electrocardioversion. In addition, the patient should be given an oxygen face mask if he or she is not intubated. Defibrillation is attempted with incremental increases in energy: 200, 300, and 360 J.

Shock

The three major classes of shock are hypovolemic, distributive, and cardiac.

Shock is defined as a physiologic state of circulatory failure resulting in inadequate tissue perfusion and tissue hypoxia. The cardinal signs of shock are simultaneous tachycardia and hypotension. The etiology of shock can be divided into three major categories: (1) hypovolemic, (2) distributive, and (3) cardiac. The two major causes of hypovolemic shock are hemorrhage and dehydration. Distributive shock is caused by a "misdistribution" of blood due to inappropriately low systemic vascular resistance. The major causes of distributive shock are septic, neurogenic, and anaphylactic. Finally, cardiac shock is due to the inability of the heart to adequately pump blood to the body owing either to intrinsic dysfunction or to extrinsic factors. Intrinsic heart dysfunction is known as cardiogenic shock or CHF. Extrinsic factors that may alter the heart's ability to adequately pump blood are pericardial effusions causing cardiac tamponade, tension pneumothorax, and massive pulmonary embolus.

Considering the various etiologies of shock, the evaluation and management of the patient in acute shock involves assessment of volume status, systemic vascular resistance (SVR), and cardiac output (see Table 2.11).

Giving fluids will worsen cardiogenic shock.

The vast majority of shock is due to hypovolemia. Consequently, in an emergency, the treatment of shock is the same as that described for hypovolemic shock. Remember, the key to treating shock is fluid resuscitation in almost all types of shock. If you do not give fluid to your patient, you are effectively making a diagnosis of cardiogenic shock.

Hypovolemic Shock

Hypovolemic shock can be due to any process that depletes intravascular volume. Hypovolemic shock is most often due to acute blood loss, dehydration, or third spacing. Identifying the source of acute blood loss is critical, especially in trauma patients, if one is to gain the upper hand in a patient with shock. If hemorrhage is suspected, the abdomen is assumed to be the source of the hemorrhage until proven otherwise. Dehydration can be due to many causes but is most commonly attributable to protracted diarrhea or vomiting, overdiuresis, or fluid restriction (e.g., in the elderly who may not be able to drink adequate fluids). Third spacing is the shift of intravascular volume into the interstitial space or other compartments (e.g., the peritoneum). Common burns, trauma, acute pancreatitis, and liver diseases are some common causes of third spacing.

Signs and Symptoms. The signs and symptoms of hypovolemic shock depend on the degree of volume loss.

- **Mild** (10–20% volume loss): The patient feels cold and exhibits orthostatic hypotension, flat neck veins, and pale and cool skin.
- **Moderate** (20–40% volume loss): The patient is thirsty, tachycardic/hypotensive, and oliguric.
- **Severe** (> 40% volume loss): The patient exhibits altered mental status

TABLE 2.11. Clinical Presentations of Shock.				
Sign/Symptom	**Condition**	**SVR**	**Skin**	**Neck Veins**
Hypovolemia	Hemorrhage	High	Cold, clammy	Flat
	Dehydration	High	Cold, clammy	Flat
	Third spacing	High	Cold, clammy	Flat
Distributive	Septic (early)	Low	Warm	Flat to normal
	Neurogenic	Low	Warm	Flat to normal
	Anaphylactic	Low	Warm	Flat to normal
Cardiac	Cardiogenic	High	Cold, clammy	Distended[a]
	Cardiac Compression	High	Cold, clammy	Distended
	Tension pneumothorax	High	Cold, clammy	Distended
Hypoglycemic	Hypoglycemia	High	Cold, clammy	Flat to normal

[a]May be flat if the patient is also hypovolemic.

(agitation leading to obtundation), severe hypotension, tachycardia, and tachypnea.

- Decreased central venous pressure (CVP); increased systemic vascular resistance.

Treatment. The goal in treating hypovolemic shock is to restore intravascular volume, treat the underlying cause of intravascular depletion, and restore tissue oxygenation. Emergency maneuvers in hypovolemic shock are as follows:

1. Place the patient in the Trendelenburg position.
2. Give the patient oxygen.
3. Place two large-bore (14G) IVs and rapidly deliver 2 L of crystalloid (bolus).
4. Reassess vitals.
5. If vitals have not improved, give 1–2 L of additional crystalloid.
6. Reassess vitals.
7. If vitals still have not improved, consider initiating IV pressors and delivering blood products.

If hemorrhage is suspected, the source of the hemorrhage should be sought while the patient is being fluid resuscitated. Hemorrhages that lead to shock are generally in one of three compartments: the abdomen, the pelvis (and retroperitoneum), or the thorax. To identify the source of hemorrhage, perform a direct peritoneal lavage (DPL) or abdominal ultrasound, place an NG tube (to rule out upper GI bleed), perform a guiac (to rule out lower GI bleed), and order a CXR (to rule out intrathoracic bleeding) and a pelvic x-ray (to rule out pelvic fracture). If a peritoneal bleed is identified, the patient must undergo emergent exploratory laparotomy. If a pelvic fracture is identified, pelvic bleed should be suspected and the patient should have angiography and embolization. If a thoracic bleed is identified, a chest tube should be placed.

Cardiogenic Shock

Cardiogenic shock, or intrinsic cardiac pump failure, can be due to arrhythmias, MI, vascular disease, myocarditis, or cardiomyopathy.

Signs and Symptoms. As with other forms of shock, symptoms of cardiogenic shock include tachycardia, hypotension, and tachypnea. In addition, a patient in cardiogenic shock will have distended neck veins and possibly peripheral edema and a third heart sound with rales. Signs of cardiogenic shock are increased CVP, increased pulmonary capillary wedge pressure, and ECG abnormalities.

Treatment. Therapy should be directed at the underlying cause and at maintaining adequate blood pressure. Be aware that fluid resuscitation may cause further failure due to fluid overload. Consider inotropes (to increase contractility), chronotropes, vasodilators (to decrease preload and afterload, which leads to decreased myocardial work), and diuretics (to decrease preload). Antiarrhythmics should also be considered. Surgical interventions include intraaortic balloon pump (which increases CO, decreases afterload, and increases myocardial perfusion).

Septic Shock

Septic shock is secondary to the systemic effects of infection. Toxins from both gram-positive and gram-negative sepsis as well as systemic inflammatory factors cause shock by vasodilation of the peripheral circulation and increased capillary permeability, leading to significantly decreased systemic vascular resistance, redistribution of cardiac output, and massive fluid loss into the tissue.

Signs and Symptoms. Early septic shock, or the hyperdynamic phase, is marked by fever, tachycardia, and hypotension in a warm and pink patient due to vasodilation. Late septic shock, or the hypodynamic phase, mimics hypovolemic shock due to increased capillary permeability and impaired cellular O_2 utilization. Signs of septic shock include leukocytosis with left shift and lactic acidosis.

Treat the underlying cause of septic shock.

Treatment. The key to treating septic shock lies in identifying and treating the source of infection with IV antibiotics, surgical drainage, and central line changes. As in hypovolemic shock, the patient will require IV fluid resuscitation, monitoring of cardiac function, pressors, and/or intubation to maintain adequate oxygenation.

Neurogenic Shock

Neurogenic shock is due to loss of vascular sympathetic tone, usually secondary to a high cervical spinal injury. Spinal anesthesia can also induce spinal shock.

Signs and Symptoms. Symptoms include hypotension; normal or slow pulse (no reflex tachycardia); warm, dry skin; and flat neck veins. Since neurogenic shock is associated with spinal trauma, patients are usually unable to wiggle their toes and have decreased rectal tone. Cardiac output and systemic vascular resistance are low.

Treatment. Other etiologies of shock must be ruled out. As with hypovolemic shock, proceed with IV fluid resuscitation, place the patient in the Trendelenburg position, and use vasoconstrictors. Protocols for spinal injury should also be followed, including high-dose steroids (a 30 mg/kg bolus of methylprednisolone, followed by 5.4 mg/kg/hr for 23 hours if steroids are initiated within three hours of injury, or for 47 hours if steroids are initiated three to eight hours after injury).

Cardiac Tamponade

Cardiac tamponade occurs as a result of the accumulation of fluid in the pericardium (i.e., pericardial effusion). The fluid accumulation prevents the heart from adequately filling or contracting efficiently, thereby decreasing stroke volume.

Signs and Symptoms. Signs of shock specific to tamponade include muffled heart sounds with pulsus paradoxus, (>10 mmHg drop in systolic BP during inspiration) hypotension, and jugular venous distention (JVD). Cardiac tamponade is confirmed by ultrasound.

Treatment. As always, treatment is aimed at the etiology of shock. Therefore, pericardiocentesis is indicated. IV fluid resuscitation is also required to increase diastolic filling, thereby increasing cardiac output.

Tension Pneumothorax

A tension pneumothorax is distinct from a pneumothorax in that the pressure in the thorax increases with every breath. This is because air can enter the pneumothorax but cannot exit. The progressive increase in thoracic pressure prevents venous return to the heart through the vena cava.

Signs and Symptoms. Signs of shock specific to tension pneumothorax include decreased breath sounds, hyperresonant chest, and tracheal deviation.

Treatment. The initial treatment is needle thoracostomy in the second intercostal space at the midclavicular line to relieve the intrathoracic pressure. Do not wait for a CXR. The diagnosis must be made clinically and the needle placed immediately. In addition, IV fluids are given to increase venous return to the heart. Subsequent chest tube placement is appropriate to resolve the pneumothorax completely.

APPENDIX

Formulas

- Mean arterial blood pressure (MAP) = DBP + ([SBP − DBP]/3) (where DBP = diastolic blood pressure and SBP = systolic blood pressure)
- A − a (arterial-alveolar) gradient $= PA_{O_2} - Pa_{O_2}$
$$= (pAtm - pH_2O) \ ^* Fi_{O_2} - (Pa_{CO_2}/RQ) - Pa_{O_2}$$
$$= (713 \ ^* Fi_{O_2}) - (Pa_{CO_2}/0.8) - Pa_{O_2}$$
Normal $Fi_{O_2} = 0.21$; normal A − a gradient 5–15 mm or upper limit of
$$\frac{age}{4} + 4$$
- Cerebral perfusion pressure (CPP) = MAP − intracranial pressure (ICP)

Electrolytes

- Osmolality = 2 * Na_{plasma} + $Glucose_{plasma}$/18 + BUN/2.8
(Normal plasma osmolality: 275–295 mOsm/kg)
- Corrected Ca = Ca_{serum} + 0.8 * [normal albumin − patient's albumin])
$$= Ca_{serum} + 0.8 \ ^* (4 - albumin_{plasma}$$
- Correct Na_{plasma} = Na_{plasma} + ($glucose_{plasma}$ − 100) * 0.0016
- Correct Na_{plasma} = Na_{plasma} + 0.2 * triglycerides (g/L)
- Correct Na_{plasma} = Na_{plasma} + 0.025 * protein (g/L)
- Change in Na_{plasma} = ($Na_{infusate}$ + $K_{infusate}$ − Na_{plasma})/(TBW + 1)
- TBW = k * weight (kg), where k = 0.6 in men and 0.5 in women
- Stool osmotic gap = stool osmolality − 2(Na_{stool} + K_{stool}), where < 50 osm consistent with secretory diarrhea, and > 125 osm consistent with osmotic diarrhea

Acid-Base Equations

- AG = Na_{plasma} − (Cl_{plasma} + $HCO_{3plasma}$)
- Urine AG = Na_{urine} + K_{urine} − Cl_{urine}
- pH = 6.1 + log (HCO_3/0.03 * P_{CO_2})

Renal Function

- Fractional excretion of sodium (FE_{Na})
= (Na_{urine}/Na_{plasma})/(Cr_{urine}/Cr_{plasma}) * 100 or
= (Na_{urine} * Cr_{plasma})/(Na_{plasma} * Na_{urine}) * 100
- Creatinine clearance (CrCl) = (Cr_{urine} * urine volume mL)/(Cr_{plasma} * time min)
- Expected CrCl = (140 − age) * wt (kg) * 0.85 for females/(72 * Cr_{plasma} [mg/dL]

Statistics

		Disease	
		+	−
Test	+	A	C
	−	B	D

Sensitivity = A/(A + B)

Specificity = D/(D + C)

False positive rate = C/(A + C)

False negative rate = B/(B + D)

Positive likelihood ratio = sensitivity / (1 − specificity)

Negative likelihood ratio = (1 − sensitivity) / specificity

Absolute risk reduction (ARR) = disease rate without intervention − disease rate with intervention

Relative risk reduction (RRR) = ARR/disease rate without intervention

Number needed to treat (NNT) = 1/ARR

*Remember **SPIN** and **SNOUT**—the higher the **SP**ecificity, the better the test for ruling **IN** a diagnosis, and the higher the **SeN**sitivity, the better the test is for ruling **OUT** a diagnosis.*

Common Abbreviations

Prescription Writing

Numbers

ī	one	
īī	two	
īīī	three	
s̄s̄	one-half	semis

Dosing Schedule

bid	twice a day	(bis in die)
hs	at bedtime	(hora somni)
tid	three times a day	(ter in die)
÷	divided doses	
q	each, every	(quaque)
q6h	every 6 hours	(quaque 6 hora)
qac	before each meal	(ante cibum)
qd	every day	(quoque die)
qh	every hour	(quiaque hora)
qid	four times a day	(quater in die)
qod	every other day	
pc	after meals	(post cibos)
prn	as needed	(pro re nata)

Routes of Administration

IM	intramuscular
inj	injection
IV	intravenous
PO	by mouth (per os)
PR	by rectum (per rectum)
SL	sublingual
SQ	subcutaneous

Medication Preparations

amp	ampule	(ampulla)
caps	capsules	(capsula)
gtt	a drop	(gute)
liq	liquid	(liquor)
sol	solution	(solutio)
supp	suppository	(suppositorium)
susp	suspension	
tab	tablet	(tabella)
ung	ointment	(unguentum)

Prepositions

$\bar{a}$	before	(ante)
$\bar{c}$	with	(cum)
$\bar{p}$	after	(post)
$\bar{s}$	without	(sine)
$\bar{x}$	except	

Miscellaneous

aa	of each	(ana)
ad	right ear	(auri dextra)
al, as	left ear	(aurio laeva, aurio sinister)
au	both ears	(aures utrae)
ad lib	at pleasure	(ad libitum)
disp	dispense	(dispensa)
NPO	nothing by mouth	(nil peros)
NTE	not to exceed	
od	right eye	(oculus dexter)
os	left eye	(oculus laevus, oculus sinister)
ou	both eyes	(oculus uterque)
qs	quantity sufficient	(quantum sufficiat)
Rx	prescription, take	(recipe)
Sig	label, or let it be printed	(signa)
stat	immediately	(statim)
ud	as directed	(ut dictum)

Although each of the chapters that follow includes a listing of top-rated books specific to that rotation or specialty, the following list outlines books that are of potential use to you on all your rotations.

GENERAL

Boards and Wards: A Review for USMLE Steps 2 & 3 $32.95
Ayala

Blackwell Science, 2000, 1st edition, 363 pages, ISBN 0632044934

A concise overview of every major rotation. Excellent for reading both before and at the beginning of each rotation. Written in outline format with great tables, charts, and algorithms. Appendices include reviews of zebras and syndromes, toxicology, and vitamins and nutrition. Fits in pocket. Not a complete resource for any specific rotation, as it lacks necessary details, but useful for a quick and comprehensive review of high-yield information for end-of-rotation written exams. The short section of clinical vignettes and practice questions included at the end of each chapter could be expanded.

The Sanford Guide to Antimicrobial Therapy $8.00
Gilbert

Antimicrobial Therapy Inc., 2001, 31st edition, 142 pages, ISBN 0933775482

The gold-standard pocket antimicrobial reference guide, updated yearly. Includes dosage, coverage, sensitivities, length of therapy, renal dosing, and drugs of choice for common and uncommon infections. Presented in table format. Small print is sometimes difficult to read. Often available free from drug reps.

Tarascon Pocket Pharmacopoeia: Classic Shirt-Pocket Edition $8.95
Green

Tarascon Publishing, 2002, 16th edition, 128 pages, ISBN 1882742214

An excellent pocket reference book of drugs indexed by generic and trade names. Includes drug class, typical dosing, metabolism, safety in pregnancy and lactation, relative cost, tables, and conversion factors. Compact and inexpensive. Also includes a short summary of ACLS protocols, emergency drug infusions, and pediatric dosing. A must-have for the wards, especially for subinterns. Often available free from drug reps.

Clinician's Pocket Drug Reference 2002 $14.95
Gomella

McGraw-Hill, 2002, 1st edition, 232 pages, ISBN 0071379347

Related to *Clinician's Pocket Reference*, this pocketbook is slightly larger than the shirt-pocket edition of Tarascon's *Pharmacopoeia* but smaller than the deluxe version. Contains information on 900 commonly used medications; includes descriptions of common uses, mechanisms of action, precautions and contraindications, and common side effects. Useful tables near the end of the book compare similar drugs.

REVIEW RESOURCES

General

Current Clinical Strategies: Diagnostic History and Physical Exam in Medicine

$12.95

Chan

Current Clinical Strategies, 2001–2002 edition, 104 pages, ISBN 1881528812

A concise outline pocketbook that contains advice on pertinent things to ask and check for on history and physical (H&P) for a particular symptom or diagnosis. Can be helpful, as you will be asked these things on rounds. Good for writing admit notes and formulating differentials. Offers limited coverage of disease, but a useful resource for its price.

Degowin's Diagnostic Examination

$39.95

Degowin

McGraw-Hill, 2000, 7th edition, 1098 pages, ISBN 0070164436

A classic handbook divided into physical exam, lab tests, and common disease patterns. Gives clear explanations of pathophysiology and provides differentials for nearly every physical finding imaginable. Includes brief discussions of the pathophysiology of abnormal lab values. The section on diagnostic clues highlights signs and symptoms along with abnormal labs found in specific diseases. Much too big to carry in pocket.

Interpretation of Diagnostic Tests

$39.95

Wallach

Lippincott Williams & Wilkins, 2000, 7th edition, 1026 pages, ISBN 0781716594

Organized by organ system with summaries of the available tests for most diseases. Discusses the interpretation of abnormal labs and differential and includes tables comparing test results from similar diseases. Similar to *Pocket Guide to Diagnostic Tests*, but larger and more comprehensive with excellent, encyclopedic coverage. Will not fit in pocket.

Pocket Guide to Diagnostic Tests

$34.95

Nicoll

McGraw-Hill, 2001, 3rd edition, 511 pages, ISBN 0838581358

A concise reference for common diagnostic tests in quick-flip table format. Discusses physiologic bases for and interpretation of lab results. Includes useful sections focusing on microbiology, drug monitoring, ECG interpretation, and diagnostic radiology. Large for pocket considering its utility, but easy to carry in backpack for quick reference.

Tarascon Pocket Pharmacopoeia: Deluxe Lab-Coat Edition $17.95

Green

Tarascon Publishing, 2002, 3rd edition, 256 pages, ISBN 1882742222

Larger and with more pages than the classic shirt-pocket text, the deluxe edition provides all the information found in the smaller version plus additional drug listings, adult versus pediatric dosages, warnings, and notes regarding adverse effects and drug interactions. Includes a table of inhibitors, inducers, and substrates of cytochrome p450 isozymes. Clear plastic slipcover fits over book; still small enough to fit comfortably in coat pocket. A discussion of mechanisms of action and an indication of the frequency of side effects would improve this larger edition.

 Clinician's Pocket Reference $34.95

Gomella

McGraw-Hill, 2001, 9th edition, 720 pages, ISBN 0838515525

A good overall orientation for the wards that makes excellent use of tables, graphs, and diagrams to explain concepts. Good reference for procedures. Includes useful algorithms, protocols for medical emergencies, interpretation of abnormal lab values, and a chapter on commonly used drugs. Practical sections on basic ECG reading and critical care medicine are also provided. However, pathophysiology is not emphasized, and there is little information regarding patient workup. General and light on coverage of diseases; too big for pocket.

 How to Be a Truly Excellent Junior Medical Student $9.95

Lederman

Tarascon Publishing, 2000, 6th edition, 124 pages, ISBN 1882742125

A comprehensive pocketbook for the beginning clinical years. Provides an introduction to the infrastructure of hospital and ward teams. Contains advice on reading charts, entering orders, writing various in-house notes, performing basic procedures, and organizing your data and presentations. Some information given is common sense. Not as useful once you become more advanced in your clinical education.

 Intern Pocket Survival Guide $7.50

Masterson

International Medical Publishing, 1992, 1st edition, 69 pages, ISBN 0963406302

A practical, small, inexpensive pocket guidebook to day-to-day chores, writing H&Ps, admissions, discharge, workup, and interventions. Includes only the most essential facts and numbers. Written for the intern, but useful for subinterns and medical students as well.

Maxwell's Quick Medical Reference   **$7.95**

Maxwell

Maxwell Publishing, 1996, 3rd edition, 32 pages, ISBN 0964519119

Compact, spiral-bound fact cards detailing ACLS algorithms, various in-house notes, normal lab values, basic formulas, the H&P, and the neurologic exam. Especially important at the beginning of the clinical years, but not as critical toward the end once you have become well acquainted with the wards. Attempts to cover a wide range of subjects, thus only superficially touching on most.

 On Call Procedures   **$28.00**

Bresnick

W. B. Saunders, 2000, 1st edition, 272 pages, ISBN 072167304X

A quick, concise resource on basic and advanced procedures, including endotracheal intubation, central line placement, and fluid taps. Includes indications, contraindications, precautions, step-by-step technique, complications, and removal. Good diagrams are provided for anatomy and approach. Although there is no substitute for actual hands-on experience, this book provides a clear picture of the invasive medical and surgical procedures one is likely to encounter on the wards.

 Blackwell's Survival Guide for Interns   **$14.95**

Hammad

Blackwell Science, 2001, 1st edition, 130 pages, ISBN 0632045892

A pocketbook written for residents and interns on the wards. Not particularly useful for junior medical students, although it may serve as a good introduction to subinternships.

 Handbook of Clinical Drug Data   **$44.95**

Anderson

McGraw-Hill, 2002, 10th edition, 1148 pages, ISBN 0071363629

A comprehensive drug guide written from primary literature; includes mechanisms of action, patient instructions, pharmacokinetics, interactions, adverse effects, drug monitoring, and abundant tables comparing each drug within a therapeutic class. A good but pricey resource for those interested in a detailed pharmacology reference. Too bulky to be used as a pocket drug manual.

B **Medi-Data**   **$9.95**

Rodriguez

Rodram Corporation, 2000, 6th edition, 58 pages, ISBN 9686277447

A small, concise pocketbook with extensive listings of normal lab values and diagnostic tests.

On Call Principles and Protocols   **$28.00**
Marshall

W. B. Saunders, 2000, 3rd edition, 478 pages, ISBN 0721650791

A practical guidebook designed for the intern or resident on call. Not as useful for the junior medical student, but may come in handy for the subintern. Attempts to cover a broad range of problems, which makes it superficial in nature. Most useful for internal medicine and surgery. Divided into phone-call management, elevator thoughts, threats to life, and bedside care.

 ## Pocket Brain of Clinical Pathophysiology   **$19.95**
Griffin

Blackwell Science, 2001, 1st edition, 115 pages, ISBN 0632046341

Organized into five broad sections with discussions of frequently encountered disorders. Each section consists of chapters that include a textual description of the diagnostic approach and clinical thinking, followed in most cases by a review and a clinical vignette. Limited number of figures and tables. Educational but oversimplified. May be too superficial to be of value by the time one reaches clinical rotations.

The Right Test   **$32.95**
Speicher

W. B. Saunders, 1998, 3rd edition, 350 pages, ISBN 0721651232

A quick-reference handbook on the pathophysiology and interpretation of abnormal laboratory values, written in question-and-answer format. Guides the student in the correct selection of tests for a particular disease or condition. A large number of primary references are given after each section. Much of the information provided can be found in larger, more detailed textbooks. *Interpretation of Diagnostic Tests* is more complete, with easier access to data. Not small enough to fit comfortably in pocket.

 ## Evidence-Based Diagnosis: A Handbook
of Clinical Prediction Rules   **$49.95**
Ebell

Springer, 2001, 1st edition, 398 pages, ISBN 0387950257

A quick reference of clinical prediction rules along with an overview of the research trials from which those rules are derived. Too technical to be of use for the medical student. Designed more for practicing physicians who wish to determine clinical probabilities or prognoses with relation to disease. CD-ROM included.

Adult History and PE-Pro

$8.75

Medical Information Systems, 2001, 2 cards, ISBN 1981953419

A thorough two-card reference set summarizing the essentials of an H&P in an expanded outline format that includes a detailed review of systems and a comprehensive physical examination section. Although most applicable to a medicine or surgery rotation, this card set also contains an extensive amount of neurology, including the Mini-Mental Status Examination, a Glasgow Coma Scale summary, and a summary of the neurologic exam. Most helpful for students beginning their clinical rotations as well as for those who seek a quick review of the H&P before their patient encounters.

Labs Card

$5.95

Rodriguez

Rodram, 2001, 1 card, ISBN 9686277757

A pocket card containing normal laboratory values for serum chemistries, hematology, urine, cerebrospinal fluid (CSF), pleural fluid, and ABGs. A nice table in the back details the differential of abnormal CSF values. Includes a bonus CD containing a clinical calculator.

ECG Pocketcard

$3.95

Börm Bruckmeier Publishing, 2001, 1 card, ISBN 1591030005

A pocket card similar to *EKG Interactive* in both scope and content. Small type is somewhat difficult to read.

EKG Interactive

$5.95

Rodriguez

Rodram, 2001, 1 card, ISBN 9686277811

A detailed pocket card containing normal ECG values, criteria for diagnosing specific ECG abnormalites, and a ruler for measuring intervals. Too advanced for the junior medical student beginning clinical rotations, as one needs prior knowledge of ECG interpretation to use the card. Would be helpful as a quick reference for the cardiology subintern. Includes a bonus CD containing a clinical calculator.

H&P Interactive

$5.95

Rodriguez

Rodram, 2001, 1 card, ISBN 9686277846

A well-organized pocket card for the H&P that includes a bonus CD containing a clinical calculator. More compact but not as detailed as *Adult History and PE-Pro*, particularly the physical exam section.

Normal Values Guide

$4.50

Medical Information Systems, 1999, 1 card, ISBN 8804950552

Contains normal lab values for electrolytes, hematology, urine, CSF, toxicology, ABGs, and protein electrophoresis. Includes a small table of fluid compositions and conversion factors. A pupil-size gauge is included in the back along with a ruler. Omits normal cardiac enzyme levels.

REVIEW RESOURCES

Pocket Cards

B ## History and Physical Exam Guide $4.50

Medical Information Systems, 2001, 1 card, ISBN 8804956658

A condensed version of *Adult History and PE-Pro,* written in an expanded outline format. Includes only a minimal description of the key features of the HPI. A disproportionate amount of the card is devoted to the cardiac exam, including the differential of heart murmurs, as compared to the other components of the physical exam.

B ## History & Physical Exam Pocketcard $3.95

Börm Bruckmeier Publishing, 2002, 1 card, ISBN 1591030056

Nice table layout with a breakdown of each section of the H&P in its own separate box. Not as comprehensive as other available cards.

B ## Normal Values-Pro $8.75

Medical Information Systems, 2002, 2 cards, ISBN 8819980096

An expanded version of *Normal Values Guide* that includes a diagram for acid-base disturbances along with more normal lab values. Not as useful as it could potentially be with the addition of an extra card. Too many lab values are listed where the normal is "negative," such as those for RPR or hepatitis C serologies.

B⁻ ## ECG Evaluation Pocketcard $3.95

Börm Bruckmeier Publishing, 2002, 1 card, ISBN 1591030013

A pocket card with one side dedicated to proper placement of leads and the other side with a systematic check-off list of steps toward ECG interpretation. Contains no normal values or criteria for diagnosing ECG abnormalities.

B⁻ ## ECG Ruler Pocketcard $3.95

Börm Bruckmeier Publishing, 2001, 1 card, ISBN 1591030021

Contains several rulers for measuring intervals and amplitudes, an example of a normal ECG waveform, and normal interval ranges. Clear plastic design allows one to overlay the rulers on top of ECGs but permits print to be on only one side of the card. Best suited to the cardiology resident or fellow.

REVIEW RESOURCES

Pocket Cards

Marriot's Practical Electrocardiography $49.95

Marriot

Lippincott Williams & Wilkins, 2000, 10th edition, 475 pages, ISBN 0683307460

A thorough ECG reference, including normal and abnormal ECG findings. May be too detailed for junior medical students as it helps to have some basic understanding before reading. Includes illustrations, literature references, ECG tracings, and glossary. Excellent for cardiology subinterns and for those interested in going to the next level of ECG interpretation. Somewhat costly.

Rapid Interpretation of EKGs $35.50

Dubin

Cover Publishing, 2000, 6th edition, 368 pages, ISBN 0912912065

Presented as a "workbook," this reference facilitates the rapid acquisition of ECG fundamentals, emphasizing active learning with fill-in-the-blanks and visual aids on each page. Includes excellent quick-reference pages at the end that you can copy and put in your coat pocket. Can be easily read in a weekend. Although its content has not changed significantly in several years, most agree this book is still considered by many to be the best basic stepping stone for the junior student. However, it is a bit short on practice ECGs and one will likely need another book for more advanced ECG interpretation.

Basic Electrocardiography in 10 days $39.95

Ferry

McGraw-Hill, 2000, 1st edition, 266 pages, ISBN 0071352929

A good discussion of how to interpret ECGs. Organized by pathology, with illustrations of the heart showing where the corresponding lesions should be located along with a vector cardiographic loop approach. Designed at an appropriate level for junior and senior medical students. Each section is followed by several ECGs for the student to diagnose.

Rapid ECG Interpretation $28.00

Khan

W. B. Saunders, 1997, 1st edition, 255 pages, ISBN 0721674682

Presents ECGs by abnormalities with explanations of the pathophysiology and differential causes of aberrant wave forms. Well organized with consistent presentation of an 11-step method for rapid ECG diagnosis.

The Only EKG Book You'll Ever Need $39.95

Thaler

Lippincott Williams & Wilkins, 1999, 3rd edition, 300 pages, ISBN 0781716675

Stresses basic electrophysiology and simple ECG interpretation organized by problems. Includes useful chapter summaries and a comprehensive review of important principles. Also includes case presentations, tables, graphs, and sample 12-lead ECGs. Concise and highly readable but could use more practice ECGs. Generally good for beginners, but too superficial for those who seek to master ECG interpretation.

150 Practice ECGs: Interpretation and Review   **$34.95**
Taylor

Blackwell Science, 2001, 2nd edition, 271 pages, ISBN 0632046236

A spiral-bound workbook with sections dedicated to basic electrophysiology and practice. Excellent for medical students wishing to practice but difficult to use, as reviews for the ECGs are randomly organized. Lacks thorough explanations of ECG pathology.

 Quick and Accurate 12-Lead ECG Interpretation   **$39.95**
Davis

Lippincott Williams & Wilkins, 2000, 3rd edition, 464 pages, ISBN 0781723272

A good introductory text for ECG interpretation. Covers basic electrophysiology and the pathophysiology of ECG findings. Not designed for more advanced reading of complex ECGs.

B **ECG Assessment and Interpretation**   **$29.95**
Lipman

F. A. Davis, 1994, 1st edition, 295 pages, ISBN 0803656467

An extensive basic review of ECG interpretation that includes discussions of etiology and treatment. Initial chapters provide a good overview of normal electrophysiology. Appendices in the back contain tables of commonly used cardiac drugs along with out-of-date ACLS algorithms. No practice ECGs are provided.

B **ECG Made Easy**   **$18.95**
Hampton

Churchill Livingstone, 1997, 5th edition, 129 pages, ISBN 0443056811

An extremely quick review of major ECG findings. Includes tables and a few rhythm strips, but does not offer practice problems or case discussions. Examples might be more informative if they showed an entire 12-lead ECG rather than just one lead and if arrows were used to point to the exact abnormalities. Can fit in coat pocket.

B **ECG Workout: Exercises in Arrhythmia Interpretation**   **$28.95**
Huff

Lippincott Williams & Wilkins, 2001, 4th edition, 368 pages, ISBN 0781731925

A practical workbook with more than 500 actual ECGs. Includes updated ACLS guidelines. Emphasizes arrhythmias with no discussion of MI, ischemia, or hypertrophy. Includes good tables, illustrations, and self-assessment problems. Best used in conjunction with a primary ECG reference. Too advanced for the junior medical student seeking to learn the basics of ECG interpretation.

Pocket Guide to ECG Diagnosis $39.95
Chung

Blackwell Science, 2001, 2nd edition, 528 pages, ISBN 0865425892

A highly technical, comprehensive pocketbook with a good introductory overview of the principles of electrophysiology. Coverage of some disorders is far too advanced for the junior medical student and likely for the subintern as well. A potential pocket reference for residents who wish to become cardiologists.

 Recognition and Interpretation of ECG Rhythms $29.95
Ochs

McGraw-Hill, 1997, 1st edition, 425 pages, ISBN 0838543235

A spiral-bound introductory manual featuring a large number of sample strips but sparse explanatory text. Contains limited coverage of topics other than dysrhythmias.

Fluid, Electrolyte, and Acid-Base Physiology $65.00

Halperin

W. B. Saunders, 1999, 3rd edition, 532 pages, ISBN 0721670725

A well-written clinical approach toward recognizing, diagnosing, and treating common metabolic abnormalities. Presented in case-based fashion with numerous clinical vignettes and clinically oriented questions. Good illustrations integrate basic science principles into the discussion of metabolic disorders.

Acid-Base, Fluids, and Electrolytes Made Ridiculously Simple $18.95

Preston

Medmaster, 2001, 1st edition, 162 pages, ISBN 0940780313

A concise, practical approach toward solving problems of acid-base, fluid, and electrolyte abnormalities. Easy to read and well organized with good use of tables, although it could use more diagrams and figures. Several questions with detailed explanations at the end of each section reinforce key principles. Fair price relative to the amount and complexity of material covered.

REVIEW RESOURCES

Fluids, Electrolytes, and Acid-Base

B+ Lecture Notes on Radiology

$39.95

Patel

Blackwell Science, 1998, 1st edition, 272 pages, ISBN 0632047585

A good general overview of diagnostic radiology presented in a disease-specific manner. A double-page-spread format with radiographs of a specific disorder on one page and a succinct explanatory text on the other allows for immediate cross-reference. The first few chapters explain the basic physics of the different radiographic forums. Basic treatment options are also provided.

B+ Radiology Secrets

$39.95

Katz

Hanley & Belfus, 1999, 1st edition, 566 pages, ISBN 1560531584

A comprehensive overview of radiology presented in a question-and-answer format typical of the *Secrets* series. Discussions are broken down by organ system and includes well-explained correlations of radiographic findings to medical disorders. Covers all imaging modalities with a large number of radiographs interspersed within the text. Too lengthy to be used as a basic introduction; more appropriate for quick reference and review for students interested in radiology.

C+ Clinical Radiology Made Ridiculously Simple

$24.95

Ouellette

MedMaster, 2000, 1st edition, 109 pages, ISBN 0940780410

Covers the essentials of the CXR, abdominal x-ray, and head CT. However, omits many other important components of clinical radiology, including ultrasound, body CT, MRI, and angiograms. Includes an inordinate number of bone films.

MD Consult
$119.95/year

www.mdconsult.com

A user-friendly Internet resource with up-to-date and comprehensive information. Provides access to several resources, including full-text journal articles, reference textbooks, practice guidelines, current research topics, and patient handouts. Some of the main journals are not provided under the service, but overall a wealth of information can be found on any medical specialty. Some medical schools offer a paid subscription for their students. Free trials are available.

 PubMed
Free

www.ncbi.nlm.nih.gov/PubMed

An excellent, free search engine made available through the National Library of Medicine. Provides specific references for and often the abstracts of the journal articles that you are trying to find. This database of essentially every medical journal article that exists is a necessity for any discussion of evidence-based medicine.

 Emedicine
Free

www.emedicine.com

A good source of up-to-date information with access to multiple medical resources, including journal articles, a differential diagnosis search engine, a medical dictionary, drug information reviews, and color illustrations. Excellent review articles are available. Not as complete with respect to online journals and textbooks as *MD Consult*, but offers at breadth of useful material.

 Harrison's Online
$99.00/year

www.harrisonsonline.com

An excellent and comprehensive online resource that contains essentially the same information as the *Harrison's* text. A subscription includes access to frequent updates to the text, interactive questions, and concise reviews and editorials. Poor search engine capability makes it difficult to navigate at times. Medical schools often pay for a subscription to this resource for their students. Free trials are available.

 New England Journal of Medicine Online
Free limited access

www.nejm.com

A great site for research offering full access to recent articles published within the *New England Journal of Medicine*. Journal articles may be printed out as they would appear in the text version. Free access is provided to a limited number of older articles. An excellent resource for students interested in internal medicine. Various subscription plans are available. Some medical schools have a paid subscription available for their students.

REVIEW RESOURCES

Internet Resources

REVIEW RESOURCES

PDA Resources

 Epocrates Rx, Version 4.0   **Free**

www.epocrates.com

A quick, accurate, and comprehensive drug resource that is updated weekly. Provides information about adult and pediatric dosing, contraindications, adverse reactions, mechanisms of action, forms of administration, and price. A multicheck feature allows one to check for drug interactions for those patients using multiple medications. Much more complete than the *Tarascon Pocket Pharmacopoeia*. Overall, an excellent, free PDA resource that is quickly becoming a popular bedside drug reference.

 2002 Griffith's 5-Minute Clinical Consult   **$64.95**

www.handheldmed.com

An excellent PDA program for the wards that provides a quick summary of both common and obscure medical conditions. Great for last-minute presentations and preparation before rounds. Well organized with an easy-to-use interface and search function. Discussions are divided into basics of disease, differential, treatment, medications, follow-up, and miscellaneous. Not a substitute for a textbook, but surprisingly comprehensive. May be combined with other products at a discounted price.

 Epocrates ID, Version 1.0   **Free**

www.epocrates.com

A good, easy-to-use companion to *Epocrates Rx* meant for providing the appropriate antibiotic coverage of infectious disease. Searchable by antibiotic, specific organism, and general site of infection. Links with *Epocrates Rx* to provide a drug interaction and side effect check. The lack of an auto-update option requires that one download the program again every few months to obtain the most recent recommendations.

 Lexi-Drugs Platinum   **$75.00**

www.lexi.com

Much more comprehensive and expensive than *Epocrates Rx,* with in-depth descriptions of mechanisms of action, side effects, drug interactions, and other pertinent drug information. An update option was recently added to product. May be combined with other products at a discounted price. Software includes one year of unlimited online updates.

MedCalc, Version 3.51   **Free**

Available from many Web sites offering free medical software, including *www.palmgear.com*

Similar in scope to *MedMath*, with the ability to personalize and save data for patients. Easy to navigate, and contains most formulas used on a regular basis.

MedMath, Version 1.2   **Free**

Available from many Web sites offering free medical software, including www.palmgear.com

An excellent program containing many frequently used formulas, including creatinine clearance, body mass index, Ranson's score, corrected electrolytes, and water deficit. Simply plug in the numbers in the appropriate sections and you will get the calculation immediately. Brief explanations of formulas are provided along with normal ranges. Contains some rarely used formulas. A great help on the wards when you can't remember how something is calculated.

 Lexi-Interact   **$75.00**

www.lexi.com

A companion to *Lexi-Drugs Platinum* that provides detailed information on drug interactions along with the relative significance of each. A review section offers clinically relevant reviews of scientific literature and a list of strategies for preventing and managing interactions. May be combined with other products at a discounted price. Software includes one year of unlimited online updates.

 2002 Tarascon ePharmacopoeia   **Free**

www.tarasconpublishing.com

A PDA version of the shirt-pocket edition of *Pharmacopoeia*. Not as comprehensive as *Epocrates Rx*.

Harrison's Principles of Internal Medicine Companion Handbook, 14th edition   **$79.95**

www.handheldmed.com

Contains good, in-depth descriptions of medical conditions, but its slow search function and poor organization make this product not as useful or cost-effective as *Griffith's 5-Minute Clinical Consult*.

 PatientKeeper Personal   **$35.00**

www.patientkeeper.com

A well-intentioned product for tracking patient data, including sections for history, physical exam, lab values, radiographic results, and assessment and plan. However, its usefulness is severely constrained by its slow PDA interface, which makes the entering of patient data a cumbersome process. This can be partially overcome by the use of a PDA keyboard, but many feel it is easier to continue tracking patient information on note cards. Some value may be found in tracking patient lab values and test results.

Patient Tracker, Version 5.1

Free

www.handheldmed.com

Similar to *PatientKeeper Personal*, this product is limited in its utility by the length
of time it takes to enter patient data

Washington Manual, 30th edition

$69.95

www.franklin.com

A PDA version of the popular internal medicine pocket handbook. Difficult to
search for topics owing to a slow interface. The paper version is faster and easier to
read with more complete coverage of medical topics, making this PDA version not
as useful as its print counterpart.

CHAPTER 3

Internal Medicine

Ward Tips
High-Yield Topics
High-Yield References
Top-Rated Books

Internal medicine
dilemmas are faced by
practitioners in all
specialties.

The internal medicine clerkship ranges from 8 to 12 weeks in duration and will broaden your scope in cardiology, pulmonology, gastroenterology, endocrinology, nephrology, rheumatology, hematology/oncology, and infectious disease in both outpatient and inpatient settings. Given the sheer scope of the field, internal medicine will serve as a strong foundation for all of your other rotations when done early and, when done later, will shore up your fund of knowledge. The internal medicine rotation is thus an invaluable experience, regardless of when it is done and what specialty you eventually choose.

WHO ARE THE PLAYERS?

Attendings. Consisting of clinical and academic faculty, the attendings are in charge of the wards team and are ultimately responsible for patient care. Attendings are also the source of most of the didactic learning that takes place during attending rounds. Your interaction with attendings consists primarily of making formal patient presentations in attending rounds and participating in didactic teaching. Thus, it is crucial to read up on your patients' problems before attending rounds, especially if you are presenting a patient.

Residents. Since residents are at least a year ahead of interns, they supervise the wards team and help formulate patients' treatment plans. Residents also serve as a major teaching resource, dispensing clinical pearls on work rounds and bringing in pertinent review articles. Your interaction with the resident will vary depending on his or her style; some remain aloof and serve only to answer questions, while others are more interactive, giving informal lectures and taking you to patients' bedsides to teach physical findings. Residents also love to pimp as a means of teaching and assessing your knowledge base. They may even take the time to give you organized lectures on ECG reading or refer you to recent journal articles that are pertinent to patients on the team.

Consult with your interns
and residents before
rounds to formulate a
plan.

Interns. Interns are the cogs that make the hospital machinery move by performing most of the primary patient care. As they will co-follow your patient, you will probably have the most interaction with your intern. All questions and management issues regarding your patient should initially be directed toward the intern. You should also remember that interns were recently medical students themselves, so they can be an invaluable resource for practical information as well as survival tips. You can use them for feedback on your progress notes and presentation style. If they have time, consult with them before rounds to discuss your plan for your patients so that you can have a more coherent plan in your mind when presenting on rounds.

HOW IS THE DAY SET UP?

The typical day on a medicine rotation starts at about 7 AM and usually runs until 4–5 PM on noncall days.

7:00–8:00 AM	Prerounds
8:00–9:00 AM	Work rounds
9:00–10:30 AM	Work time
10:30–12:00 noon	Attending rounds
Noon–1:00 PM	Noon conference
1:00 PM–?	Work time, student conferences

WHAT DO I DO DURING PREROUNDS?

Please refer to "Prerounds" in "A Typical Medicine Day" in Chapter 1.

HOW DO I DO WELL IN THIS ROTATION?

Learning the material well does not always correlate with doing well on the clerkship. Often, your grade will depend on subjective forces beyond your control, such as whether your personality matches that of your residents. However, the following tips will help stack the deck in your favor.

Know your patient. You should know the latest clinical information on your patient, be it the most recent laboratory values, the planned studies of the day, or simply how the patient is feeling. Relay this information to the intern so that management plans can adapt. Keep on top of consults and tests you have ordered. Speak with the consulting service about their recommendations: Consultants can give you valuable information and may even have time to give you a short tutorial on your patient's disease process. Another important part of knowing your patient is a daily check of the nurses' log of medications given. This check will allow you to ensure that the antibiotics you ordered were given (which is not always the case) as well as to gauge whether the patient is receiving symptomatic relief. For example, is the patient's pain well controlled, or is he or she asking for a lot of pain medication? You should also be aware of a patient's social situation so that you can keep the family up to date regarding his or her progress. Finally, be aware of special circumstances to be considered on discharge (e.g., getting a hotel room or transportation for a homeless patient).

Develop a differential. The search for the etiology of a patient's problem begins with knowing the differential diagnosis. Therefore, a critical goal of this rotation is to learn the basic differentials of common patient signs and symptoms. The differential can often be broken into three groups: common etiologies, uncommon etiologies, and etiologies you don't want to miss (because they're either highly treatable or life threatening). Mastering the differentials of common problems will serve you well in any specialty.

You should know the latest clinical information on your patient.

You cannot diagnose what is not in your differential diagnosis.

Medicine is more than a 9-to-5 job.

Care about your patients. Perhaps the single most important thing you can do on *any* rotation is to be genuinely concerned about your patients. Nothing will elicit more respect from faculty and your team. Don't simply leave at 5:00 PM if your patient is crashing. Remember why you decided to go to medical school in the first place.

Get along with your team. It is critical to remember that you are part of a team. Even though you may be low on the totem pole, you still have an integral role to play and are a genuine asset to your team. In addition, medical students who make life easier for the interns and residents through diligent and efficient work will be rewarded in their evaluations. It is thus important to be personable and enthusiastic to ensure that the members of your team can work as a cohesive unit. By contrast, a surefire way to effectively shoot yourself in the foot is to openly conflict with others on your team. If you feel uncomfortable with another team member or sense any kind of personality problem developing, it is crucial to nip the problem in the bud as early as possible. If you are unable to smooth things over, do whatever it takes to avoid conflicts so that the team can continue to work together without problems. A serious rift in the team is an uncommon situation, but when it does occur, it can be devastating to patient care, team morale, and your workup.

Be early. Never underestimate the importance of punctuality. Attendings and residents probably won't take notice when you show up on time, but they *will* remember if you walk in late.

Work independently. Try to work as independently as your talent permits. The easier you make your intern's life, the more he or she will appreciate you. If you can call the consults, order the lab tests, collect lab and radiology results, and determine if the patient is comfortable, you will go a long way. Expect to be highly dependent on others initially; this is perfectly normal. But as you become more experienced, you will feel the desire—and have the confidence—to work more independently.

Read, read, read. Keep both a pocket manual and a home reference book handy. As a third-year student, you have a responsibility to read about your patients and all their issues. This will save you when the inevitable pimping starts. Reading will also help you ask intelligent questions about the diagnosis and treatment of your patient and will ultimately move you in the direction of making management decisions. Performing searches for current literature and reading hallmark papers pertaining to your patient's problem are also important. You will have to gauge how many searches you can do in accordance with your time constraints.

Ask for feedback. Midway through the course, have the attending and resident set aside time so that they can give you feedback. "You're doing fine" is not an acceptable response. Be persistent and ask about your weaknesses. This will help you identify areas needing improvement and will also notify them that you are a responsible student.

If you are sincerely interested in pursuing a career in internal medicine, you need to take additional steps. First, let the members of your team know of your interests. They may make a special effort to teach and help you. However, don't lie; insincerity is easily sensed and is definitely looked down upon. Second, the status of your attending becomes crucial; it is ideal to have at least one block of your clerkship with a senior attending (i.e., a big shot). In residency applications, the person writing your letter of recommendation is often almost as important as what is said about you in the letter. Performing well will virtually assure you of a good letter of recommendation from a senior faculty member. Talk to your resident and the course scheduler to see if you can work with a senior faculty member in at least one block of your clerkship.

PRESENTATIONS

Work rounds. Presentations during work rounds consist of an oral version of your SOAP note. During these presentations, the team will focus on brevity and efficiency, with emphasis on the assessment and plan. A well-thought-out assessment and plan takes extra time during prerounds, so start early and discuss your ideas with your intern. Do not be discouraged if your assessment and plan is completely wrong—you are there to learn, and the team will appreciate the fact that you are trying. It is better to come up with a well-thought-out plan that is incorrect than to simply say "I don't know" when you are asked about your next move in patient management.

Attending rounds. This is your time in the spotlight, when you really need to shine. Your attending will probably want a more lengthy formal oral presentation than the ones you give on work rounds. Although attendings will primarily want to learn about your patient, they will also observe your presentation style and note how well you understand that patient's problems. One key means of demonstrating your knowledge is to include pertinent positives and negatives relating to your patient's condition. This is not easy at first, especially since it requires an understanding of the presentation of the other possibilities in the differential. It is okay, however, if you leave out something from the history, since the attending will simply ask for additional information if it is important. Don't panic if your attending asks you several additional questions about your patient; instead, make a mental note of the specific tidbits that your attending likes to hear so that you can include them in your next presentation. You should also make sure you understand why the attending considers certain pertinent positives or negatives to be relevant to your patient.

Remember that your attending's comments weigh heavily in your final grade. Formal oral patient presentations constitute a large part of how the attending perceives you, so you will want to shine in this arena. Ask the attending how he or she would like you to present the patient. Practice your presentation before attending rounds, even running it by your resident for feedback.

KEY NOTES

Admit notes and SOAP notes are key to your medicine rotation. Please review the sample notes in Chapter 1.

SOAP note—

Subjective
Objective
Assessment
Plan

KEY PROCEDURES

Explanations for the basic procedures that follow can be found in any pocket ward manual, such as Gomella's *Clinician's Pocket Reference to Patient Care*.

- Phlebotomy
- Musculoskeletal injection
- IV line placement
- Arterial line
- Arterial blood gas placement
- Foley placement

If you're lucky, your resident may allow you to perform the following advanced procedures on your patient:

- Thoracocentesis
- Paracentesis
- Lumbar puncture

WHAT DO I CARRY IN MY POCKETS?

Checklist
- ❑ Stethoscope
- ❑ Eye chart
- ❑ Tuning fork (512 and/or 1028 Hz)
- ❑ Penlight
- ❑ Reflex hammer
- ❑ Tongue blades
- ❑ Current pharmacopoeia and antibiotic guide
- ❑ Calipers for ECG reading and an ECG summary card
- ❑ Index cards and/or patient summary sheets tracking vital signs and tests over hospital stay
- ❑ Normal-lab-value reference card

HIGH-YIELD TOPICS

ROTATION OBJECTIVES

Because internal medicine covers so many domains, you should set achievable goals in your bid to attain a solid fund of knowledge. The following is a list of common diseases that you may want to review during the rotation. Remember, you will face these diseases regardless of the specialty you choose, so learn away. (Disease entities that are discussed in this chapter are listed in italics.)

Cardiology
- *Angina pectoris, unstable angina,* and *Prinzmetal's (variant) angina*
- *Acute myocardial infarction*
- Arrhythmias (e.g., bradyarrhythmias, tachyarrhythmias, and *atrial fibrillation*)

- Cardiomyopathies
- *Congestive heart failure*
- *Hypertension*
- Infective *Endocarditis,* myocarditis, and pericarditis
- *Syncope*
- *Valvular heart disease*

Pulmonology
- Acute respiratory failure
- Asthma (refer to Pediatrics, Chapter 6)
- *Chronic obstructive pulmonary disease*
- *Bronchogenic carcinoma*
- *Chronic cough*
- Interstitial lung disease
- *Pleural effusion*
- *Pneumonia*
- *Pneumothorax*
- *Pulmonary embolism*
- Pulmonary nodules and masses

Nephrology
- Acid-base disturbances
- *Acute renal failure*
- Chronic renal failure and uremia
- *Glomerular Disease*
- Electrolyte disorders (e.g., *hyponatremia* and hypernatremia, hypo- and hyperkalemia)
- *Nephrolithiasis*

Gastroenterology
- *Abdominal pain*
- Hepatic disease (e.g., *cirrhosis* and *hepatic encephalopathy, hepatitis,* portal hypertension)
- *Diarrhea*
- Disorders of swallowing (e.g., achalasia, esophageal cancer)
- *Gastritis*
- *Gastroesophageal reflux disease*
- *Peptic ulcer disease*
- Gastrointestinal bleeding (refer to Surgery, Chapter 4)
- Gastrointestinal cancer
- Inflammatory bowel disease (e.g., Crohn's disease, ulcerative colitis; refer to Surgery, Chapter 8)
- *Irritable bowel syndrome*
- Malabsorption
- Pancreatitis (refer to Surgery, Chapter 8)

Hematology
- *Anemia,* including hemolytic anemias
- *Coagulation disorders* (e.g., *bleeding disorders and hypercoagulable states*)
- Neutropenic fever

Oncology
- Breast cancer
- Leukemias
- Lymphadenopathy
- Lymphomas
- Paraneoplastic syndromes
- Prostate cancer

Endocrinology
- Adrenal disorders (e.g., hyperaldosteronism, hypoaldosteronism, Addison's disease, Cushing's disease)
- Diabetes insipidus (central and nephrogenic)
- *Diabetes mellitus (types 1 and 2),* including *diabetic ketoacidosis*
- Hyper- and hypocalcemia
- Hyperlipidemias (e.g., familial hypercholesterolemia)
- Gonadal disorders (e.g., testicular feminization, 5α-reductase deficiency)
- Nutritional disorders (e.g., osteomalacia, scurvy, pellagra, beriberi)
- Pituitary disorders (e.g., acromegaly)
- Thyroid disorders (e.g., Graves' disease, Hashimoto's thyroiditis)

Infectious Disease
- Animal-borne diseases (e.g., Lyme disease, rabies, malaria)
- CNS infections (e.g., meningitis, encephalitis; refer to Neurology, Chapter 4)
- *Fever of unknown origin*
- *HIV and AIDS*
- Intra-abdominal infections (e.g., spontaneous bacterial peritonitis)
- Respiratory tract infections (e.g., pneumonia, URI)
- Sexually transmitted diseases (e.g., chlamydia, syphilis, gonorrhea, herpes)
- *Tuberculosis*
- *Urinary tract infections*

Rheumatology
- Fibromyalgia
- Gout and pseudogout
- Osteoarthritis
- Rheumatoid arthritis
- Sarcoidosis
- Septic arthritis
- Seronegative spondyloarthropathies (e.g., ankylosing spondylitis)
- *Systemic lupus erythematosus*
- Vasculitis (e.g., polyarteritis nodosa, temporal arteritis)

General Medicine

- *Cancer screening*
- Health maintenance issues
- Medical ethics issues
- Outpatient management

Cardiology

ANGINA PECTORIS

Angina pectoris refers to substernal chest pain that originates from myocardial ischemia (increased oxygen demand or decreased oxygen supply), is associated with exertion, and is relieved with rest or nitroglycerin. Major risk factors include those associated with coronary artery disease (CAD): age, gender, hypertension, dyslipidemia, diabetes, smoking, and family history. Other risk factors include cocaine and/or amphetamine use, a history of previous MI, obesity, elevated homocysteine, and lipoprotein (a). Having a "Type A" personality might also play a role. Males are affected more frequently than females. Prinzmetal's (variant) angina mimics angina pectoris but is caused by vasospasm of the coronary vessels. It often affects young women and classically occurs at rest in the early morning.

Signs and Symptoms. Classic symptoms include exertional substernal chest pressure that radiates to the lower jaw, left shoulder, or left arm (Levine's sign) and may be associated with nausea, vomiting, and dyspnea. Signs include elevated blood pressure (BP), tachycardia, diaphoresis, and an S4 heart sound due to a stiff left ventricle. Be aware that the elderly, diabetics, and postoperative patients may suffer from "silent ischemia" or angina without chest pain. Stable angina lasts less than 30 minutes and is promptly relieved by rest or through the administration of nitroglycerin.

Differential. The differential includes the following:

- **Life threatening:** Tension pneumothorax (PTX), aortic dissection, pulmonary embolism (PE), unstable angina, and MI.
- **Others:** Costochondritis (Tietze's syndrome), esophagitis, gastroesophageal reflux disease (GERD), peptic ulcer disease (PUD), cholecystitis, pericarditis, pneumonia, and intercostal neuritis (e.g., from herpes zoster and diabetes mellitus [DM]).

Workup. An ECG and a troponin-I or CK-MB level every eight hours for 24 hours should be obtained to rule out MI. The ECG may show ST-segment depression or T-wave flattening (see Figure 3.1). Look for electrocardiographic or scintigraphic evidence of ischemia during pain or stress testing once an MI has been ruled out (see Key Cardiac Diagnostic Exams). In Prinzmetal's angina, the ECG shows ST-segment elevation (not depression). The diagnosis is confirmed by a coronary angiogram that is free of significant stenotic lesions and that displays coronary vasospasm when the patient is given ergonovine.

Major risk factors for CAD:

Age

Gender

Dyslipidemia

Diabetes mellitus

Hypertension

Smoking

Family history

HIGH-YIELD TOPICS

Internal Medicine

Deadly causes of chest pain—

TAPUM

Tension pneumothorax
Aortic dissection
Pulmonary embolism
Unstable angina
Myocardial infarction

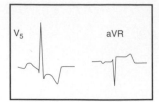

FIGURE 3.1. ST depression typical of ischemia. Note that the ST elevation in aVR is really depression, as it goes in the opposite direction of the QRS. (Reprinted, with permission, from Nicoll D et al. *Pocket Guide to Diagnostic Tests,* 2nd ed. Stamford, CT: Appleton & Lange, 1997: 294.)

Treatment

- **Initial treatment:** The initial treatment of angina assumes possible infarction. Therefore, the patient should receive aspirin (ASA), oxygen, beta blockers, telemetry monitoring, and possibly anticoagulation with heparin. Therapy for Prinzmetal's angina consists of coronary vasodilators (nitrates, possibly intracoronary calcium-channel blockers).
- **Medical:** Sublingual nitroglycerin, long-acting nitrates, beta blockers, and calcium-channel blockers decrease myocardial O_2 demand by reducing cardiac work.
- **Coronary revascularization:** Coronary artery bypass grafting (CABG) and percutaneous transluminal coronary angioplasty (PTCA) increase oxygen delivery to the myocardium by increasing blood flow.
- **Risk factor modification:** The patient must quit smoking and adhere to dietary changes and exercise recommendations. Treat underlying hypertension, diabetes, and hypercholesterolemia.

UNSTABLE ANGINA

Angina is considered "unstable" if it does one of three things:

1. It is new.
2. It is accelerating—it occurs with less exertion, lasts longer, or is less responsive to medications (e.g., nitrates).
3. It occurs at rest.

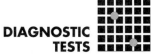

DIAGNOSTIC TESTS

KEY CARDIAC DIAGNOSTIC EXAMS

Exercise Electrocardiography

The patient's ECG is monitored while exercising. Exercise often takes the form of a treadmill according to the Bruce protocol: treadmill speed and elevation are increased every three minutes. Angina, ST-segment changes on ECG, exercise intolerance, or decreased systolic blood pressure indicate myocardial ischemia. A positive test should be further evaluated with cardiac catheterization.

Myocardial Perfusion Scintigraphy

Radionuclides (e.g., thallium, Tc-MIBI) are injected into the blood. The amount of radionuclide uptake by the myocardium is directly related to the amount of blood flow; areas of diminished uptake indicate relative hypoperfusion. With exercise or dipyridamole (Persantine)-induced vasodilation, coronary vessels vasodilate, giving the most blood flow to those vessels without lesions. If no areas of hypoperfusion are observed, the test is negative. If defects are observed, a resting scan is done to determine if perfusion defects are reversible. Defects that normalize at rest indicate reversible ischemia, whereas fixed defects signify areas of dead tissue (i.e., post-MI). Areas of reversible ischemia may be rescued with PTCA or CABG surgery.

Echocardiography

A real-time ultrasound of the heart, the echocardiogram ("echo") reveals abnormal wall motion due to ischemia or infarction. Echo gives the additional benefits of assessing left ventricular (LV) function and estimating the ejection fraction (EF), an important predictor of prognosis. A normal EF is approximately 55%.

Coronary Angiography

An invasive procedure that visualizes the coronary vasculature by injecting dye into the vessels, coronary arteriography is the definitive diagnostic procedure for CAD. Stenotic lesions in the vessels will be visualized and quantified with respect to the extent of obstruction (most lesions causing symptoms are greater than 70% stenotic) as well as their location. While this procedure gives anatomical information, it does not indicate whether any given stenosis is clinically significant; that is, a 50% stenotic lesion may be the cause of the patient's symptoms as opposed to the 70% lesion in another vessel. This procedure also gives an estimate of the EF. Catheterization is typically used to (1) confirm the presence and map the extent of CAD, and (2) define the method of revascularization (PTCA vs. CABG) if indicated.

Unstable angina is worrisome because it often signifies a transient vessel occlusion (i.e., disruption of an atherosclerotic plaque and/or vasospasm in the area of a plaque) and an area of myocardial ischemia that can acutely progress to complete occlusion and MI.

Treatment. Management consists of admission to the hospital for aggressive treatment similar to that for MI. Therapy includes nitrates, beta blockers, morphine, O_2, ASA, and heparin. After the patient is stable, his or her coronary vasculature should be evaluated by the diagnostic methods discussed above. If the patient still has angina despite the above measures, he or she should be considered for urgent coronary arteriography and revascularization. As in stable angina, the patient should be administered an ACE inhibitor (ACEI) and statins.

ACUTE MYOCARDIAL INFARCTION

Myocardial infarction is usually caused by an occlusive thrombus or prolonged vasospasm in a coronary artery. The most common cause is an acute thrombus on a ruptured atherosclerotic plaque. The time course and extent of vessel occlusion are key, as collateral circulation might help preserve some myocardial function. Risk factors are similar to those for angina. Males are affected more frequently than females, although the incidence in women increases following

> **Treatment of unstable angina and MI—**
>
> **MONA has Hep B**
> **M**orphine
> **O**xygen
> **N**itrates (e.g., nitroglycerin)
> **A**spirin
> **Hep**arin
> **B**eta blockers

the onset of menopause. Twenty percent of MI patients present with sudden death due to a lethal arrhythmia (often ventricular fibrillation). The best predictor of survival is left ventricular EF. Coronary anatomy is summarized in Figure 3.2.

Signs and Symptoms. Pain is similar to that of angina (i.e., pressure or tightness that can radiate to the left arm, neck, or jaw) but is much more severe, lasts for more than 30 minutes, and does not resolve with nitroglycerin. In addition to prolonged chest pain, patients may complain of nausea and vomiting, light-headedness, dyspnea, anxiety, and an "impending sense of doom." Signs that may be present include diaphoresis, tachycardia, pulmonary rales, heart failure, hypotension, gallop rhythms (especially an S4), and mitral regurgitation secondary to papillary muscle dysfunction. Elderly, diabetic, and postoperative patients are particularly susceptible to "silent MIs."

Differential. The differential is similar to that for angina. Be sure to evaluate for the deadly causes of chest pain.

Elderly, diabetic, and postoperative patients are particularly susceptible to "silent MIs."

CLINICAL ANATOMY

CORONARY ARTERY DISTRIBUTION

- **Left anterior descending:** Supplies the anterior left ventricle (LV) and interventricular septum.
- **Left circumflex:** Supplies the anterolateral and posterolateral LV.
- **Right coronary:** Supplies the interventricular septum, the right ventricle (RV), the posteroinferior LV, and the sinoatrial (SA) and atrioventricular (AV) nodes.

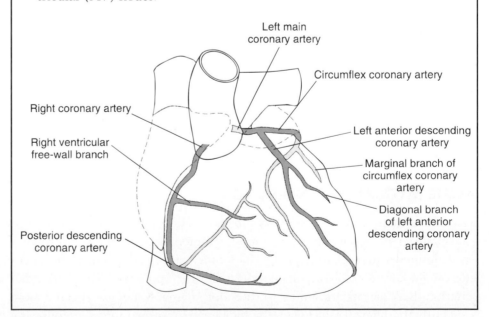

FIGURE 3.2. Coronary arteries and their principal branches. (Reprinted, with permission, from Stobo JD et al. *Principles and Practice of Medicine,* 23rd ed. Stamford, CT: Appleton & Lange, 1996:17.)

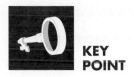
Q-WAVE VS. NON-Q-WAVE MI

A Q wave on ECG in the presence of infarction indicates that the infarction extends through the full thickness of the myocardial wall (transmural).

A non-Q-wave MI (NQWMI) involves the subendocardium, not the full thickness. NQWMIs are dangerous in the sense that the patient is still at risk for a full-thickness infarct in that area.

Workup

- **ECG:** ECG changes in acute MI generally follow a specific sequence (see Figure 3.3):

  Peaked T waves → T-wave inversion → ST-segment elevation → Q waves → ST-segment normalization → T waves return to upright

  ECG changes in the anterior leads (V_1–V_4) usually indicate an anterior MI, whereas changes in leads II, III, and aVF are consistent with an inferior MI.

- **Cardiac enzymes:** The death of myocardium releases cardiac enzymes into the blood that can be measured: troponin-I, CK-MB, and lactate dehydrogenase (LDH). Refer to Figure 3.4 for the time course of the various enzyme elevations. Troponin-I appears the earliest and is the most sensitive and specific of all the enzymes for the detection of MI. CK-MB appears next, followed by LDH. LDH levels remain elevated for three to six days.

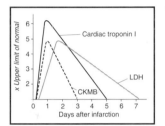

FIGURE 3.4. Myocardial enzymes. The time course of serum enzyme concentrations after a typical MI. (Reprinted, with permission, from Harvey AM et al. (eds). *The Principles and Practice of Medicine*, 23rd ed. Stamford, CT: Appleton & Lange, 1988.)

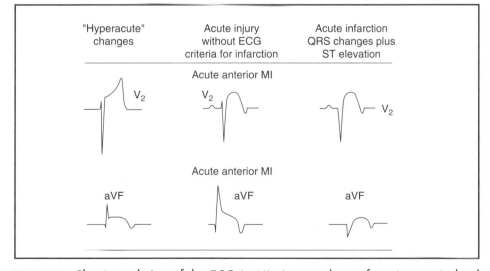

FIGURE 3.3. Classic evolution of the ECG in MI. A normal waveform is seen in lead V_2. Follow the ECG change from left to right. Note the elevated ST segments and peaked T waves that evolve into rounded "tombstones" with new Q waves and T-wave inversions. (Reprinted, with permission, from Nicoll D et al. *Pocket Guide to Diagnostic Tests*, 2nd ed. Stamford, CT: Appleton & Lange, 1997:291, 296.)

Treatment

- **Increase O$_2$ supply:** Give supplemental O$_2$, emergent angioplasty vs. thrombolytics.
- **Decrease O$_2$ demand:** Treat with bed rest, pain meds (e.g., morphine), stool softeners, beta blockers (shown to decrease mortality), nitrates, ACEIs (shown to decrease mortality), and anxiolytics.
- **Cholesterol management:** Administer statins to decrease low-density lipoprotein (LDL) < 100 post-MI (shown to decrease mortality).
- **Thromboprophylaxis:** ASA (shown to decrease mortality) and heparin to prevent stenotic lesions from enlarging.
- **Thrombolytics:** Also known as "clot busters," thrombolytics dissolve thrombotic plaque. Thrombolytics (e.g., tissue plasminogen activator [tPA] and streptokinase) yield the greatest benefit early (achieving 50% mortality reduction one to three hours after chest pain) but are still effective up to ten hours after chest pain onset (10% mortality reduction). Thrombolytics are indicated in patients less than 80 years old who present within 6 to 12 hours of chest pain and with ECG evidence of infarct (ST elevation > 1 mm in two contiguous leads). Intracerebral hemorrhage can complicate up to 1% of all cases using thrombolytics.
- **Emergent angioplasty:** Balloon angioplasty has been shown to be as good as or better than thrombolytics. However, it is more costly and is a technically more difficult procedure. Intracerebral hemorrhage can complicate up to 1% of all cases using thrombolytics.

KEY POINT

GO FOR THE GUSTO

GUSTO was a randomized trial that compared four thrombolytic strategies for acute MI. This study, which involved 41,000 patients, demonstrated a modest increase in survival with accelerated tPA followed by IV heparin compared to streptokinase regimens.

Complications. Infarct extension (especially in NQWMI and those treated with thrombolytics), arrhythmias (e.g., V-tach and V-fib), acute CHF, cardiogenic shock, pericarditis (fibrinous or hemorrhagic), papillary muscle rupture, ventricular rupture, LV aneurysm, mural thrombus, and cardiac tamponade are all potential complications of an MI. Those with cardiac tamponade exhibit the classic Beck's triad (hypotension, distant heart sounds, elevated jugular venous pressure [JVP]), pulsus paradoxus (> 10 mm fall in BP during systole), and electrical alternans (beat-to-beat QRS height alteration).

ATRIAL FIBRILLATION

Atrial fibrillation (AF) is the most common arrhythmia. It is an irregularly irregular rhythm (i.e., one characterized by irregular RR intervals) and is marked by an absence of P waves prior to each QRS complex on the ECG.

The atrial rate of 400–600 beats per minute (bpm) induces an irregularly irregular ventricular response rate of 80–160 bpm. The risk of developing AF doubles with each decade over the age of 55. By the age of 80, the prevalence of AF approaches 8–10%. The prevalence in men is slightly greater than that in females. The Framingham Heart Study showed that patients with AF have an increased risk of cardiovascular mortality as well as a 3- to 13-fold increase in the risk of embolic stroke. The etiologies are summarized by the mnemonic "PIRATES."

Signs and Symptoms. The clinical presentation of AF can vary from asymptomatic to severely symptomatic. Fatigue and nonspecific findings are generally the most common, but patients can report palpitations, exertional fatigue, tachypnea, dyspnea, light-headedness, "skipped beats," a "racing heart," angina, syncope, and an alteration in cognitive function. On exam, the classic irregularly irregular rhythm will be palpated. Irregular heartbeats of varying loudness can be heard on cardiac auscultation.

Differential. A number of cardiac rhythms can yield an irregular heartbeat. These include frequent paroxysmal atrial contractions (PACs), paroxysmal ventricular contractions (PVCs), multifocal atrial tachycardia (MAT), and atrial flutter with variable AV conduction. These can be differentiated with a thorough analysis of the ECG. A complete description of arrhythmias can be found in Chapter 2.

Workup. The ECG will be your primary diagnostic tool. You should see a narrow complex rhythm (QRS < 120 msec) with no consistent interval between the QRS complexes. There is a conspicuous absence of P waves (see Figure 3.5). The workup should be directed toward the suspected etiologies described above and can include a CBC, thyroid-stimulating hormone (TSH), troponin-I, and echocardiogram.

Causes of atrial fibrillation—

PIRATES
Pulmonary disease (e.g., COPD, PE)
Ischemia
Rheumatic heart disease
Anemia/**A**trial myxoma
Thyrotoxicosis
Ethanol ("holiday heart")
Sepsis

HIGH-YIELD TOPICS

Internal Medicine

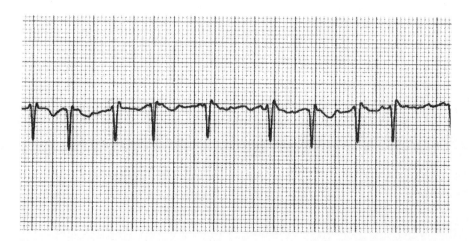

FIGURE 3.5. Atrial fibrillation in V_1. Note the absence of P waves and the irregularly irregular rhythm. (Reprinted, with permission, from Stobo JD et al. *Principles and Practice of Medicine*, 23rd ed. Stamford, CT: Appleton & Lange, 1996:78.)

Treatment

- **Control ventricular rate:** Emergent rate control with a calcium-channel blocker (diltiazem IV) or a beta blocker (metoprolol IV) is indicated to ensure adequate LV filling and sufficient cardiac output. Consider nonemergent rate control with digoxin (in an outpatient setting) if the patient is tolerating the arrhythmia. Hypotension is an emergency that may require immediate DC cardioversion.
- **Cardiovert rhythm:** Cardioversion to sinus rhythm is the ultimate treatment goal in AF. Amiodarone is quickly becoming the treatment of choice for most patients. Prerequisites to successful treatment include recent onset (< 12 months) and lack of severe left atrial dilation (chamber measures < 45 mm by echocardiography). Electrocardioversion (initially start with 100 J DC) should also be considered, as it is the most successful form of cardioversion. If the arrhythmia has been present for more than 48 hours, the patient must either be anticoagulated with warfarin for three to four weeks before cardioversion or receive transesophageal echocardiography (TEE) to exclude an atrial thrombus. Patients are always anticoagulated for three to four weeks after cardioversion.
- **Prevent embolization:** The lack of coordinated atrial contraction increases the risk of thrombogenesis. If cardioversion is unsuccessful, prophylaxis with warfarin (or ASA in younger patients) is appropriate.

CONGESTIVE HEART FAILURE

Congestive heart failure (CHF) occurs when the heart is unable to pump sufficient amounts of blood to meet the oxygen requirement of the heart and other body tissues. Nearly 10% of Americans older than 70 will have CHF; approximately 400,000 new cases are diagnosed each year. Overall, the mortality rate approaches 20%, with those who have the most severe degrees of CHF sustaining a 50% annual mortality. Mortality in men is greater than that in women. Risk factors for developing CHF include infarction, hypertension, valvular heart disease (e.g., mitral stenosis, right-sided endocarditis), pericardial disease, cardiomyopathy, pulmonary hypertension, and, most commonly, CAD (which causes 50–75% of cases). Factors that worsen CHF in previously stable patients are summarized in the mnemonic "FAILURE."

There are various classification systems for CHF, including functional (severity), systolic versus diastolic, and left versus right. The New York Heart Association (NYHA) has defined the functional classification for CHF.

In systolic dysfunction, the decreased EF (< 40%) results in increased preload (increased left ventricular end-diastolic pressure, or LVEDP) and, ultimately, in an increased systolic contractility according to the Frank-Starling law. These compensatory mechanisms are only temporarily effective and eventually lead to hypertrophy, ventricular dilation, and increased myocardial work. In CAD, this is problematic in that the increased work (with limited O_2 supply) can lead to further ischemia and possibly MI.

Causes of CHF exacerbation include

FAILURE—
Forgot medication
Arrhythmia/**A**nemia
Ischemia/**I**nfarct/**I**nfection
Lifestyle (too much Na+ intake) = most common cause
Upregulation (increased CO) = pregnancy, hyperthyroidism
Renal failure→fluid overload
Embolus (pulmonary)

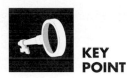
NYHA FUNCTIONAL CLASSIFICATION OF CHF

- Class I: No limitation of activities; no symptoms with normal activities.
- Class II: Slight limitation of activities; comfortable at rest or with mild exertion.
- Class III: Marked limitation of activity; comfortable only at rest.
- Class IV: Confined to complete rest in bed or chair as any physical activity brings on discomfort; symptoms present at rest.

Diastolic dysfunction, by contrast, is characterized by a decrease in compliance with a normal contractile function. The ventricle is either unable to actively relax or unable to passively fill properly (i.e., increased stiffness, decreased recoil, concentric hypertrophy). Again, there is an increased LVEDP but with normal contractile function; cardiac output remains essentially normal, and the EF is either normal or slightly increased. Activation of the renin-angiotensin-aldosterone system (RAAS) is not prominent, but increased hydrostatic pressure can cause pulmonary congestion (see Table 3.1).

Signs and Symptoms. Signs and symptoms depend on whether the left or right heart has CHF. In LV failure, early symptoms include dyspnea on exertion (DOE) and decreased exercise tolerance. Subsequently, the patient may develop orthopnea, dyspnea at rest, paroxysmal nocturnal dyspnea (PND), chronic cough, nocturia (volume overload is diuresed at night), pulmonary congestion (i.e., pulmonary rales, pleural effusion, "cardiac wheeze," tachypnea), diaphoresis, cool extremities, and a laterally displaced point of maximal impulse (PMI). Patients with right-sided failure will complain of anorexia (due to hepatic congestion), cyanosis, and fatigue; a physical exam may yield an elevated JVP, pulsatile hepatomegaly (with possible transaminitis), peripheral edema, ascites, and an abnormal hepatojugular reflex. Signs that are common to both include a ventricular heave, tachycardia, atrial fibrillation, and additional heart sounds (S3 is present with systolic dysfunction; S4 is present with hypertension, CAD, and diastolic dysfunction).

Differential. Causes to consider include PE, acute MI, myocarditis, pneumonia, and high-output CHF. In high-output CHF, the cardiac output is elevated, despite inadequate tissue oxygenation. Causes include thyrotoxicosis, severe anemia, Paget's disease, beriberi, and arteriovenous (AV) fistulas.

Workup. CBC, BUN, creatinine, and TSH can rule out severe anemia, renal failure, and thyrotoxicosis, respectively, as underlying causes. CXR may show cardiomegaly and pulmonary vascular congestion (dilated vessels, interstitial or alveolar edema, Kerley-B lines). Echocardiography provides information on the size and function of both ventricles and valves and can be useful in pinpointing an underlying cause (e.g., ischemia [segmental wall motion abnormalities], valvular disease). If ischemic heart disease is suspected, MI should be ruled out; cardiac catheterization may indicate whether CABG is an option.

The most common cause of right-sided heart failure is left-sided heart failure.

HIGH-YIELD TOPICS

Internal Medicine

TABLE 3.1. Causes of Systolic and Diastolic Dysfunction in CHF.

Causes	Related Condition
Systolic dysfunction	
Decreased contractility	Ischemic heart disease (most common), myocardial dysfunction
	Dilated cardiomyopathy: decreased contractile functioning without pressure or volume overload (**PIPED** causes: **P**ost-myocarditis, **I**diopathic, **P**eripartum, **E**thanol, **D**rugs [cocaine, heroin])
	Myocarditis
	"Hypertensive burnout," valvular heart disease (both cause diastolic dysfunction first, but when the myofibrils stretch, the heart dilates and the EF decreases)
Increased afterload	Increase in systolic pressure: hypertension, aortic stenosis
	Increased chamber radius: dilated cardiomyopathy, valvular regurgitation
Diastolic dysfunction	
Abnormal active relaxation	Ischemia
	Disorders that cause left ventricular hypertrophy, or LVH (e.g., hypertension, aortic stenosis, hypertrophic obstructive cardiomyopathy [HOCM])
Abnormal passive filling	Restrictive cardiomyopathy: infiltrative disorders (e.g., amyloidosis, scleroderma, hemochromatosis) that increase the stiffness of the ventricle to restrict filling and compliance
	Concentric hypertrophy due to hypertension

Treatment

Although systolic and diastolic dysfunction often coexist, the treatment of CHF depends on the primary mechanism of failure. The treatment of diastolic dysfunction rests on trying to restore the original relaxation and filling properties of the heart; control of hypertension is paramount. Pharmacologically, diuretics, calcium-channel blockers (to induce bradycardia and facilitate myocardial relaxation), beta blockers (to induce mild bradycardia and inhibit remodeling), antianginals (e.g., nitroglycerin), and antiarrhythmics (if needed) should be used.

ACEIs, beta blockers, and diuretics form the cornerstones of the treatment of systolic dysfunction. ACEIs (e.g., enalapril) have been shown to decrease mortality and hospitalization in patients with Class II–IV CHF. Angiotensin receptor blockers (ARBs) seem equivalent to their ACEI predecessors. Beta blockers (e.g., carvedilol) have similarly been shown to decrease mortality and hospitalizations in the same CHF classes. Diuretics are useful for symptomatic improvement but have not been shown to have a survival benefit. Recently, however, spironolactone has been shown to decrease the risk of mortality in patients with Class III and IV CHF by 30% when given with ACEIs, diuretics, and digoxin. Digoxin has similarly yielded symptomatic relief in CHF patients and also seems to decrease the number of hospitalizations but has no significant effect on mortality. The combination of hydralazine and isosorbide nitrate has proven beneficial in increasing survival among patients with symptomatic CHF. However, there has been no mortality benefit shown with the use of calcium-channel blockers, and long-term use of vasodilators may increase mortality. Antiarrhythmics (e.g., amiodarone) with anticoagulation are recommended when an arrhythmia is present and causes clinical deterioration.

HYPERTENSION

Hypertension is an extremely common disease in both ambulatory and inpatient internal medicine. The pathophysiology of hypertension is important, although the key to your rotation lies in understanding the algorithm for stratifying the severity and treating the disease (see Tables 3.2 and 3.3). More than 95% of patients with hypertension have primary ("essential") hypertension with no identifiable cause. However, it is important to rule out secondary causes of hypertension, including renovascular disease (fibromuscular dysplasia in young females or atherosclerotic disease in men), renal parenchymal disease, coarctation of the aorta, medications (e.g., oral contraceptives), and endocrine disorders (e.g., Cushing's syndrome, hyperaldosteronism, pheochromocytoma, hyperthyroidism, hyperparathyroidism, acromegaly).

TABLE 3.2. Classification of Blood Pressure for Adults > 18 Years Old.

Category	Systolic (mmHg)	Diastolic (mmHg)	Follow-up Recommendations
Optimal	< 120	< 80	Recheck in two years
Normal	< 130	< 85	Recheck in two years
High to normal	130–139	85–89	Recheck in one year
Stage I hypertension	140–159	90–99	Confirm within two months
Stage II hypertension	160–179	100–109	Evaluate or refer within one month
Stage III hypertension	≥180	N ≥ 110	Evaluate or refer immediately or within one week

Taken from the Sixth Report of the Joint National Committee on Prevention, Detection, Workup, and Treatment of High Blood Pressure. *Arch Intern Med* 1997;157:2413–2439.

TABLE 3.3. Hypertensive Management Indications.ᵃ	
Manifestation	**Treatment**
DM with proteinuria	ACEIs
CHF	ACEIs with diuretics (including spironolactone; see CHF section)
Isolated systolic hypertension	Diuretics are preferred; long-acting dihydropyridine calcium-channel blockers
MI	Non–intrinsic sympathomimetic activity (non-ISA) beta blockers, ACEIs
Osteoporosis	Thiazide diuretics
Benign prostatic hypertrophy (BPH)	α-antagonists

ᵃBegin with lifestyle management (diet, exercise); BP goal in uncomplicated hypertension is < 140/< 90; BP goal in renal disease with proteinuria is < 130/< 85 (< 125/< 75 if possible) and in DM patients < 130/< 75. Diuretics and beta blockers have been shown to have a mortality benefit in uncomplicated hypertension and are first-line treatments unless there is a comorbid condition requiring another medication.

INFECTIVE ENDOCARDITIS

Infective endocarditis (IE) is the most common endovascular infection, with 10,000 to 15,000 new cases seen each year. Men are affected more frequently than women, with a mean age of onset at 60 years. The mortality rate is approximately 25%. Infectious etiologies are numerous, but infection of the endothelial lining generally results from four factors: (1) local hemodynamic abnormalities; (2) the presence of endothelial damage; (3) the presence of bacteria; and (4) the status of the host's immune system. Those with rheumatic heart disease, mitral valve prolapse (MVP), congenital valve abnormalities, the presence of foreign bodies (e.g., pacemakers, prosthetic valves), senile calcification, HOCM, or a history of intravenous drug use (IVDU) are particularly at risk.

Acute endocarditis is an infection of normal heart valves, most commonly with *Staphylococcus aureus*, that results in a rapid decline in valve function and death. Subacute endocarditis, on the other hand, is caused primarily by *Streptococcus viridans* infecting abnormal heart valves and has a more insidious course and gradual decline. A more complete list of etiologies is included in Table 3.4.

Signs and Symptoms. Patients generally present with fever, chills, malaise, night sweats, anorexia, and weight loss. Arthralgias and myalgias may also be present. On exam, patients will have fever, a new or changing murmur, splenomegaly, and the classic findings outlined in the Duke criteria. Complications include CHF, embolization (especially from left-sided disease), glomerulonephritis, anemia, and myocardial abscess formation.

TABLE 3.4. Microbiologic Causes of Infective Endocarditis.

Type of Endocarditis	Common Etiologic Organisms
Culture-negative endocarditis	HACEK organisms—*Haemophilus*, *Actinobacillus*, *Cardiobacterium*, *Eikenella*, *Kingella*
Prosthetic valve endocarditis (PVE)	Early PVE is caused by perioperative seeding of *Staphylococcus epidermidis*, and late PVE is generally caused by the same organisms as NVE
Endocarditis due to IVDU	Most common cause is *Staphylococcus aureus*; consider this if tricuspid valve is involved.
Native valve endocarditis (NVE)	Most common causes are *Streptococcus viridans*, *S. bovis*, *Enterococcus*
GU and GI surgery patients	Most common causes are gram-negative bacteria
Miscellaneous causes	Less common, but include fungi (*Candida*, *Aspergillus*, especially with indwelling catheter), *Rickettsia*, and *Chlamydia*

IE Findings Not To Miss
- **Roth's spots:** retinal hemorrhages.
- **Janeway lesions:** painless lesions on the palms and soles.
- **Osler's nodes:** painful nodes on the tips of fingers or toes.

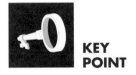
KEY POINT

Differential. Endocarditis should always be suspected in patients with fever of unknown origin (FUO) and IVDU. For those who fulfill the Duke criteria, the differential is limited to IE and other endovascular abnormalities, including septic thromboemboli and mycotic aneurysms.

Workup. The Duke criteria constitute the standard for making a clinical diagnosis of endocarditis. A complete exam should consist of funduscopy, a cardiac exam, a skin exam, at least two sets of blood cultures, echocardiography (TEE has 90% sensitivity for mitral valve pathology in comparison to the 60% sensitivity of transthoracic echocardiography [TTE]), and various labs, including a CBC (an elevated WBC is seen in acute endocarditis and moderate anemia in subacute endocarditis), erythrocyte sedimentation rate, or ESR (elevated), urinalysis, or UA (proteinuria and hematuria with glomerulonephritis), and rheumatoid factor (positive).

Treatment. IE requires four to six weeks of high-dose IV antibiotics. Treatment consists of an anti-staphylococcal β-lactam (e.g., nafcillin) with an aminoglycoside (e.g., gentamicin). In areas with high methicillin-resistant *Staphylococcus aureus* (MRSA) prevalence or in the presence of coagulase-negative staphylococcus infection, vancomycin can be substituted for the β-lactam. Surgery for IE is indicated if the patient has severe, refractory CHF

> ## DUKE CRITERIA FOR INFECTIVE ENDOCARDITIS
>
> ### Major Criteria
>
> - Persistently positive blood cultures (two or more positive cultures separated by at least 12 hours, three or more cultures at least one hour apart, or 70% of cultures positive if four are drawn)
> - Echocardiographic evidence of endocardial disease
>
> ### Minor Criteria
>
> - Fever
> - Vascular phenomena (arterial emboli, Janeway lesions, pulmonary emboli, mycotic aneurysm)
> - Immunologic phenomena (Osler's nodes, Roth's spots, glomerulonephritis, positive rheumatoid factor)
> - Predisposing heart abnormality
> - Positive blood cultures not meeting major criteria
> - Positive echocardiogram not meeting major criteria
>
> To make a diagnosis of IE, two major criteria, one major plus three minor criteria, or five minor criteria must be fulfilled.

due to IE, treatment-resistant IE, infection of a prosthetic valve, suspected fungal infection, recurrent embolic events, and/or progressive intracardiac spread of infection. For patients with valvular abnormalities, prophylactic amoxicillin or clarithromycin is recommended one hour prior to dental, GU, or GI surgeries.

SYNCOPE

The causes of SYNCOPE—

Situational
Vasovagal
Neurogenic
Cardiac
Orthostatic hypotension
Psychiatric
Everything else

Syncope is a sudden, transient loss of consciousness and postural tone due to inadequate cerebral blood flow that resolves promptly and spontaneously; patients usually have preceding light-headedness. More than 30% of people will have a syncopal episode at some point in their lives. Causes are summarized in the mnemonic "SYNCOPE." Situational causes include syncopal episodes due to the Valsalva maneuver, defecation, cough, micturition, carotid sinus hypersensitivity (syncope with head turning, tight collars, or shaving), or subclavian steal (syncope with arm exercise). Vasovagal syncope, or the "common faint," is most frequently found in young patients and is usually precipitated by a stressful or emotional situation; this type is due to excessive vagal tone or impaired reflex control of the peripheral circulation. Symptoms such as diaphoresis, pallor, and abdominal discomfort might precede the syncopal episode. Neurogenic causes include transient ischemic attacks (TIAs) of the vertebrobasilar circulation. Cardiac causes include cardiac arrhythmias or conduction disturbances (e.g., sick sinus syndrome, second- or third-degree

AV heart block, torsades de pointes, ventricular tachycardia, ventricular fibrillation), inflow/outflow obstruction (e.g., valvular stenosis, HOCM, PE, pulmonary hypertension, myxoma), and/or cardiac ischemia/decreased contractility. Orthostatic hypotension can be caused by hypovolemia or, in patients with DM, by autonomic insufficiency; systolic blood pressure will decrease at least 20 mmHg when the patient changes from supine to standing. "Everything else" (nearly 50% of cases) includes idiopathic causes as well as drugs and medications that can cause vasodilation and orthostasis.

Workup. Workup is tailored to those causes that seem most likely on the basis of the complete history and physical exam. Workup should include orthostatic vitals, a tilt table test, and an ECG. Unless a metabolic abnormality is sought, routine blood work is not extremely helpful. Further tests may include a Holter monitor (detects 20–50% of arrhythmias), echocardiography, an exercise treadmill, and cardiac catheterization. A subclavian ultrasound or angiography can be helpful if subclavian steal is suspected; carotid sinus massage may help elucidate carotid sinus hypersensitivity.

Treatment. Treatment is etiology specific, but if a cardiac condition is present, its treatment is of primary importance. Patients with orthostasis should have their volume repleted and underlying problems (e.g., anemia) corrected. Those with subclavian steal should be referred to a vascular surgeon. Those with vasovagal syncope may benefit from beta blockers. Carotid artery hypersensitivity can be treated with anticholinergics (e.g., diphenhydramine) or a pacemaker. Neurologic causes should be referred to a specialist.

VALVULAR HEART DISEASE

Valvular diseases can be divided into two general types: stenotic lesions and regurgitant lesions. Most valvular heart disease presents in the seventh decade of life; the exception is mitral stenosis, which presents in the fourth and fifth decades. Until recently, the most common cause of valvular heart disease in adults was rheumatic fever; however, as treatment of streptococcal infections has assumed prominence and as the incidence of rheumatic fever in the United States has significantly decreased, the leading cause of valvular heart disease in adults has become mechanical degeneration due to normal "wear and tear." Childhood valvular lesions are most likely caused by congenital abnormalities. Refer to Table 3.5 for a summary of major valvular lesions.

TABLE 3.5. Valvular Heart Lesions.

Valvular Lesion	Risk Factors	Symptoms	Murmur	Physical Exam	Treatment
Aortic stenosis	Rheumatic heart disease, congenital aortic stenosis, bicuspid valve, "senile degeneration" beginning with aortic sclerosis.	Classic triad, including exertional dyspnea, angina (35–50% of patients), and syncope. Can lead to CHF and death (50% of those with CHF die within one to two years if not corrected).	Midsystolic crescendo-decrescendo (diamond-shaped) murmur heard best at second intercostal space; radiates to carotids and apex (Gallavardin's phenomenon); + systolic ejection click.	"Pulsus parvus and tardus" (weak and delayed carotid upstroke), sustained apical beat; S4, and single, soft S2.	Avoid afterload reducers and beta blockers. Curative therapy is valve replacement; balloon valvuloplasty is palliative for poor surgical candidates.
Aortic regurgitation	Rheumatic heart disease, IE, ventricular septal defect (VSD), congenital bicuspid valve, Marfan's syndrome, aortic dissection, collagen vascular diseases, syphilitic aortitis, idiopathic aortic root dilation.	LVH, angina (due to reduced diastolic coronary filling), left heart failure (LHF) due to volume overload, leading to dyspnea, orthopnea, and paroxysmal nocturnal dyspnea (PND).	Three murmurs: 1. High-pitched, blowing diastolic murmur at left sternal border (LSB) → loudest when leaning forward. 2. Austin-Flint → low-pitched mid-diastolic rumble similar to mitral stenosis without opening snap. 3. Midsystolic murmur at base (due to high volume flow).	Increase in stroke volume and widened pulse pressure, laterally displaced PMI secondary to LVH, pulsus bisferiens. Look for classic signs of aortic regurgitation.	Curative treatment is aortic valve replacement. If not possible, treat with afterload reducers (vasodilators, ACEIs), diuretics, and/or digitalis.
Mitral stenosis	Rheumatic heart disease.	LHF (DOE, orthopnea, PND), right heart failure (RHF) (edema, ascites, hepatospleno-megaly, increased JVP), hemoptysis.	Mid-diastolic rumble with opening snap at apex; no change with inspiration (vs. tricuspid stenosis, which increases with inspiration).	AF, pulmonary rales, increased intensity of S1 and P2, RV heave, signs of left or right CHF.	Avoid inotropic agents. Use diuretics, anticoagulants, digitalis, balloon valvuloplasty, and, for refractory disease, valve replacement.

TABLE 3.5 (continued). Valvular Heart Lesions.

Valvular Lesion	Risk Factors	Symptoms	Murmur	Physical Exam	Treatment
Mitral valve prolapse (MVP)	Found in 7% of population, especially in young women.	Usually benign, asymptomatic.	Late systolic murmur with mid-systolic click (Barlow's syndrome). Valsalva makes the murmur earlier and longer.	Can progress to mitral regurgitation (MR).	Generally not necessary unless symptomatic or progressive in severity.
Mitral regurgitation (MR)	Rheumatic heart disease, MI (i.e., ruptured chordae tendineae; papillary muscle dysfunction), severe MVP, endocarditis.	LHF (DOE, orthopnea, PND) that can progress to RHF.	High-pitched, holosystolic murmur at apex and radiating to the axilla; + systolic thrill.	Laterally displaced PMI with LV heave, S3, AF, signs of LHF and possibly RHF, fatigue.	ACEIs, vasodilators, diuretics, digitalis, anticoagulation, and, in chronic or severe MR, valve repair and/or replacement.
Hypertrophic obstructive cardiomyopathy (HOCM)	Idiopathic, although half of all patients have evidence of autosomal-dominant transmission; the hypertrophied IV septum is apposed against the anterior leaflet of the mitral valve during systole, resulting in LV outflow obstruction.	Many are asymptomatic or mildly symptomatic. Often the first manifestation is sudden death. Symptomatic patients complain of dyspnea, angina, syncope, and symptoms of CHF.	Systolic, diamond-shaped, harsh murmur at the apex and LSB, poorly transmitted to carotids (vs. aortic stenosis); earlier and longer with decreased LV size (Valsalva and standing); decreases with increased LV size (squatting).	Spike and dome carotid upstroke, LVH, arrhythmias including AF, S4, signs of CHF.	Avoid competitive sports and strenuous activity owing to risk of sudden death; digitalis is contraindicated. Propranolol decreases HR and outflow gradient; verapamil decreases outflow gradient but should not be used in CHF. Surgical treatment is first line and involves myomectomy, mitral valve replacement, pacemakers, or septal infarction (experimental).

HIGH-YIELD TOPICS

Internal Medicine

CHRONIC OBSTRUCTIVE PULMONARY DISEASE

Chronic obstructive pulmonary disease (COPD) is a progressive disease characterized by a decrease in lung function due to airflow obstruction. COPD is generally due to cigarette smoking and is subdivided into chronic bronchitis and emphysema. Chronic bronchitis is a clinical diagnosis of excessive bronchial secretion with productive cough for at least three months per year over two consecutive years. Emphysema is a pathologic diagnosis of terminal airway destruction that is due to smoking (centrilobular) or to an inherited α-1 antitrypsin deficiency (panlobular). Most patients exhibit components of both chronic bronchitis and emphysema, and nearly all are smokers. In contrast to asthma, COPD is not reversible. COPD is the fourth most common cause of death in the United States.

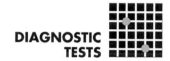

DIAGNOSTIC TESTS

PULMONARY FUNCTION TESTS

Pulmonary function tests (PFTs) consist of spirometry, diffusion capacity for carbon monoxide (DL_{CO}), and arterial blood gases (ABGs). They are used primarily to detect the presence and to quantify the severity of obstructive and restrictive pulmonary disease (see Table 3.6).

- **Obstructive dysfunction:** Decreased expiratory airflow and increased air trapping in the lung secondary to obstructed airways. Seen in asthma, chronic bronchitis, emphysema, and bronchiectasis.

- **Restrictive dysfunction:** Decreased lung volume. Seen in extrapulmonary (chest wall disorders, neuromuscular disease, pleural disease) and pulmonary diseases (pulmonary infiltrates and diffuse interstitial lung disease).

Signs and Symptoms. Signs and symptoms of COPD are often absent until the disease is significantly advanced (with loss of > 50% of lung function). Emphysema patients are classically described as "pink puffers" who exhibit decreased breath sounds, minimal cough, DOE, pursed lips, weight loss, rare cyanosis, and hypercarbia/hypoxia late in disease. Patients with chronic bronchitis are described as "blue bloaters" with severe (usually sterile) productive cough, rhonchi, early onset of hypercarbia/hypoxia and cyanosis, weight gain, lethargy, peripheral edema (due to CHF), and late-onset dyspnea. In both disorders, patients may present with a barrel chest from high lung volumes, muscle use, accessory chest jugular venous distention (JVD), end-expiratory wheezing, prolonged expiration and/or muffled breath sounds.

Differential. The differential of COPD includes asthma, bronchiectasis, cystic fibrosis (CF), CHF, congenital heart abnormalities, and pulmonary hypertension.

TABLE 3.6. PFTs in Obstructive and Restrictive Lung Disease.

Measurement[a]	Obstructive	Restrictive
Spirometry		
FEV_1	↓	N or ↓
FEV_{25-75}	↓	N or ↓
FEV_1/FVC	↓	N or ↑
Lung volumes		
FVC	N or ↓	↓
VC	N or ↓	↓
TLC	N or ↓	↓
RV	↑	N, ↓, or ↑

[a]FEV_1 = forced expiratory volume in 1 second; FEV_{25-75} = forced expiratory flow between 25% and 75% of vital capacity; FVC = forced vital capacity; VC = vital capacity; VC = vital capacity; TLC = total lung capacity; RV = residual volume.
Adapted, with permission, from Tierney LM et al. *Current Medical Diagnosis & Treatment 1997*, 36th ed. Stamford, CT: Appleton & Lange, 1997:239.

Workup. CXR, PFTs, ABGs, and electrolytes are the mainstay of the workup. In emphysema, the CXR shows hyperinflation, hyperlucency, loss of the capillary-alveolar surface area, a flattened and depressed diaphragm, widened retrosternal air space, and an increased anterior-posterior (AP) diameter (see Figure 3.6). Parenchymal bullae or subpleural blebs are pathognomonic for emphysema. There are no specific findings for chronic bronchitis on CXR or PFTs except those associated with the comorbid emphysema. Spirometry is diagnostic and consistent with the patterns summarized in Table 3.6. For both disorders, an ABG during an acute exacerbation could show hypoxemia with an acute respiratory acidosis (increased PCO_2; patients with COPD have a baseline increased PCO_2) as well as an increased A-a gradient. Blood and sputum cultures (with Gram stain) are warranted in the presence of fever or increased purulent sputum production.

Treatment. The management of COPD is akin to that of asthma and is similar for both emphysema and chronic bronchitis. Acute exacerbations are treated with O_2, hydration, IV steroids, anticholinergics (ipratropium is the first line in COPD), nebulized beta agonists (albuterol), and, if infectious, antibiotics (e.g., trimethoprim-sulfamethoxazole [TMP-SMX], cefuroxime). When the patient is stable, PFTs can assess the severity of the COPD. Chronic management includes smoking cessation, anticholinergics, inhaled beta agonists, influenza and pneumococcal vaccines, and, if indicated, home O_2 therapy. The benefit of mucokinetics in chronic bronchitis has not been conclusively established, but they can be used. As with asthma, prophylactic antibiotics do not seem to be of use in preventing exacerbations; however, corticosteroids, while used in COPD, do not seem to yield the same symptomatic benefit. Patients with α_1-antitrypsin deficiency should be given appropriate supplementation.

Anticholinergics are first-line treatment for COPD.

HIGH-YIELD TOPICS

Internal Medicine

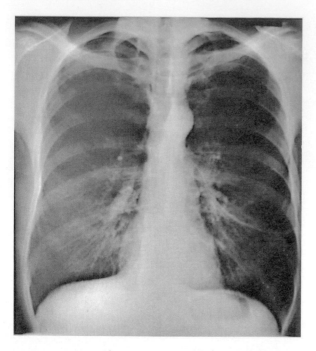
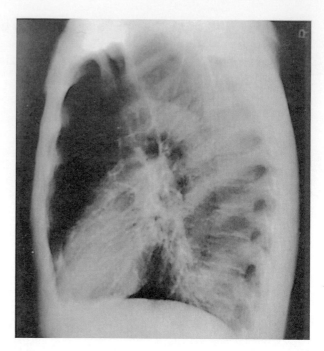

FIGURE 3.6. CXR with COPD. Note the hyperinflated and hyperlucent lungs, flat diaphragm, increased AP diameter, and narrow mediastinum. (Reprinted, with permission, from Stobo JD et al. *Principles and Practice of Medicine*, 23rd ed. Stamford, CT: Appleton & Lange, 1996:135.)

KEY POINT

Beware of "CO_2 retainers" who occasionally do worse with supplemental O_2 because they lose their hypoxemic drive to hyperventilate and acutely increase their P_{CO_2}.

Lung cancer is the leading cause of cancer death in men and women.

INDICATIONS FOR HOME OXYGEN

- $P_{O_2} < 55$ mmHg or $SaO_2 < 88\%$
- P_{O_2} 55–59 mmHg with symptoms of hypoxia (mental status changes, RHF from cor pulmonale, polycythemia).

Complications

- **Chronic respiratory failure:** Chronic hypoxemia with a compensated respiratory acidosis (high P_{CO_2})
- **Destruction of pulmonary vasculature:** Leads to pulmonary hypertension and eventually to RHF (cor pulmonale)
- **Pneumonia**
- **Bronchogenic carcinoma**

BRONCHOGENIC CARCINOMA

Lung cancer is the most common cause of cancer death in the United States. Most patients present between 50 and 70 years of age. Smoking is the most important risk factor in both men and women in all types except bronchoalveolar, although exposure to secondhand smoke, asbestos, and other environmental agents is also important. The incidence, location, and risk factors associated with each tumor subtype are summarized in Table 3.7.

TABLE 3.7. Lung Tumors and Their Characteristics[a]

Tumor Type	Frequency	Location	Association with Smoking	Paraneoplastic Diseases
Small cell (oat cell)	18%	Central hilum	++ (99% are smokers)	Cushing's syndrome, syndrome of inappropriate diuretic hormone (SIADH), peripheral neuropathy, Lambert-Eaton syndrome
Squamous cell	29%	Central hilum	++	Hypercalcemia (parathyroid hormone–related peptide [PTHrP]), hypertrophic pulmonary osteoarthropathy
Adeno-carcinoma	32%	Lung periphery, subpleura	Most frequent type in nonsmokers	Hypertrophic pulmonary osteoarthropathy, thrombophlebitis
Broncho-alveolar	3%	Lung periphery, alveoli	–	
Large cell	9%	Lung periphery	+	Gynecomastia, hypertrophic pulmonary osteoarthropathy

[a]All forms of lung cancer can exhibit dermatomyositis, anemia, disseminated intravascular coagulation (DIC), eosinophilia, thrombocytosis, and acanthosis nigricans.

Signs and Symptoms. Patients often present with cough, dyspnea, hemoptysis, chest pain, and constitutional symptoms (fever, chills, weight loss, malaise, and night sweats). Only 10–25% of patients are asymptomatic at the time of diagnosis. Physical examination may reveal decreased breath sounds, crackles, increased fremitus with postobstructive pneumonitis, and pleural effusion. Physical exam may also reveal a "SPHERE" of bronchogenic carcinoma complications.

Differential. Tuberculosis (TB) and other granulomatous diseases, fungal disease (aspergillus, histoplasmosis), lung abscess, metastasis, benign tumor (bronchial adenoma), hamartoma, and carcinoid should be considered.

HIGH-YIELD TOPICS

Internal Medicine

SPHERE of lung cancer complications—

Superior vena cava syndrome
Pancoast's tumor
Horner's syndrome
Endocrine (paraneoplastic)
Recurrent laryngeal symptoms (hoarseness)
Effusions (pleural or pericardial)

Workup. Initial workup should include CXR, CBC with differential, electrolytes, liver function tests (LFTs), and calcium. Lung cancer is usually first noted as a nodule on CXR. CXR may show hilar and peripheral masses, atelectasis, infiltrates, or pleural effusion (see Figure 3.7). A CT scan (or MRI) of the chest can better characterize involvement of the parenchyma, pleura, and mediastinum. A histologic diagnosis from fine-needle aspiration (FNA), bronchoscopy with biopsy, lymph node biopsy, thoracocentesis, mediastinoscopy, or thoracotomy is necessary, as the treatment and prognosis for small cell lung carcinoma (SCLC) and non–small cell lung carcinoma (NSCLC) differ.

Treatment. Treatment depends on the type and extent of the lung cancer and includes surgery, chemotherapy, and radiation therapy. Surgical resection followed

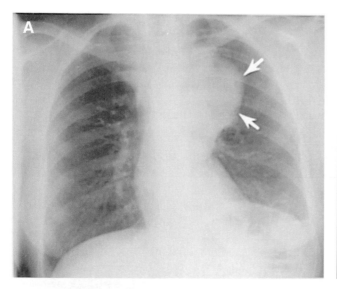

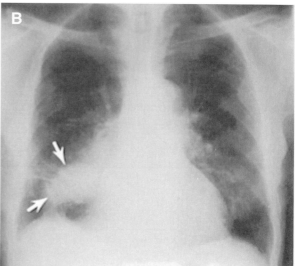

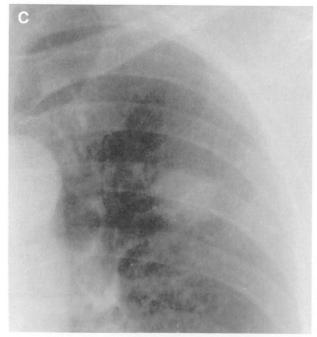

FIGURE 3.7. CXRs in lung cancer. (A) Small cell cancer in the left hilum. Note the left hemidiaphragm paralysis secondary to phrenic nerve involvement. (B) Squamous cell cancer in the right lower lobe. (C) Adenocarcinoma in the left upper lobe. (Reprinted, with permission, from Stobo JD et al. *Principles and Practice of Medicine,* 23rd ed. Stamford, CT: Appleton & Lange, 1996:180.)

by radiation/chemotherapy is the treatment of choice in NSCLC. SCLC is not resectable but responds to combination and radiation therapy; however, recurrence is common, and the median survival rate is lower than that for NSCLC.

CHRONIC COUGH

Chronic cough is a cough that is present for more than three weeks. For nonsmokers, the prevalence is 14–23%; for smokers, the prevalence rises with the number of packs smoked, increasing from 25% with half a pack per day to 50% in those who smoke more than two packs per day. Ninety percent of cases are caused by the five most common etiologies: smoking, postnasal drip, asthma, GERD, and chronic bronchitis. However, other causes to consider include medication-induced cough (e.g., ACEI), airway hyperresponsiveness secondary to upper respiratory infection (URI), cancer, TB, aspiration, foreign bodies, occupational irritants, psychogenic factors, CHF, and irritation of cough receptors in the ear. Chronic cough may often have more than one etiology.

Most Common Causes of Chronic Cough:

Smoking

Postnasal drip

Asthma

GERD

Chronic bronchitis

Signs and Symptoms. Patients can present with a variety of symptoms. If the cough is asthma related, the patient might complain of coughing that worsens at night, a family history of eczema/dermatitis/allergy, audible wheezes, or coughing due to specific irritants (e.g., pollen, smoke, temperature). Wheezing may be absent in "cough-variant asthma." If GERD is the culprit, the patient might complain of a sour mouth, heartburn, or worsened symptoms while supine. Postnasal drip might present, with mucus draining from the nose or down the throat and, on exam, cobblestone mucosa. If malignancy is suspected, inquire about constitutional symptoms such as fever, chills, weight loss, malaise, and night sweats.

Workup and Treatment. The workup of a chronic cough should begin with a complete history and should include a thorough head, neck, heart, and lung exam. The patient should avoid suspected irritants (e.g., medications, allergies). If the patient has had a recent URI, he or she should be given an antihistamine with a decongestant or steroids. The recommended workup should proceed in a stepwise manner to rule out the various causes of chronic cough:

- Treat postnasal drip with a combination antihistamine/decongestant; if symptoms persist, consider adding a steroid and/or performing a CT of the sinuses.
- Evaluate and treat for asthma (see Pediatrics, Chapter 6)
- If postnasal drip and asthma are ruled out, treat for GERD with H_2 blockers or proton pump inhibitors (PPIs); consider endoscopy or 24-hour pH monitoring if refractory.
- If all of the above are negative, consider bronchoscopy and treat the specific etiology.

PLEURAL EFFUSION

Pleural effusion is defined as an abnormal accumulation of fluid in the pleural space. It is normally classified as transudative or exudative.

- **Transudative effusion:** Intact capillaries lead to protein-poor pleural fluid that is an ultrafiltrate of plasma due to increased hydrostatic pressure and/or a decreased oncotic pressure. Primary causes include CHF, cirrhosis, nephrotic syndrome, peritoneal dialysis, superior vena cava obstruction, myxedema, urinothorax, protein-losing enteropathy, and PE.
- **Exudative effusion:** Inflammation leads to leaky capillaries, resulting in a protein-rich fluid. Common causes include TB, bacterial infection (parapneumonic effusion and empyema), viral infection, neoplasm, PE with infarct, collagen vascular disease, pancreatitis, hemothorax, sarcoidosis, uremia, asbestosis exposure, pericardial disease, chylothorax, and traumatic tap.

Signs and Symptoms. The patient may complain of dyspnea and pleuritic chest pain but is often asymptomatic. On physical exam, there may be decreased breath sounds, dullness to percussion, and decreased tactile fremitus.

Differential. The causes of effusion can generally be categorized according to the type of pleural effusion that is present.

Workup. CXR may show blunting of the costophrenic angles. A decubitus CXR can determine whether the fluid is free flowing or loculated. The definitive diagnostic test is thoracocentesis. Pleural fluid should be sent for the following:

- **CBC with differential:** Evaluate for signs of infection or trauma (e.g., increased RBCs).
- **Protein and LDH:** Helps differentiate exudates and transudates.
- **Amylase:** High amylase suggests esophageal rupture, pancreatic pleural effusion, or malignancy.
- **pH:** The normal pleural pH is 7.60; a pH < 7.30 suggests empyema, rheumatoid pleurisy, TB pleurisy, or malignancy.
- **Glucose:** Glucose < 60 mg/dL suggests bacterial infection, rheumatoid pleuritis, or malignancy.
- **Gram stain.**
- **Cytology:** Can reveal malignant cells.

A needle biopsy of pleura diagnoses TB effusion. Definitive diagnosis is made by thoracocentesis or open biopsy.

Treatment. Treat transudative effusion by addressing the underlying condition; perform a therapeutic lung tap when massive effusion leads to dyspnea.

KEY POINT

DEFINING FEATURES OF AN EXUDATE

- Pleural fluid protein/serum protein > 0.5.
- Pleural fluid LDH/serum LDH > 0.6.
- Pleural fluid LDH > 2/3 upper normal limit for serum LDH.

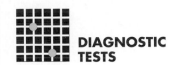

PLEURAL FLUID TIP-OFFS

- **Bloody:** Neoplasm, TB, traumatic tap, pulmonary embolus, hemothorax
- **Low glucose:** Neoplasm, TB, empyema, rheumatoid arthritis (extremely low glucose)
- **Lymphocytic:** Viral infection, TB, malignancy
- **Milky (triglyceride-rich):** Chylothorax

Treatment for exudative effusion is as follows:

- **Malignant:** In malignant effusion, malignant cells from an unresectable tumor invade the pleural surface and fluid. Consider pleurodesis (injection of an irritant such as talc into the pleural cavity to scar the two pleural layers together) in symptomatic patients who are unresponsive to chemotherapy and radiation therapy. Therapeutic thoracocentesis, pleuroperitoneal shunting, and surgical pleurectomy are alternatives.
- **Parapneumonic:** This is a pleural effusion in the presence of pneumonia. If you suspect infected or "complicated" parapneumonic effusion, you should consider immediate drainage via a chest tube. Signs of a "complicated" effusion include puslike appearance, a positive Gram stain, low pH (< 7.3), low glucose (< 40 mg/dL), and high LDH (> 1000 IU/L).
- **Hemothorax:** Place a chest tube to control bleeding by the apposition of pleural surfaces, determine the amount of blood loss, and assess the risk of infection and fibrothorax.

All parapneumonic effusions need a diagnostic tap.

PNEUMONIA

Pneumonia is an infection of the bronchoalveolar unit with an inflammatory exudate. Causes are often broadly categorized as "typical," or caused by bacteria from the nasopharynx, and "atypical," or caused by organisms (bacteria, viruses, fungi) inhaled from the environment. Atypical organisms are often difficult to visualize on Gram stain and are not susceptible to antibiotics that act on the cell wall (e.g., β-lactams). *Streptococcus pneumoniae* is the most common cause of community-acquired pneumonia.

Pneumococcus is the most common cause of community-acquired pneumonia.

Signs and Symptoms. Classic symptoms are productive cough (purulent yellow or green sputum or hemoptysis), dyspnea, fever/chills, night sweats, and pleuritic chest pain. Atypical pneumonia may present with a more gradual onset of symptoms, dry cough, myalgias, headaches, sore throat, and pharyngitis. Physical exam may show decreased or bronchial breath sounds, crackles, wheezes, dullness to percussion, egophony, and tactile fremitus. Elderly patients and those with COPD or DM may have minimal signs on exam. Table 3.8 summarizes pulmonary exam differences between pneumonia, pleural effusion, and pneumothorax.

HIGH-YIELD TOPICS

Internal Medicine

TABLE 3.8. Pulmonary Diagnostic Tips.

Physical Exam Finding	Pneumonia	Pleural Effusion	Pneumothorax
Breath sounds	Decreased	Decreased	Decreased
Abnormal sounds	Inspiratory rales	Egophony (E → A changes)	None
Percussion	Dull	Dull	Hyperresonant
Tactile fremitus	Increased	Decreased	Decreased

Workup.

- **CBC:** Leukocytosis and left shift (immature form of WBCs present) with bands are typically seen.
- **CXR:** Look for lobar consolidation or patchy or diffuse infiltrates (see Figure 3.8).
- **Sputum Gram stain and culture:** Identifies the pathogenic organism as well as an organism's susceptibility to antibiotics. A good sputum sample has many PMNs and few epithelial cells. Otherwise, suspect contamination by oral flora.
- **Blood culture:** If the patient appears very ill, suspect sepsis from pneumonia.
- **ABGs:** Poor oxygen saturation and acid-base disturbance will be observed in an ill patient.

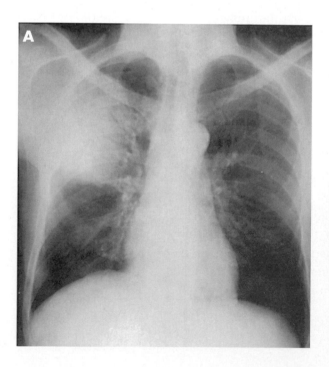
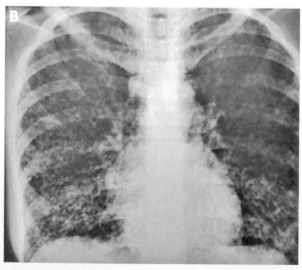

FIGURE 3.8. Typical CXRs in pneumonia. (A) Acute lobar pneumonia in right upper lobe. (B) Interstitial (atypical) pneumonia. (Reprinted, with permission, from Stobo JD et al. *Principles and Practice of Medicine*, 23rd ed. Stamford, CT: Appleton & Lange, 1996:127.)

- For persistent, recurrent infections, consider the underlying causes of lung injury, obstruction, or decreased immune protection, such as bronchogenic carcinoma, lymphoma, Wegener's granulomatosis, or unusual obstruction (TB, *Nocardia, Coxiella burnetii, Aspergillus*).
- Consider disease-specific clues such as rust-colored sputum (pneumococcus), "currant-jelly" sputum *(Klebsiella)*, cold agglutinins *(Mycoplasma)*, CD4+ < 200, and/or elevated LDH *(Pneumocystis carinii* pneumonia, or PCP).

Treatment. The initial choice of antibiotics will be directed against what you judge to be the most likely pathogens affecting the host given his or her risk factors and environmental exposures. Patients should fall into one of the five categories listed in Table 3.9. Once Gram stains, cultures, and sensitivities return, antibiotic coverage can be adjusted accordingly.

Consider hospitalization in patients more than 65 years or in those with comorbidities, immunosuppression, altered mental status, aspiration, malnutrition, alcohol abuse, tachypnea, hypotension, sepsis, hypoxemia, or multilobar involvement.

Any patient sick enough to be admitted likely warrants IV antibiotics. However, if a patient is afebrile for more than 24 hours, consider switching to an oral antibiotic. If the patient remains afebrile on the oral antibiotic, he or she

Rust-colored sputum = pneumococcus

Currant-jelly sputum = Klebsiella

Alcoholic? Think anaerobes.

COPD? Think H. flu.

TABLE 3.9. Treatment of Pneumonia.

Patient Type	Suspected Pathogens	Initial Coverage
Outpatient community-acquired pneumonia, ≤ 60 years old, otherwise healthy	*Streptococcus pneumoniae, Mycoplasma pneumoniae, Chlamydia pneumoniae, Haemophilus influenzae*, viral	Erythromycin, tetracycline. Consider clarithromycin or azithromycin in smokers to treat *H. flu.*
As above except ≥ 60 years old or with comorbidity (COPD, heart failure, renal failure, diabetes, liver disease, EtOH abuse)	*S. pneumoniae, H. flu*, aerobic gram-negative rods (GNRs—*Escherichia coli, Enterobacter, Klebsiella*), *Staphylococcus aureus, Legionella*, viruses	Second-generation cephalosporin (cefuroxime), TMP/SMX, amoxicillin. Add erythromycin if atypicals *(Legionella, Mycoplasma, Chlamydia)* are suspected.
Community-acquired pneumonia requiring hospitalization	*S. pneumoniae, H. flu*, anaerobes, aerobic GNRs, *Legionella, Chlamydia*	Second- or third-generation cephalosporin (cefotaxime or ceftriaxone) or a beta lactam with beta lactamase inhibitor. Add erythromycin if atypicals are suspected.
Severe community-acquired pneumonia requiring hospitalization (generally needs ICU care)	*S. pneumoniae, H. flu*, anaerobes, aerobic GNRs, *Mycoplasma, Legionella, Pseudomonas*	Erythromycin, or other macrolide, a third-generation cephalosporin with anti-pseudomonal activity (or another anti-pseudomonal agent), and an aminoglycoside.
Nosocomial pneumonia—patient hospitalized > 48 hours or in a long-term care facility > 14 days	GNRs, including *Pseudomonas, S. aureus, Legionella*, and mixed flora	Third-generation cephalosporin with anti-pseudomonas activity and an aminoglycoside (gentamicin).

may be able to finish the course of antibiotics (7 to 14 days total) as an outpatient. While the patient is in the hospital, think about incentive spirometry, chest physical therapy, hydration, and ambulation to loosen consolidation and improve aeration.

PNEUMOTHORAX

Pneumothorax is a collection of air in the pleural space that can lead to pulmonary collapse; causes can be primary, secondary, or tension type.

- **Primary (spontaneous):** This may involve rupture of subpleural apical blebs; most commonly seen in thin, tall young males.
- **Secondary:** Causes include COPD, asthma, TB, trauma, and PCP, or may be iatrogenic (thoracocentesis, subclavian central line placement, positive-pressure mechanical ventilation, bronchoscopy).
- **Tension PTX:** This is a deadly variant in which a pulmonary or chest wall defect acts as a one-way valve, drawing air into the chest during inspiration but trapping it during expiration. Etiologies include penetrating trauma, infection, CHF, and positive-pressure mechanical ventilation. Tension PTX proceeds to shock and death unless it is immediately recognized and treated.

Signs and Symptoms. Patients report unilateral pleuritic chest pain and dyspnea. Examination can reveal tachycardia as well as pulmonic areas with diminished/absent breath sounds, hyperresonance to percussion, and decreased tactile fremitus. Suspect tension PTX if you also see respiratory distress, falling O_2 saturation, hypotension, distended neck veins, and tracheal deviation away from the side of the PTX. Don't forget—a patient with a PTX may be asymptomatic!

Differential. Suspect other deadly causes of chest pain (TAPUM) as well as pneumonia, pleural effusion, and pericardial tamponade.

Workup. CXR reveals a visceral pleural line and/or lung retraction from the chest wall (best seen with end-expiratory film in an upright position). Don't delay treatment while waiting for the CXR if you suspect tension PTX.

Treatment. Small PTXs are allowed to resolve spontaneously and may be treated with 100% O_2 by face mask. Large, severely symptomatic PTXs are treated with a chest tube and/or pleurodesis. A tension PTX requires immediate needle decompression if the patient is unstable: a large-bore needle (14-gauge angiocath) is inserted into the second or third intercostal space at the midclavicular line on the side of the PTX. A hissing sound signals the decompression of the PTX. A chest tube (thoracostomy tube) can then be placed.

PULMONARY EMBOLISM

Pulmonary embolism (PE) is an occlusion of the pulmonary vasculature, typically by a blood clot. Ninety-five percent of the time, the embolus originates from a DVT above the calf. PEs often lead to pulmonary infarction, RHF, and tissue hypoxia. Risk factors for DVTs and PEs include Virchow's triad:

Deadly causes of chest pain—

TAPUM

Tension pneumothorax
Aortic dissection
Pulmonary embolism
Unstable angina
Myocardial infarction

- **Blood stasis:** Immobility, obesity, CHF, and surgery.
- **Venous endothelial injury:** Surgery of the pelvis/lower extremity, trauma, surgery, and recent fracture.
- **Hypercoagulable states:** Pregnancy or postpartum, oral contraceptive use, coagulation disorder (see Coagulation Disorders section), malignancy, and severe burns.

Signs and Symptoms. Patients often report sudden-onset dyspnea, pleuritic chest pain, low-grade fever, cough, anxiety, and, rarely, hemoptysis, hypotension, or syncope. Physical exam findings include tachycardia, tachypnea, low-grade fever, a loud P2, and with RHF, prominent jugular "a" waves. If DVTs are present, the patient will commonly have an erythematous, edematous, tender, warm lower extremity with a positive Homans' sign (calf pain on forced dorsiflexion, which is neither sensitive nor specific for PE).

Workup. Although PE is a difficult diagnosis to make because of the nonspecific signs and symptoms with which it is associated, you should always have a high clinical suspicion for PE because it is life threatening. Table 3.10 outlines the diagnostic tests for PE.

TABLE 3.10. Diagnostic Tests for PE.

Test	Findings/Comments
CXR	Usually normal. Hampton's hump (wedge-shaped infarct) and Westermark's sign (decreased vascular markings in embolized lung zone) are rarely seen.
ECG	Usually sinus tachycardia and/or nonspecific ST-T-wave changes. An S1Q3T3 pattern is pathognomonic.
ABG	Respiratory alkalosis ($\uparrow$ pH, $\downarrow$ P_{CO_2}), P_{O_2} less than 80 mm (90% sensitive).
D-dimer	Includes the latex agglutination and enzyme-linked immunosorbent assay (ELISA) D-dimer tests, the latter being more sensitive. A low D-dimer might help rule out a low suspicion PE. Neither assay is specific, as D-dimers increase in MI, sepsis, and other systemic illnesses. However, the ELISA D-dimer will be elevated (> 500 ng/mL) in more than 90% of patients with a PE.
Pulmonary angiogram	Gold standard. However, invasive and inherently risky.
V/Q scan	A segmental area or areas of mismatch in the lung (i.e., well ventilated but not perfused) suggest PE (see Figure 3.9). Results reported as normal or low/intermediate/high probability of PE: ■ Normal result rules out PE. ■ High probability: 85–90% incidence of PE. ■ Low probability: does not rule out PE (14–31% incidence).
Spiral CT	Helical (spiral) CT (with IV contrast) is sensitive to PE in the proximal pulmonary arteries but less so in the distal segmental arteries.
Doppler ultrasound	Helps determine if DVTs are present in the lower extremities.

Adapted, with permission, from Tierney LM et al. *Current Medical Diagnosis & Treatment 1997*, 36th ed. Stamford, CT: Appleton & Lange, 1997:292.

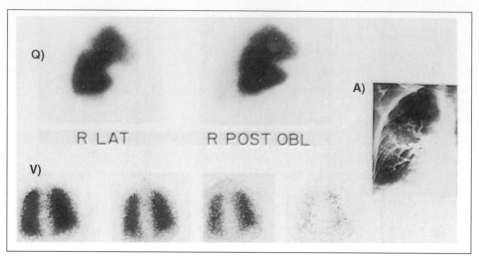

FIGURE 3.9. V/Q scan shows unmatched defects in the right midlung. The perfusion scan (Q) of the right lung (seen from the right lateral view and the right posterior oblique view) shows defects in the right anterior midlung, while the ventilation scan (V) is normal. Pulmonary angiogram (A) of the right lower lobe shows an embolus to the right midlung field. (Reprinted, with permission, from Stobo JD et al. *Principles and Practice of Medicine,* 23rd ed. Stamford, CT: Appleton & Lange, 1996:174.)

Sudden onset of dyspnea in the setting of a clear CXR is suspicious for PE.

The PIOPED study is a classic paper that studied the use of ventilation-perfusion (V/Q) scans and clinical suspicion in the diagnosis of PE. Data from that study have been used to develop diagnostic algorithms (see Figure 3.9). Trust your clinical judgment. Even a patient with a low-probability V/Q scan still has a 40% chance of having a PE if the clinical suspicion is high.

Treatment

- **Anticoagulation:** Give heparin (for a partial thromboplastin time [PTT] of 60–90) to prevent clot extension and then warfarin (international normalized ratio [INR] goal of 2–3) for long-term anticoagulation (usually lasting three to six months).
- **DVT prophylaxis:** Treat with intermittent pneumatic compression of the lower extremities, low-molecular-weight heparin (LMWH), and early ambulation.
- **Inferior vena cava (IVC) filter (Greenfield filter):** Consider if anticoagulation is contraindicated or if PEs continue despite anticoagulation.
- **Surgical embolectomy:** Usually not successful and attempted only if the patient is crashing.

Nephrology

ACUTE RENAL FAILURE

Acute renal failure (ARF) is an abrupt decrease in renal function leading to the retention of creatinine and BUN. You should learn this disease well because (1) the clinical manifestations are often nonspecific, (2) it can become rapidly fatal, and (3) it can usually be reversed if recognized early and managed properly.

The etiologies of ARF are categorized as prerenal, intrinsic, and postrenal. Prerenal failure is caused by decreased renal plasma flow and decreased GFR. Injury to the nephron causes intrinsic (renal) ARF. Postrenal ARF results from obstruction of the kidney's urinary outflow (see Table 3.11).

Signs and Symptoms. Patients may complain of malaise, fatigue, anorexia, oliguria, and nausea secondary to uremia. Physical examination may reveal a pericardial friction rub, asterixis, hypertension, and/or decreased urine output. Hypovolemia suggests prerenal failure, whereas hypervolemia is consistent with renal or postrenal failure. Other signs and symptoms reflect the underlying cause (see Table 3.12).

Workup. A history (about comorbid conditions and recent medication use), physical examination, CBC, electrolyte panel (hyperkalemia can be life threatening), BUN:creatinine ratio, urine output (oliguria is an output of <

TABLE 3.11. Causes of Acute Renal Failure.

Prerenal	Renal (Intrinsic)	Postrenal
Hypovolemia (hemorrhage, dehydration)	Acute tubular necrosis (ATN)	Prostate disease
Severe GI or renal fluid loss	Prolonged renal ischemia	Nephrolithiasis
Fluid sequestration (e.g., extensive burns)	Glomerular disease (e.g., glomerulonephritis, nephritic syndrome, vasculitis)	Pelvic tumors
Bilateral renal artery stenosis	Acute interstitial nephritis (AIN)	Recent pelvic surgery
Systemic vasodilation (e.g., sepsis, anaphylaxis)	Nephrotoxic drugs/ substances (e.g., NSAIDs, aminoglycosides, radiocontrast, acetaminophen, myoglobin)	Neurogenic bladder
Low cardiac output (e.g., cardiogenic shock, CHF)	Hyperviscous state (e.g., multiple myeloma)	Urethral stricture
Cirrhosis	Renovascular obstruction (e.g., thromboembolism)	Congenital abnormalities
Nephrotic syndrome Drugs (e.g., ACEIs, NSAIDs)		

TABLE 3.12. Physical Exam Findings in Acute Renal Failure.

Prerenal	Renal (Intrinsic)	Postrenal
Weight loss, or weight gain in heart disease	Weight gain	Enlarged prostate
Poor skin turgor	Obtundation	Weight gain
Orthostatic changes	Hypotension changing to hypertension	Bladder distention
Ascites or edema	Increased JVD and pulmonary congestion	Pelvic mass
Renal artery bruits	Muscle trauma and ischemia Infected IV and arterial lines and surgical wounds	

Adapted, with permission, from Stobo JD et al. *Principles and Practice of Medicine*, 23rd ed. Stamford, CT: Appleton & Lange, 1996:383.

400 mL/day), UA, urine osmolality, and urine electrolytes are indicated (see Tables 3.13 and 3.14). Foley placement with postvoid residual measurement also helps rule out an obstructive etiology and facilitates tracking of urine output. Renal ultrasound is useful in ruling out obstruction and in differentiating acute from chronic renal failure; a renal biopsy is rarely indicated.

Treatment. Postrenal ARF should be treated with Foley catheterization, percutaneous nephrotomy, or ureteral stent; with postobstructive diuresis, replete fluids and electrolytes. Hypovolemic prerenal ARF patients need fluid repletion in small, defined boluses; do give excess fluid repletion in patients who are already fluid overloaded (e.g., CHF). Treatment of renal ARF is etiology dependent, but in general, patients should be on fluid restriction with medications adjusted for renal impairment. Those with ATN, the most common cause of ARF, should be given furosemide with fluid replacement. The "AEIOU" mnemonic summarizes the criteria for initiating dialysis.

> **Indications for dialysis—**
>
> **AEIOU**
> **A**cidosis
> **E**lectrolyte abnormalities (K > 6.5 mEq/L)
> **I**ngestions
> **O**verload (fluid)
> **U**remic symptoms (e.g., pericarditis, encephalopathy)

TABLE 3.13. Urine Sediment Findings in Acute Renal Failure.

Urine Sediment (UA)	Etiology
Hyaline casts	Prerenal ARF
Red cell casts, RBCs	Glomerulonephritis (intrinsic)
WBCs, white cell casts, +/− eosinophils	Allergic tubulointerstitial nephritis (intrinsic)
"Muddy," granular casts, renal tubular epithelial cells	Acute tubular necrosis (intrinsic)

TABLE 3.14. Urine Indices in Prerenal, Renal, and Postrenal Acute Renal Failure.

Index	Prerenal	Renal (Intrinsic)
Urine specific gravity	> 1.020	~1.010
BUN/creatinine ratio	> 20	< 10-20
Urine Na^+ (mEq/L)	< 20	> 40
FE_{Na}[a]	< 1%	> 2%
Urine osmolality (mOsm/kg)	> 500	< 350

[a]FE_{NA} = fractional excretion of sodium.

GLOMERULAR DISEASE

Glomerular disease encompasses a broad differential of diseases that all result in injury to the glomerulus, impaired GFR, and the appearance of protein and/or blood cells in the urine. The two general categories are nephrotic and nephritic syndromes.

Nephrotic syndrome is characterized by severe proteinuria (> 3.5 g protein in the urine per day), generalized edema, hypoalbuminemia, and hyperlipidemia. Hyperlipiduria and hypercoagulability may also be seen. The common causes of nephrotic syndrome are outlined in Table 3.15. In general, patients will present with complaints of generalized edema and foamy urine; there is also an increased risk of thromboembolism and infection. Laboratory workup will show proteinuria (best with a 24-hour urine collection), lipemia, and decreased albumin (< 3 g/dL). A renal biopsy might help elucidate the etiology. Treatment is etiology dependent, but protein and salt restriction, diuretics, anticoagulants, and antihyperlipidemics are indicated. Steroids may be necessary for severe disease.

Nephritic syndrome is an inflammatory disorder characterized by the acute onset of oliguria (urine output < 400 mL/day) and ARF. Hematuria (smoky-colored urine due to RBCs and RBC casts), subnephrotic-range proteinuria, hypertension, and edema are also present. Typical causes of nephritic syndrome are included in Table 3.16. Symptoms are characteristic of the syndrome: smoky-colored urine, decreased urine output, hypertension, and edema in dependent areas (including the periorbital and scrotal regions). Workup will yield hematuria and some degree of proteinuria on the routine UA; as nephritic syndromes cause ARF, there will also be decreased GFR with elevated BUN and creatinine. Complement, antinuclear antibody (ANA), antineutrophil cytoplasmic antibody (ANCA), and antiglomerular basement membrane (anti-GBM) antibodies should be measured. Renal biopsy may be useful for histologic workup (e.g., rapidly progressive glomerular nephritis [RPGN, from Goodpasture's or Wegener's] has characteristic crescents made of monocytes in Bowman's space). Treatment is again etiology dependent, but it is necessary to treat the hypertension, fluid congestion, and uremia through

125

TABLE 3.15. Causes of Nephrotic Syndrome.

Disease	Description	History/PE	Labs and Histology	Treatment
Minimal change disease	Common in children; generally idiopathic.	Tendency toward infections and thrombotic events.	Lipid-laden renal cortices; fusion of epithelial foot processes.	Steroids; excellent prognosis.
Focal segmental glomerular sclerosis	Idiopathic or secondary to drug use (e.g., heroin), HIV infection.	Refractory hypertension; typical patient is a young black male.	Microscopic hematuria, requires renal biopsy—sclerosis in capillary tufts of deep juxtaglomerular (JG) apparatus.	Supportive care, prednisone, cytotoxic therapy for refractory patients.
Membranous glomerulo-nephritis	Most common adult nephropathy; immune complex disease.	Associated with hepatitis B, syphilis, and malaria.	"Spike and dome" appearance of the basement membrane and subepithelial deposits; granular IgG and C3 deposits.	Prednisone and cytotoxic therapy for severe disease.
Membrano-proliferative glomerulo-nephritis	Can also be a nephritic syndrome.	Slow progression to renal failure.	"Tram-track" double-layered basement membrane. Type I has subendothelial deposits; type II involves a C3 nephritic factor and decreased C3.	No regimen has been proven to be safe and effective, but corticosteroids with a cytotoxic agent might help.
Diabetic nephropathy	Most common cause of chronic renal failure; 50% of type 1 and 20% of type 2 diabetics.	15–20 years of uncontrolled DM; retinopathy is often present.	Increased thickness of basement membrane and mesangium; diffuse and nodular forms; Kimmelstiel-Wilson nodules are pathognomonic.	Prevention is key: tight glucose and blood pressure control, protein restriction, and ACEIs.
Renal amyloidosis	Primary (plasma cell dyscrasia) and secondary (infectious or inflammatory) are the most common forms.	Additional organ involvement common; diagnosis made with abdominal fat aspirate.	Subendothelial and mesangial amyloid deposits seen with Congo red.	No specific treatments, although colchicine, melphalan, and prednisone may help.
Lupus nephritis	Can be the presenting symptom of systemic lupus erythematosus (SLE); found in 85–90% of SLE patients.	Suspect in young woman with nephrotic syndrome and decreased complement level.	Five classes; the worst form is diffuse proliferative glomerulonephritis (class IV); wire-loop appearance with extensive granular subendothelial deposits.	Classes I and II do not require treatment; corticosteroids with cytotoxic agents required for classes IV and V.

TABLE 3.16. Causes of Nephritic Syndrome.

	Description	History and PE	Labs and Histology	Treatment
Postinfectious glomerulonephritis	Often associated with recent streptococcal infection (group A β-hemolytic), but may follow a variety of infections.	Oliguria, edema, hypertension, smoky-brown urine.	Low serum C3, ↑ ASO titer, lumpy-bumpy immuno-fluorescence.	Supportive. Prognosis: very good.
IgA nephropathy (Berger's disease)	Associated with URI or GI infection; etiology unknown. Most common worldwide glomerulonephritis.	Gross hematuria.	Increased serum IgA level, renal biopsy is standard for diagnosis.	Glucocorticoids for acute flares. Prognosis: 20% progress to end-stage renal disease.
Wegener's granulomatosis	Granulomatous inflammation of the respiratory tract with necrotizing vasculitis of small and medium-sized vessels.	Fever, malaise, weight loss, hematuria, respiratory symptoms with nodular lesions that cavitate and bleed.	Presence of cANCA, cell-mediated immune response is present.	High-dose cortico-steroid and cytotoxic agents Prognosis: frequent relapses after remission.
Goodpasture's syndrome	Glomerulonephritis with pulmonary hemorrhage; peak incidence in men in their mid-20s.	Hemoptysis, dyspnea, possible respiratory failure	Iron-deficiency anemia, hemosiderin-filled macrophages in sputum, pulmonary infiltrates on CXR.	Plasma exchange therapy, pulsed steroids. Prognosis: variable; may progress to end-stage renal failure.

Reprinted, with permission, from Le T et al. *First Aid for the USMLE Step 2*, 3rd ed. New York: McGraw-Hill, 2001:431.

salt and water restriction. Diuretics, dialysis, and steroids should be administered if necessary.

HYPONATREMIA

Hyponatremia is, in general, an excess of body water in relation to serum sodium. To qualify, serum sodium must be < 135 mEq/L. Causes are multiple, and the differential diagnosis can be narrowed in a systematic fashion as outlined in Figure 3.10. See Chapter 2 for more details.

Signs and Symptoms. Mild hyponatremia may be asymptomatic. As the hyponatremia becomes more marked, confusion, muscle cramps and twitching, nausea, lethargy, seizures, status epilepticus, and eventually coma can ensue.

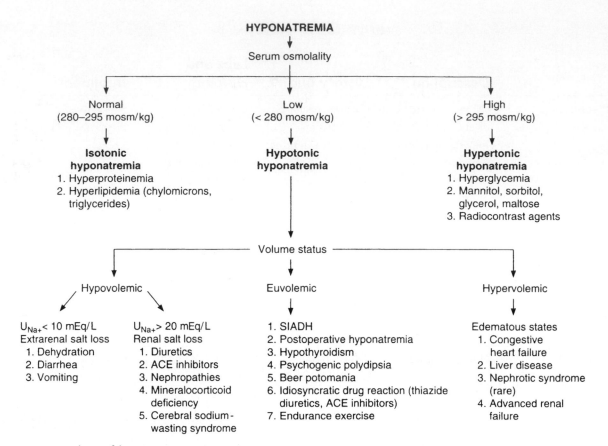

FIGURE 3.10. Workup of hyponatremia. (Reprinted, with permission, from Tierney LM et al. *Current Medical Diagnosis & Treatment 2002*, 41st ed. New York: McGraw-Hill, 2002:893.)

Workup. Plasma and urine osmolality, plasma and urine electrolytes, and urine volume must be measured. FE_{Na} can then be calculated, and hyponatremia can be classified as seen in Figure 3.10.

Treatment. As always, treat the underlying etiology. Hypotonic hyponatremic treatment methods vary by volemic status:

- **Hypovolemic:** replete volume with normal saline
- **Euvolemic:** salt and water restriction
- **Hypervolemic:** salt and water restriction

NEPHROLITHIASIS

Nephrolithiasis, commonly known as kidney stones, occurs most commonly in men, with a peak age of onset in the 20s and 30s. Stones can be composed of calcium (75–80% of all stones are calcium phosphate or calcium oxalate), uric acid, cystine, or struvite (more common in females, from urinary tract infections (UTIs) with urease-producing bacteria such as *Proteus*).

Signs and Symptoms. Patients generally present with progressive flank pain that radiates to the inguinal region. Associated symptoms can include hematuria, nausea, vomiting, and occasionally dysuria and tenesmus. The physical exam generally yields costovertebral tenderness.

Differential. The differential diagnosis includes renal infarct, lumbar disk disease, aortic dissection, renal malignancy, pyelonephritis, trauma, and glomerulonephritis.

Workup. Workup includes a physical exam, a urinalysis (to evaluate pH and the presence of bacteria, blood, and crystals), an abdominal x-ray (90% of kidney stones are radiopaque; uric acid stones are radiolucent), and, if necessary, a spiral CT scan (which can also help differentiate the various causes of the flank pain).

Treatment. Treatment varies by stone type, but patients should increase fluid intake; stones > 5 mm require more invasive procedures such as extracorporeal shock-wave lithotripsy (ESWL), retrograde ureteroscopy (for mid-ureteral stones), or percutaneous nephrolithotomy. Even with treatment, recurrence within a decade is common.

Gastroenterology

ABDOMINAL PAIN

The differential diagnosis of abdominal pain is extremely broad. When evaluating abdominal pain, the differential might be narrowed by evaluating the pain in terms of (1) pain quality, (2) pain location, and (3) physical exam findings.

Visceral and parietal pain presents with different qualities and can help localize the source of pain to various anatomic locations. Visceral pain involves distention of a hollow organ or viscus and is dull and crampy, poorly localized, and vague. By contrast parietal pain involves the parietal peritoneum, is sharp and stabbing, and is well localized. The location of the pain can also indicate not only the organs but also the possible pathophysiologic processes that might be occurring (see Table 3.17).

Finally, physical exam findings might help localize and categorize the severity of the pain. Key findings indicating that the patient's abdominal pain needs immediate attention include absent bowel sounds (e.g., pancreatitis, ischemia, acute abdomen), high-pitched bowel sounds (e.g., obstruction), rebound tenderness, and pulsatile masses. Attention should also be paid when patients have point tenderness, a positive Murphy's sign, and palpable masses. Diagnostic workup and treatment should correspond to the organs and disease processes considered in the most likely differential.

CIRRHOSIS

Cirrhosis is the irreversible destruction of normal hepatic architecture with characteristic diffuse fibrosis and regenerative nodules. Causes include alcohol

TABLE 3.17. Characterization of Abdominal Pain by Location.

Abdominal Quadrant	Organs	Possible Disease Entities
Right upper quadrant (RUQ)	Liver, gallbladder, kidney	Hepatitis, cholelithiasis, choledocholithiasis, cholecystitis, biliary colic, primary sclerosing cholangitis (PSC), primary biliary cirrhosis (PBC), pyelonephritis, hepatic tumors/abscesses, pneumonia, MI, pericarditis, and perforated ulcer
Epigastric	Stomach, duodenum, pancreas, abdominal aorta	Cardiac disease, gastritis, peptic ulcer disease, pancreatitis (pain decreases when sitting forward), and abdominal aortic aneurysm
Left upper quadrant (LUQ)	Spleen, kidney	Splenomegaly, splenic infarct, splenic rupture, pyelonephritis, pneumonia, MI, pericarditis, and perforated ulcer
Periumbilical	Abdominal aorta, small bowel, appendix (early)	Abdominal aortic aneurysm or dissection, ischemic bowel (abrupt, episodic midline pain, worsens with food, out of proportion to exam), small-bowel obstruction (crampy, episodic pain worse with food), umbilical hernia, appendicitis, and gastroenteritis
Right lower quadrant (RLQ)	Appendix, ovary, fallopian tubes, kidney, ureter, intestines, testes	Nephrolithiasis, pyelonephritis, appendicitis, Meckels diverticulum, right-sided diverticulitis, Crohn's disease, ovarian cyst, ovarian torsion, pelvic inflammatory disease (PID), ectopic pregnancy, testicular torsion, and epididymitis
Suprapubic	Bladder, uterus, ovaries, fallopian tubes	UTI, bladder cancer, PID, endometriosis, menstrual cramp/Mittelschmerz, ovarian cysts, and ectopic pregnancy
Left lower quadrant (LLQ)	Ovary, fallopian tubes, kidney, ureter, intestines, testes	Nephrolithiasis, pyelonephritis, left-sided diverticulitis, inflammatory bowel disease, ovarian cyst, ovarian torsion, PID, ectopic pregnancy, testicular torsion, and epididymitis

abuse (the most common cause in the United States), chronic hepatitis B (HBV, the most common cause worldwide) or hepatitis C (HCV), metabolic diseases (e.g., Wilson's disease, hemachromatosis, α_1-antitrypsin deficiency), drugs and toxins (e.g., isoniazid [INH], methyldopa, acetaminophen, methotrexate, carbon tetrachloride), biliary diseases (e.g., primary biliary cirrhosis or chronic biliary obstruction), cardiac cirrhosis, or impaired venous drainage of the liver (e.g., inferior vena cava or hepatic vein [Budd-Chiari] occlusion).

Signs and Symptoms. Patients often present with fatigue, malaise, and peripheral edema. The stigmata of liver disease, summarized in Figure 3.11, are usually present on physical examination. Hepatic encephalopathy and/or hepatorenal syndrome can ensue. The etiology of hepatic encephalopathy remains unclear, although ammonia levels are elevated in the blood. With more severe forms, asterixis, confusion, and coma are evident. Hepatorenal syndrome is marked by oliguria, low FE_{Na}, and failure of the azotemia to respond to fluid bolus; mortality approaches 90%.

Differential. Nephrotic syndrome, CHF, constrictive pericarditis, abdominal malignancy, and peritoneal tuberculosis should be ruled out.

Workup. Cirrhosis severity is defined by the Child-Pugh criteria (see Table 3.18), which are based on abnormalities in bilirubin, albumin, and prothromin time (PT). Additional abnormalities can include elevated ammonia, decreased BUN (due to decreased protein production), hyponatremia, anemia, thrombocytopenia, and possibly abnormal transaminases and alkaline phosphatase. Additional tests are etiology dependent: decreased ceruloplasmin indicates Wilson's disease, elevated α-fetoprotein indicates hepatocellular carcinoma, increased ferritin and total iron-binding capacity (TIBC) indicate hemachromatosis, and the absence of α-globulin on electrophoresis indicates α_1-antitrypsin deficiency. The serum ascites-albumin gradient (SAAG) from a paracentesis is the most specific test for differentiating the causes of ascites; SAAG > 1.1 suggests cirrhosis (see Table 3.19).

Treatment. Abstinence from alcohol is the most important aspect of management. Physicians must also manage all complications. For ascites, management involves sodium restriction, potassium-sparing diuretics, and large-volume paracentesis; a transjugular intrahepatic portosystemic shunt (TIPS) that connects the portal vein to the IVC is effective in refractory ascites. Treat-

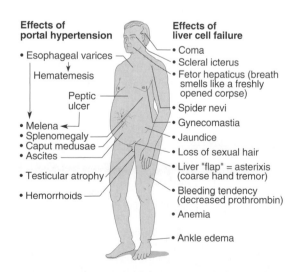

Effects of portal hypertension
- Esophageal varices
  - Hematemesis
- Peptic ulcer
- Melena
- Splenomegaly
- Caput medusae
- Ascites
- Testicular atrophy
- Hemorrhoids

Effects of liver cell failure
- Coma
- Scleral icterus
- Fetor hepaticus (breath smells like a freshly opened corpse)
- Spider nevi
- Gynecomastia
- Jaundice
- Loss of sexual hair
- Liver "flap" = asterixis (coarse hand tremor)
- Bleeding tendency (decreased prothrombin)
- Anemia
- Ankle edema

FIGURE 3.11. Signs and symptoms of cirrhosis and portal hypertension. (Adapted, with permission, from Chandrasoma P, Taylor CE. *Concise Pathology*, 3rd ed. Stamford, CT: Appleton & Lange, 1998:654.)

TABLE 3.18. Child-Pugh Criteria for the Classification of Cirrhosis.[a]

Factor	1	2	3
Serum bilirubin, μmol/L (mg/dL)	< 34 (< 2.0)	34–51 (2.0–3.0)	> 51 (> 3.0)
Serum albumin, g/L(g/dL)	> 35 (> 3.5)	30–35 (3.0–3.5)	< 30 (< 3.0)
Ascites	None	Easily controlled	Poorly controlled
Neurologic disorder	None	Minimal	Advanced coma
Prothrombin time (second prolonged) (INR)	0–4 < 1.7	4–6 1.7–2.3	> 6 > 2.3

[a] The Child-Pugh score is calculated by adding the scores of the five factors and can range from 5 to 15. The Child-Pugh class is either A (a score of 5 to 6), B (7 to 9), or C (10 and above). In general, "decompensation" indicates cirrhosis with a Child-Pugh score of ≥ 7 (Child-Pugh class B), and this level is the accepted criterion for applying for liver transplantation.
Reprinted, with permission, from Braunwald E et al (eds). *Harrison's Principles of Internal Medicine*, 15th ed. New York: McGraw-Hill, 2001:1711.

ment of esophageal varices can include nonselective beta blockers (to prevent initial bleeding), IV vasopressin (with nitroglycerin), IV somatostatin, endoscopic sclerotherapy or band ligation, and, finally, balloon tamponade. Management of hepatic encephalopathy includes protein restriction, lactulose (to promote ammonia excretion), and neomycin (to decrease ammonia-producing bacteria in the colon). Consider liver transplantation for refractory patients.

HEPATITIS

Acute or chronic liver inflammation can be due to a number of agents, most notably hepatic viruses and alcohol. Risk factors include IVDU (HBV, HCV), unprotected sexual intercourse (HBV), alcohol use, and travel where fecal-oral transmission of viruses is common (hepatitis A and E [HAV, HEV]). See Table 3.20 for a comparison of hepatic viruses.

TABLE 3.19. Serum Ascites-Albumin Gradient (SAAG) Values and Their Differentials.

SAAG > 1.1	SAAG < 1.1
Cirrhosis	Nephrotic syndrome
CHF	Tuberculosis
Alcoholic hepatitis	Pancreatic disease
Hepatic metastases	Malignancy and peritoneal mets
Budd-Chiari syndrome	

TABLE 3.20. Hepatic Viruses.

Hepatic Virus	Virus Type	Mode of Transmission	Onset; Mean Incubation	Complications
HAV	RNA; picornavirus	Fecal-oral (e.g., shellfish)	Abrupt; 30 days	Does not cause chronic hepatitis or cancer
HBV	DNA; hepadnavirus	Blood-borne: percutaneous, sexual, perinatal, possibly oral	Insidious; 8 days	Chronic hepatitis, cirrhosis, and hepatocellular carcinoma; vaccine available
HCV	RNA; flavivirus	Blood-borne: percutaneous (important in IVDU), possibly perinatal	Insidious; 50 days	Chronic hepatitis (more than HBV), cirrhosis, and hepatocellular carcinoma
HDV	Defective RNA virus	Percutaneous, sexual; coinfection or superinfection with HBV	Insidious; requires HBV infection	More severe form of hepatitis—more chronic and fulminant cases
HEV	RNA, related to calicivirus	Fecal-oral (especially water-borne)	Abrupt; 40 days	Fulminant hepatitis in pregnant women; does not cause chronic state or malignancy

Signs and Symptoms. Acute hepatitis often starts with a viral prodrome (malaise, fatigue, URI symptoms, nausea, vomiting, joint pain), followed by jaundice, fever, diarrhea, and fatigue. The physical exam can yield jaundice, scleral icterus, hepatomegaly, splenomegaly, lymphadenopathy, and RUQ tenderness. Chronic hepatitis, which occurs in roughly 80% of those infected with HCV and 10% of those with HBV, presents with symptoms of chronic liver disease such as jaundice and cirrhosis. Nearly 30% of patients with HCV and 40% of those with HBV will develop cirrhosis; 3–5% of those with chronic HBV will develop hepatocellular carcinoma.

Differential. Various causes of hepatitis (viral, alcohol, autoimmune, granulomatous, drug-induced), "shock" liver due to hypoperfusion, neoplasm, abscess, toxoplasmosis, rickettsial diseases, and systemic viral illnesses such as mononucleosis should be considered.

Workup. Acute hepatitis workup includes a CBC and LFTs, which will show elevated transaminases (AST:ALT > 2:1 indicates alcoholic hepatitis). Hepatic serology confirms the diagnosis (see Figure 3.12). Workup for chronic hepatitis includes hepatic serologies, a liver biopsy, and transaminases, which

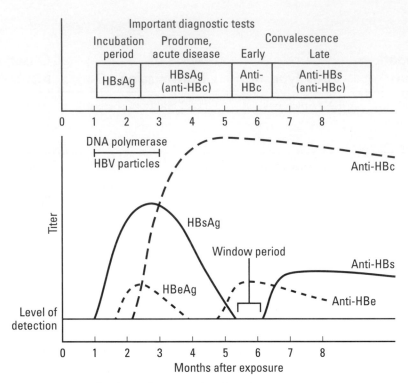

FIGURE 3.12. Serum antibody and antigen levels in hepatitis B.

must be elevated for more than six months; there can also be an increase in alkaline phosphatase and, in severe cases, PT.

Treatment. The treatment of acute hepatitis includes rest, assessing sick contacts, and, in HBV and HCV, possibly α-interferon; steroids can be used for severe alcoholic hepatitis. Treatment for chronic HBV includes α-interferon and lamivudine; α-interferon and ribavirin are used for chronic HCV. A major contraindication to the use of α-interferon is comorbid depression.

DIARRHEA

Acute diarrhea is usually infectious, often has a sudden onset, and lasts less than three weeks. Chronic diarrhea has a broader differential, often waxes and wanes, and generally persists more than three weeks.

Diarrhea is the excretion of > 250 g of stool per day.

The basic mechanisms of diarrhea include increased secretion of water and electrolytes, increased osmotic load in the colonic lumen, malabsorption, altered colonic motility, and exudative inflammation of colonic mucosa. Secretory diarrhea occurs when secretagogues—endogenous endocrine products (vasoactive intestinal polypeptide-secreting tumors [VIPomas], serotonin), endotoxins or infection (cholera), and GI luminal substances (e.g., bile acids, fatty acids, laxatives)—stimulate increased levels of fluid transport across the epithelial cells into the intestinal lumen. Osmotic diarrhea, on the other hand, is due to the presence of poorly absorbed substances that retain water in the intestinal lumen. This can be due to the ingestion of excess osmoles (e.g., mannitol, sorbitol ingestion), ingestion of substrate that is subsequently converted to excess osmoles, or the presence of a genetic enzyme deficiency for a particular diet (e.g., lactase deficiency). Malabsorptive diarrhea is due to the inability to digest or absorb a particular nutrient, which can in turn be attributable to bacterial overgrowth, pancreatic enzyme deficiency, or altered motility/anatomy.

Workup. The differential might be better refined with a complete history about sick contacts, recent travel, immune status, recent antibiotic use, and homosexuality. Weight loss, malnutrition, vitamin deficiency, and dehydration may be evident. Secretory diarrhea may be watery, while that from osmotic causes may be greasy or bulky. Acute diarrhea does not require laboratory investigation unless the patient has a high fever, bloody diarrhea, or diarrhea lasting more than four to five days. In this case, stool should be sent for fecal leukocytes (Wright's stain), bacterial culture, *Clostridium difficile* toxin, and ova and parasites (O & P). Consider sigmoidoscopy in patients with severe proctitis, bloody diarrhea, or possible *C. difficile* colitis. The workup for chronic diarrhea is based on the differentiation of osmotic versus secretory forms, which can be distinguished in two ways. First, an osmotic diarrhea will improve with fasting, whereas a secretory diarrhea will not. Second, a stool osmotic gap > 50 mOsm/kg H_2O suggests an osmotic diarrhea. For a complete chronic diarrhea workup, see Figure 3.13.

Treatment. Acute diarrhea should be treated with oral or IV fluids and electrolyte replacement. Antidiarrheal agents (e.g., loperamide or bismuth salicylate) may improve symptoms but are contraindicated in patients with bloody diarrhea, high fever, or systemic toxicity (e.g., *Escherichia coli* O157:H7, *Salmonella*). Antibiotic use is controversial, but for certain organisms (e.g., *C. difficile*) antibiotics are beneficial; for others, including *Salmonella* and *E. coli* O157:H7, the use of antibiotics can exacerbate the disease state. Chronic diarrhea treatment should be aimed at the underlying causes and can also include loperamide, opioids, clonidine, octreotide, cholestyramine, enzyme supplements, and/or avoidance of dietary substances that contribute to the diarrhea.

GASTRITIS

Gastritis, or inflammation of the gastric mucosa, can be divided into acute and chronic types. Acute or "stress" gastritis involves superficial lesions that evolve rapidly; the most common causes include NSAID use, alcohol, and stress from severe illness (e.g., Curler's ulcers in burn patients). Chronic (nonerosive) gastritis is of two types. Type A gastritis is fundal gastritis secondary to autoantibodies to parietal cells; it accounts for < 10% of chronic gastritis and is often comorbid with pernicious anemia, thyroiditis, and other autoimmune disorders. Type B gastritis accounts for > 90% of chronic gastritis cases and is found in the antrum. In contrast to type A, these are caused by NSAIDs (the most common cause), *Helicobacter pylori*, cytomegalovirus (CMV), and herpes. Although usually asymptomatic, patients can present with indigestion, nausea, vomiting, anorexia, and GI bleeding (hematemesis,

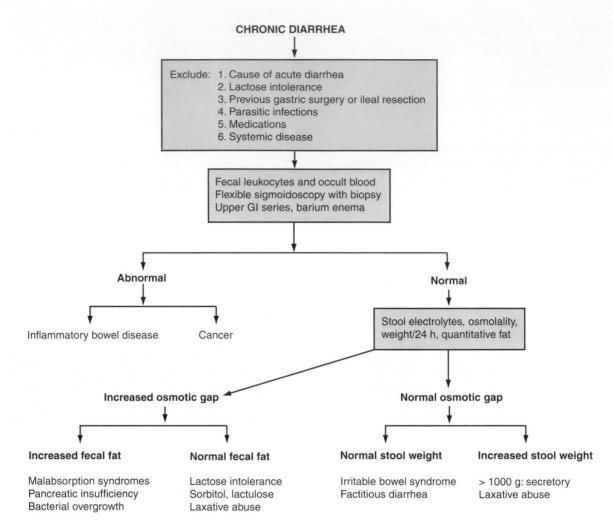

FIGURE 3.13. Decision diagram for the diagnosis of causes of chronic diarrhea. (Reprinted, with permission, from Tierney LM et al. *Current Medical Diagnosis & Treatment 2002*, 41st ed. New York: McGraw-Hill, 2002:585.)

melena). Complications of type B gastritis include an increased risk of PUD and gastric cancer. Workup involves upper endoscopy and biopsy and testing for *H. pylori*. Treatment depends on the underlying cause. The basic intervention includes decreased intake of offending agents, antacids, H_2 blockers, PPIs, and/or antibiotics for *H. pylori*. Patients at risk for stress ulcers (e.g., ICU patients) should be given prophylactic H_2 blockers on admission.

GASTROESOPHAGEAL REFLUX DISEASE

Gastroesophageal reflux disease (GERD) is the backflow of gastric contents into the esophagus, resulting in symptomatic tissue irritation and damage. Transient lower esophageal sphincter (LES) relaxation is the most common etiology of GERD. However, GERD can also be due in part to an incompetent LES, abnormally acidic gastric contents, disordered gastric motility, delayed gastric emptying, and hiatal hernia. Its prevalence ranges from 36% to 44% in American adults; predisposing risk factors include obesity, pregnancy, and scleroderma/Raynaud's disease. Alcohol, caffeine, nicotine, chocolate, and fatty foods can reduce LES tone and increase reflux.

Signs and Symptoms. Patients most commonly present with heartburn (substernal burning) that typically occurs 30 to 90 minutes after a meal, frequently worsens with reclining, and often improves with antacids, standing, or sitting. Other symptoms include sour taste ("water brash"), regurgitation, dysphagia, epigastric pain, halitosis, morning cough, laryngitis, chronic cough, and wheezing/dyspnea (which can mimic or exacerbate asthma).

Differential. Peptic ulcer disease (PUD), CAD, infectious (CMV, candidal) or chemical esophagitis, gallbladder disease, achalasia, esophageal spasm (most common in adults; resembles a corkscrew), and pericarditis should be considered.

Workup. Physical exam is typically normal unless GERD is secondary to systemic disease (e.g., scleroderma); diagnosis is usually made on the basis of clinical history. Upper endoscopy should be performed if the patient has long-standing symptoms or to identify and grade esophagitis or Barrett's esophagus. Workup may also include abdominal x-ray (AXR), CXR, barium swallow (of limited usefulness, but can help diagnosis hiatal hernia and possibly motility problems), esophageal manometry, and 24-hour pH monitoring.

Treatment. Treatment involves lifestyle modification (weight loss, head-of-bed elevation, avoiding late meals), pharmacologic management (H_2 blockers, PPIs, promotility agents), and surgical intervention (Nissen fundoplication or hiatal hernia repair if severe). Upper endoscopy with biopsy is useful in monitoring Barrett's esophagus and esophageal adenocarcinoma.

Complications. Esophageal ulceration, esophageal stricture, aspiration of gastric contents, upper GI bleeding, and Barrett's esophagus (columnar metaplasia of the distal esophagus secondary to chronic acid irritation; associated with increased risk of esophageal adenocarcinoma) can result.

> **BARRett's—**
>
> **B**ecomes
> **A**denocarcinoma;
> **R**esults from
> **R**eflux

PEPTIC ULCER DISEASE

Peptic ulcer disease (PUD) is a break that occurs in the gastric or duodenal mucosa (and in some cases the submucosa). Duodenal ulcers (DUs) are five times more common than gastric ulcers (GUs). DUs are associated with excess gastric acid production; GUs are associated with impaired mucosal defenses without acid hypersecretion. The three major causes of PUD are NSAID use, chronic *pylori* infection, and acid hypersecretory states such as Zollinger-Ellison syndrome. *H. pylori* plays a causative role in > 90% of DUs as well as in 60–70% of GUs. Other risk factors include male gender, stress, steroid use, NSAID or ASA use, alcohol or tobacco consumption, and a family history of DU. The lifetime incidence of PUD is 5–10%.

Signs and Symptoms. Patients with PUD usually present with a chronic or periodic burning/gnawing/dull/aching epigastric pain that is often temporarily alleviated with eating and antacids (especially with DU) but usually recurs roughly three hours later. Pain from GUs can worsen with food, leading to weight loss. Less common symptoms of PUD include nausea, hematemesis ("coffee-ground" emesis), blood in the stool, early satiety, or pain radiating to the back.

Rule out Zollinger-Ellison syndrome with serum gastrin levels in cases of GERD and PUD that are refractory to treatment.

Differential. Consider GERD, perforation, gastric cancer, gastritis, pancreatitis (acute or chronic), cholecystitis, choledocholithiasis, irritable bowel syndrome (IBS), esophageal rupture, ureteral colic, nonulcer dyspepsia, Zollinger-Ellison syndrome, CAD, angina, MI, aortic aneurysm, and, depending on temporal onset and pain severity, other causes of acute abdomen.

Workup. Physical exam will yield varying degrees of epigastric tenderness and, if active bleeding is present, a positive stool guaiac. A "succussion splash" (the sound of air and fluid in a distended stomach) can also be seen as a result of gastric outlet obstruction about three hours after eating. The definitive diagnosis of PUD is made with upper endoscopy and concurrent biopsy of the lesion; this tool can be used to rule out active bleeding and determine the presence of malignancy (10% of GUs have adenocarcinoma). *H. pylori* can be detected by endoscopic biopsy with a direct, rapid urease test (CLO test), urease breath tests, or serum IgG (which is less expensive but less sensitive, indicating only exposure, not active infection); all have a sensitivity > 90%. A barium upper GI series can also be used to diagnose PUD, and a gastrin level can rule out Zollinger-Ellison syndrome. GUs are associated with an increased risk of gastric carcinoma and should thus be biopsied.

Treatment. Treatment of PUD focuses on protecting the mucosa, decreasing acid production, and eradicating *H. pylori* infection (if indicated) in order to relieve symptoms and speed the recovery of the mucosa. All exacerbating agents (NSAIDs, nicotine, alcohol) should be discontinued. Antacids, H_2 blockers (e.g., cimetidine, ranitidine, famotidine), PPIs (e.g., omeprazole, lansoprazole), and sucralfate are used. PUD treatment traditionally involves four to six weeks of an H_2 blocker or a PPI with an antacid. Concurrent antibiotic treatment for *H. pylori* infection has proven extremely beneficial in preventing the recurrence of ulcers (see Table 3.21). All patients with symptomatic GUs for more than two months despite therapy must undergo endoscopy with biopsy to rule out gastric adenocarcinoma. Refractory cases may require a surgical procedure such as vagotomy (proximal gastric vagotomy, preferred) or a highly selective truncal vagotomy with antrectomy.

*PUD **perforates** into the peritoneal space and **penetrates** into adjacent organs.*

Complications. Complications of PUD include hemorrhage (erosion into the gastroduodenal artery), gastric outlet obstruction, perforation (usually anterior ulcers), penetration, and intractable disease.

IRRITABLE BOWEL SYNDROME

Irritable bowel syndrome is an idiopathic, functional disorder characterized by continuous or recurring symptoms of abdominal pain and irregular bowel habits. Patients most commonly present in their teens and 20s, but since this syndrome is chronic, they can present at any age. There is a two- to threefold increased prevalence in females, and nearly 50% of all patients who seek medical care have comorbid psychiatric disorders (e.g., depression, anxiety). The etiology is still unknown but most likely involves a disruption in normal colonic motility.

TABLE 3.21. Treatment of *H. pylori* Infection.

Treatment Regimen	Comments
Tetracycline (or amoxicillin) + metronidazole + bismuth subsalicylate for 14 days	First-line "triple therapy" yields 84–89% eradication.
Amoxicillin (or metronidazole) + clarithromycin + omeprazole for 14 days	88–92% eradication rate.
Ranitidine, bismuth citrate, clarithromycin, and amoxicillin, metronidazole, or tetracycline for 14 days	
Ranitidine (or omeprazole) + amoxicillin + metronidazole for 12 days	89–90% eradication rate.
Omeprazole + amoxicillin for 14 days	80% eradication rate.
Clarithromycin + omeprazole for 14 days	More expensive and slightly less effective than "triple therapy," but may yield more compliance with fewer side effects.

Signs and Symptoms. Patients present with at least three months of continuous or recurrent abdominal pain/irritation that is relieved by a bowel movement, has a change in frequency, or has a change in consistency. Additional symptoms include mucus in the stools, a feeling of abdominal distention or bloating, or altered stool passage (e.g., urgency, incomplete voiding).

Differential. Inflammatory bowel disease, mesenteric ischemia, diverticulitis, PUD, colonic neoplasia, infectious/pseudomembranous colitis, and gynecologic disorders should be considered.

Workup. The physical exam is often unremarkable except for mild abdominal tenderness. The Rome II criteria for IBS diagnosis require at least 12 total weeks of abdominal pain (continuous or recurrent) that is relieved with bowel movement, a change in bowel frequency, and/or a change in bowel form (primarily diarrhea, primarily constipation, or alternating diarrhea and constipation). Additional requirements for an IBS diagnosis are summarized in Table 3.22. However, other causes of disease must be ruled out. Labs include CBC, electrolytes, TSH, ESR, stool cultures, abdominal films, and barium contrast studies. Manometry may be used to assess sphincter function.

Treatment. Patients with IBS, especially the type associated with constipation, are encouraged to increase their fiber/psyllium intake and decrease their intake of foods that increase intestinal gas (e.g., legumes). At meals, cholestyramine might be helpful in the diarrhea-type IBS. Pharmacologically,

Abdominal Pain/Discomfort	and	Two or More at Least 25% of the Time
Relieved with defecation *and/or* With change in stool frequency *and/or* With change in stool consistency		Change in stool frequency Change in consistency Difficult stool passage Sense of incomplete evacuation Presence of mucus in stool

[a]Symptoms must have been present for more than three months.
Reprinted, with permission, from Braunwald E et al (eds). *Harrison's Principles of Internal Medicine,* 15th ed. New York: McGraw-Hill, 2001:1692.

antidiarrheals (loperamide), antispasmodics (anticholinergics such as dicyclomine and hyoscyamine), and antidepressants (tricyclic antidepressants or selective serotonin reuptake inhibitors) may be indicated. Alosetron is approved for women with diarrhea-predominant IBS. Psychologically, patients need assurance from their physicians.

Hematology

ANEMIA

Anemia is a reduced number of total RBCs, a decrease in hemoglobin, or a decrease in hematocrit. Etiologies are numerous (see Figure 3.14) but can be distinguished according to the following general mechanisms: decreased production (macrocytic, microcytic, normocytic), increased destruction (e.g., hemolysis, which can be intracorpuscular or extracorpuscular and intravascular or extravascular), and increased blood loss. The first two mechanisms have an increased reticulocyte count; the final mechanism has a decreased reticulocyte count.

Signs and Symptoms. Patients are usually asymptomatic or present with complaints of fatigue, dyspnea, dizziness, and/or exertional angina. On exam, mildly anemic patients will have a normal exam, but those with moderate to severe anemia can have pallor of the skin and conjunctiva, a flattened jugular vein, tachycardia, and systolic flow murmur. Depending on the cause, there may be other physical manifestations of disease:

- **B_{12} deficiency:** Peripheral neuropathy with loss of position and vibratory sense.
- **Blood loss (e.g., malignancy):** A positive fecal occult blood test.
- **Hypothyroidism:** Menorrhagia, dry and coarse skin and hair, personality change, loss of lateral eyebrows, periorbital edema.
- **Severe iron deficiency:** Angular cheilitis, atrophic glossitis, weak nails, and koilonychias.

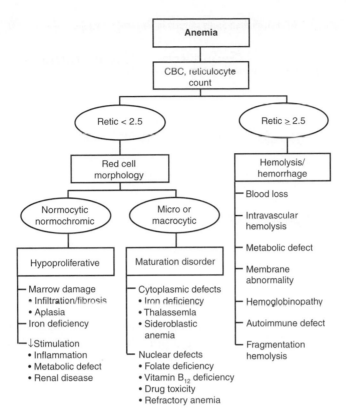

FIGURE 3.14. The physiologic classification of anemia. (Reprinted, with permission, from Braunwald E et al. *Harrison's Principles of Internal Medicine,* 15th ed. New York: McGraw-Hill, 2001:352.)

- **Genetic causes of anemia (e.g., sickle cell anemia, hereditary spherocytosis, thalassemia):** A family history of similar symptoms.
- **Folate deficiency:** Medication (e.g., methotrexate, TMP/SMX, sulfa drugs) can be responsible.

Workup. Workup consists of a complete physical exam and a CBC. If anemia is discovered, iron studies (serum iron, TIBC, and serum ferritin [see Table 3.23]), serum B_{12} (or methylmalonyl), serum folate, reticulocyte count, and possibly a peripheral blood smear can be ordered. If B_{12} deficiency is found, a Schilling test will help differentiate whether the cause is inadequate diet, lack of intrinsic factor (pernicious anemia), bacterial overgrowth, or an ileal disease. If hemolysis is found on the peripheral smear, a Coombs' test with PT and PTT measurements will help differentiate the different causes of normocytic, hemolytic anemias. It is important to rule out other causes of anemia, such as hypothyroidism (TSH), GI bleed (fecal occult blood), liver disease (LFTs), chronic renal disease (BUN and creatinine), and multiple myeloma (serum protein electrophoresis [SPEP], urine protein electrophoresis [UPEP]). Bone marrow biopsies are indicated if the patient presents with pancytopenia, macrocytic anemia with an unknown etiology, or a myelophthisic process.

TABLE 3.23. Iron Study Results in Microcytic Anemia.

Disorder	Serum Iron	Serum Ferritin	TIBC
Iron deficiency anemia	↓	↓	↑
Anemia of chronic disease	↓	↑	↓
Thalassemia	N	N	N
Sideroblastic anemia	↑	N/↑	N

COAGULATION DISORDERS

Coagulation disorders include bleeding and hypercoagulable diseases. Bleeding disorders can be further classified as problems with platelets (number or function) or with coagulation (coagulation factor inhibitors or deficiencies). Petechiae or ecchymoses suggest platelet problems; hemarthroses or delayed bleeding after trauma indicate a factor abnormality. Inquire about a family history of coagulation disorders (e.g., hemophilia A or B, von Willebrand's disease), medication history (e.g., heparin, warfarin, ASA), and comorbid medical conditions (e.g., liver failure, vitamin K deficiency, DIC, HIV). Labs should include a platelet count, PT, PTT, thrombin time (TT), bleeding time, LFTs, INR, and, if suspected, a von Willebrand's or DIC screen. To detect a specific coagulation factor defect, the patient's plasma can be added to normal plasma (50:50 mixing study). If the PT and PTT normalize, the coagulation factor is missing; deficiencies in factors VIII, IX, and XI are the most common. If the PT and PTT do not normalize, the patient has a factor inhibitor; factor VIII inhibitor is the most common. Treatment is etiology dependent: give IM vitamin K for vitamin K deficiency or warfarin overdose, platelet transfusions for thrombocytopenia, and plasma products with specific factors for missing factors.

**KEY
POINT**

KEY FACTOR DEFICIENCIES AND THEIR PT AND PTT ABNORMALITIES

- PT↑ —VII
- PTT↑ —VII, IX, XI, XII
- PT and PTT↑ —II, V, X, fibrinogen
- TT↑ —dysfibrinogenemia

WEPT—

Warfarin
Extrinsic pathway
PT lab abnormality

Hypercoagulable disorders are clinically important because they increase the risk of thromboembolic events. These states should be suspected in patients with multiple embolic events, embolic events at an early age, thrombi at unusual locations, and repeated spontaneous abortions. Etiologies are numerous; the most common causes are antiphospholipid syndrome, deficiencies or alterations in protein C, protein S, factor V (factor V Leiden), antithrombin III, heparin-induced thrombocytopenia (HITT), and homocystinuria. Workup is similar to that for bleeding disorders and should also include an anticardiolipin antibody, lupus anticoagulant, VDRL, homocysteine level, and quantitative assays for the factors that might be altered. Treatment includes anticoagulation (potentially lifelong), repletion of missing factors, and possibly an IVC filter.

Endocrinology

DIABETES MELLITUS

Although diabetes mellitus (DM) is occasionally diagnosed on admission when it presents as diabetic ketoacidosis (DKA) or as hyperosmolar hyperglycemia nonketotic coma (HHNK), it will most often be seen as a chronic medical issue. DM is a metabolic syndrome of abnormal hyperglycemia secondary to an absence of insulin and in type 2, an abnormality in insulin secretion and resistance. DM can be classified into two types:

- **Type 1:** Formerly known as insulin-dependent diabetes mellitus (IDDM), type 1 DM accounts for 15% of cases and is most commonly diagnosed in juveniles. It is characterized by a lack of insulin, thus necessitating exogenous insulin. It is strongly associated with HLA-DR3 and HLA-DR4, is generally not associated with obesity, has a weak genetic predisposition, and commonly presents initially with DKA.
- **Type 2:** Formerly known as non-insulin-dependent diabetes mellitus (NIDDM), type 2 DM comprises more than 85% of DM cases and usually occurs in obese patients more than 40 years old. Most type 2 DM is the result of increasing insulin resistance in peripheral tissues, hyperinsulinemia to compensate for the resistance, and eventual burnout by the pancreatic islet cells, resulting in decreased insulin. Because the initial problem is not a lack of insulin but an insufficient amount relative to need, oral hypoglycemics are the initial treatment of choice. There is a strong genetic predisposition, and although DKA can occur in type 2 DM, HHNK is more common.

Signs and Symptoms. Type 1 and symptomatic type 1 DM patients commonly present with polydipsia, polyuria (including nocturia), and polyphagia. Type 1 is also commonly associated with rapid or unexplained weight loss. Type 2 DM patients typically have a more insidious onset of symptoms, and at the time of diagnosis they may already have end-organ damage. Patients may complain of fatigue, candidal infections, poor wound healing, or blurred vision due to a change in the hydration status of the lens.

Differential. Consider pancreatic diseases (e.g., chronic pancreatitis, hemachromatosis), hormonal abnormalities (e.g., glucagonoma, Cushing's syndrome, acromegaly), medications (e.g., corticosteroids, thiazide diuretics, phenytoin), gestational DM, stress, and diabetes insipidus (central or nephrogenic).

Workup. The National Diabetes Data Group (NDDG) and the World Health Organization (WHO) Criteria for the Clinical Diagnosis of Diabetes

Mellitus suggest that a patient satisfy one of the three following criteria in order to be diagnosed with DM:

- Random plasma glucose > 200 mg/dL together with the presence of the classic symptoms of diabetes, or
- Fasting plasma glucose > 125 mg/dL on two separate occasions (normal < 100; impaired glucose tolerance 110–125), or
- Two-hour postprandial plasma > 200 mg/dL on 75-g oral glucose tolerance test (OGTT) on two separate occasions.

The presence of urine glucose and urine ketones and an elevated hemoglobin A_{1C} also support the diagnosis of DM. The latter is used to monitor the efficacy of and compliance with therapy over the preceding three months. Tight control of serum glucose has been shown to slow the development and progression of retinopathy, nephropathy, and neuropathy in type 1 diabetes, but it is unclear if the same effect is seen in type 2 patients (see Table 3.24). The presence of urine microalbumin or elevated creatinine indicates renal involvement.

Treatment. Type 1 DM should be treated with a regular regimen of insulin injections (see Figure 3.15). Patients must be taught to monitor their blood glucose at home, as research has shown that tight control of glucose in type 1 DM reduces end-organ damage. Patients should be carefully monitored for end-organ damage.

The initial treatment of choice for type 2 DM is lifestyle modification; weight loss, diet, and exercise can help increase insulin sensitivity in target tissues. If this fails, patients with type 2 DM should be started on oral hypoglycemic monotherapy. Metformin, the first-line treatment, is an insulin sensitizer that increases the peripheral uptake of glucose and inhibits hepatic gluconeogenesis; the most serious side effect is fatal lactic acidosis. Sulfonylureas (e.g., glyburide, glipizide, tolbutamide) increase pancreatic β-cell secretion of insulin, with side effects including weight gain and hypoglycemia. The glitazones increase insulin sensitivity in the muscle and liver, but with the hepatotoxicity associated with troglitazone, LFTs must be monitored. α-glucosidase inhibitors (acarbose) decrease intestinal absorption of carbohydrate by inhibiting the breakdown of oligosaccharides; the major complication is GI upset.

Infectious Disease

FEVER OF UNKNOWN ORIGIN

Fever of unknown origin is one of the more vexing dilemmas in internal medicine. It is defined as a fever of at least 38.3°C (101°F) for at least three weeks that is undiagnosed after one week of study in the hospital. In adults, infections and cancer account for > 60% of cases of FUO; autoimmune diseases account for approximately 15%.

TABLE 3.24. Complications of Diabetes Mellitus.

Complications of Treatment	Description
Somogyi effect	Nocturnal hypoglycemia causing elevated morning glucose due to release of counterregulatory hormones (reduce insulin to treat).
Dawn phenomenon	Early-morning hyperglycemia caused by reduced effectiveness of insulin at that time.
Acute complications	
Diabetic ketoacidosis (DKA)	Hyperglycemia-induced crisis that occurs most commonly in Type 1 diabetics. It is often precipitated by stress, including infections, MI, alcohol, drugs (e.g., corticosteroids, thiazide diuretics), or pancreatitis, or by noncompliance with insulin therapy. Patients often present with abdominal pain, vomiting, Kussmaul respirations (slow, deep breaths), and a fruity, acetone odor. Patients are severely dehydrated with many electrolyte abnormalities (e.g., hypokalemia, hypophosphatemia, increased anion gap metabolic acidosis) and may also develop mental status changes. Treatment includes fluids, potassium, and insulin to correct electrolyte abnormalities and treatment of initiating event.
Hyperosmolar hyperglycemic nonketotic coma	Presents as profound dehydration, mental status changes, and an extremely high plasma glucose (> 600 mg/dL) without acidosis; occurs most commonly in Type 2 diabetics, is precipitated by acute stress, and is often fatal. Treatment includes aggressive rehydration, insulin, and aggressive fluid and electrolyte replacement.
Chronic complications	
Retinopathy	Appears when diabetes has been present for at least three to five years. Preventive measures include control of hyperglycemia and hypertension and laser therapy for neovascularization.
Diabetic nephropathy	Characterized by glomerular hyperfiltration followed by microalbuminuria. Begin therapy with an ACEI control hyperglycemia; control hypertension.
Neuropathy	Peripheral, symmetric, sensorimotor neuropathy leading to foot trauma and diabetic ulcers. Treat with preventive foot care, analgesics, and tricyclic antidepressants.
Macrovascular complications	Cardiovascular, cerebrovascular, peripheral vascular disease. Cardiovascular disease is the most common cause of death in diabetic patients. Goal BP is < 130/< 76; lower LDL to < 130. In the presence of known CAD, lower LDL to < 100 and triglycerides to < 200 mg/dL.

Reprinted, with permission, from Le T et al. *First Aid for the USMLE Step 2*, 3rd. ed. New York, McGraw-Hill, 2001:113.

FUO can be divided into five etiologic categories:

1. **Infectious:** TB and endocarditis (e.g., HACEK organisms) are the most common systemic infections causing FUO, while a occult abscess is the most common cause of localized infections.
2. **Neoplastic:** Leukemias and lymphomas are the most common cancers that cause FUO; hepatic and renal cell carcinomas are the most common solid tumors.
3. **Autoimmune:** Still's disease, temporal arteritis, rheumatoid arthritis, SLE, and polyarteritis nodosa are the most common causes, although many rheumatologic diseases can cause FUO.

HIGH-YIELD TOPICS

Internal Medicine

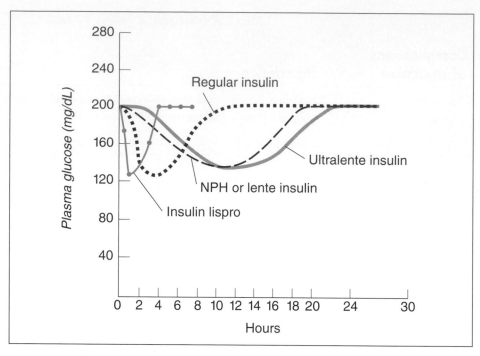

FIGURE 3.15. Effects of various insulins in a fasting diabetic patient. (Reprinted, with permission, from Tierney LM et al. *Current Medical Diagnosis & Treatment 2002*, 41st ed. New York: McGraw-Hill 2002:1220.)

4. **Miscellaneous:** This category includes drug fever, cirrhosis, alcoholic hepatitis, granulomatous hepatitis, sarcoidosis, hyperthyroidism, Addison's disease, Whipple's disease, recurrent PE, factitious fever, and IBD, among others.
5. **Undiagnosed** (10–15%).

Workup. The workup of FUO should initially include a complete history and physical, CBC with differential, ESR, LFTs, and multiple blood cultures. Depending on the clinical presentation and suspicion of malignancy or abscess, imaging studies may include CXR, CT, or MRI. Additional testing might include echocardiogram (e.g., TEE), bone marrow biopsy, skin biopsy, lymph node biopsy, liver biopsy, and, as a last resort, exploratory laparotomy.

Treatment. Broad-spectrum antibiotics are usually started empirically in severely ill patients but should be discontinued if the fever does not respond. Avoid empiric steroids unless vasculitis is suspected. The Naprosyn test is useful in distinguishing infectious from neoplastic events.

HIV

Since HIV infection is spread almost exclusively through the transmission of bodily fluids, risk factors for HIV infection include unprotected anal, oral, and vaginal sex and needle sharing. Infants of HIV-positive mothers, health care workers accidentally stuck with a needle containing blood from an HIV-positive patient (or with mucocutaneous exposure), and patients receiving multiple transfusions of blood and blood products are also at risk. Symptomatic disease usually presents around age 30; HIV is more prevalent in males than females, but as transmission via heterosexual contact increases, the incidence in women is likewise increasing.

Signs and Symptoms. Although many HIV-infected individuals are initially asymptomatic, 50–60% of HIV-positive patients may present with flulike symptoms (fever, malaise, rash, headache, generalized lymphadenopathy) during acute seroconversion. Most patients will recover from the initial retroviral syndrome and enter the latency phase, during which they are asymptomatic despite high levels of viral replication. Eventually, the patient's immune system cannot control the infection, the CD4 counts fall, and AIDS and opportunistic infections ensue. AIDS is defined as either a CD4 count < 200 cells/mm³ or the presence of an AIDS-defining illness. AIDS-defining illnesses include CMV, *Mycobacterium avium-intracellulare* (MAI), progressive multifocal leukoencephalopathy (PML), herpes simplex virus (HSV), candidal esophagitis, AIDS wasting syndrome (i.e., cachexia), invasive fungal infection, toxoplasmosis, PCP, Kaposi's sarcoma, lymphoma (CNS), TB, and pneumococcal pneumonia. Additional opportunistic infections include candidal vaginitis, varicella-zoster virus (VZV), oral hairy leukoplakia, and chronic diarrhea from *Cryptosporidium*, *Microspora*, and *Isospora*.

Workup. The ELISA test is a general HIV screening measure that detects the presence of anti-HIV antibodies in the bloodstream. The test has high sensitivity but moderate specificity, resulting in numerous false positives. Those with a positive ELISA test must have a follow-up Western blot to confirm HIV infection. If both the ELISA and Western blot are positive, then check a viral load (the number of viral RNA copies per milliliter of blood), CD4 count, PPD with controls, VDRL, and antibodies against CMV, toxoplasmosis, HBV, HAV, and HCV. Additional tests include a CBC, electrolytes, LFTs, creatinine, a CXR, and a Pap smear for women.

Treatment. The treatment of HIV-positive patients depends primarily on CD4 count, viral load, and the presence of HIV complications; the general guidelines are to begin antiretroviral therapy if the CD4 count is < 500 cells/mm³ or if the patient has an AIDS-defining illness. Treatment regimens for HIV are evolving rapidly, but treatment currently centers on HAART (highly active antiretroviral therapy) regimens. The most commonly used regimen includes a protease inhibitor (e.g., saquinavir, ritonavir, indinavir) and two nucleoside analogues (e.g., AZT, ddI, 3TC, D4T).

In addition, the prophylaxis and treatment of various opportunistic infections is indicated if CD4 counts fall below particular levels or if symptoms are present (Table 3.25). Prophylaxis can be discontinued when the CD4 count increases adequately.

AIDS is defined as either a CD4 count < 200 cells/mm³ or the presence of an AIDS-defining illness.

CD4 count is a marker for the extent of the disease, while viral load indicates the rate of disease progression.

HIGH-YIELD TOPICS

Internal Medicine

TABLE 3.25. Opportunistic Diseases in AIDS and Treatment Options.

Disease	Indications for Prophylaxis	Treatment Options
Pneumocystis carinii pneumonia	CD4 < 200, oral candidiasis, or unexplained fever for more than two weeks	TMP-SMX, dapsone, aerosolized pentamidine, dapsone + pyrimethamine + leucovorin, atovaquone, prednisone
Toxoplasma gondii	CD4 < 100 + IgG to toxoplasmosis	TMP-SMX, dapsone + pyrimethamine + leucovorin, atovaquone; if encephalitis, can use sulfadiazine (or clindamycin) + pyrimethamine + leucovorin
Mycobacterium avium-intracellulare	CD4 < 75	Clarithromycin or azithromycin with at least one of the following: ethambutol, rifabutin, clofazimine, ciprofloxacin
Cytomegalovirus	CD4 < 50 + IgG to CMV	Ganciclovir, foscarnet (second options are cidofovir, fomivirsen)
Candida	CD4 < 50	Fluconazole, ketoconazole
Cryptococcus neoformans	CD4 < 50	Fluconazole, amphotericin B, itraconazole
Histoplasma capsulatum	CD4 < 50 in endemic areas	Itraconazole, amphotericin B
Coccidioides immitis	CD4 < 50 in endemic areas	Fluconazole, amphotericin B, itraconazole
Mycobacterium tuberculosis	Skin test > 5 mm, active TB contact, or prior positive skin test without treatment	For prophylaxis, INH + pyridoxine or rifampin (or rifabutin) + pyrazinamide. For treatment, INH + pyridoxine + rifampin (rifabutin) + ethambutol
Herpes simplex virus	Prophylaxis not recommended	Acyclovir, famciclovir, foscarnet for treatment
Varicella-zoster virus	Significant exposure without history of disease or vaccination	Varicella-zoster immune globulin for prophylaxis; acyclovir, famciclovir, or foscarnet for treatment
Influenza	All patients	Influenza vaccine
Streptococcus pneumoniae	All patients	Pneumococcal vaccine
Hepatitis B	Susceptible anti-HBcAg-negative patients	HBV vaccine
Hepatitis A	Susceptible anti-HAV-negative patients	HAV vaccine
Kaposi's sarcoma	Prophylaxis not recommended	Cutaneous—observation, intralesional vinblastine; severe cutaneous—systemic chemotherapy, α-interferon, radiation; visceral disease—combination chemotherapy
Lymphoma	Prophylaxis not recommended	Combination chemotherapy, radiation therapy, and dexamethasone (for CNS lymphoma)

Adapted, with permission, from Fanci, AS and Lane C. *Harrison's Principle of Internal Medicine*, 15th ed. Mc-Graw Hill, 2001: 1881–1884 (Table 309-11).

TUBERCULOSIS

After declining in the 1980s, tuberculosis is once again increasing in prevalence. Risk factors for TB include immunosuppression (e.g., HIV, solid organ transplantation, carcinoma), alcoholism, preexisting lung disease (e.g., silicosis), diabetes, chronic renal failure/dialysis, old age, homelessness, malnourishment/low body weight, and crowded living conditions with poor ventilation (e.g., military barracks). Immigrants from developing countries and persons with known exposure to infected patients are also at risk.

Signs and Symptoms. Symptoms of active pulmonary TB include productive cough, hemoptysis, weakness, anorexia, weight loss, malaise, night sweats, and fever. Symptoms can resemble bacterial pneumonia. The physical exam may yield dullness to percussion with decreased tactile fremitus if effusions are present. Extrapulmonary manifestations can include scrofula (cervical lymphadenopathy) and spine pain (Pott's disease). TB is a common cause of FUO, and the kidney is the most common extrapulmonary site of tuberculosis infection.

Differential. Pneumonia (bacterial, fungal, viral), other atypical mycobacterial infections, HIV infection, HIV-related opportunistic infections (e.g., PCP), UTI, lung abscess, lung cancer, and sarcoidosis should be considered.

Workup. CXR findings in active pulmonary TB include enlarged, calcified mediastinal lymph nodes and calcified pulmonary granulomas (Ghon complex) in the apical and posterior areas of the upper lobes of the lungs bilaterally; apical pleural scarring and cavitary lesions may be present as well. Most cases of TB are presumptively diagnosed with a positive acid-fast stain of the sputum, since it may take several weeks to culture TB from sputum given its slow incubation period. A positive PPD test is indicative only of previous exposure to *Mycobacterium tuberculosis* and may not be present in immunocompromised individuals (e.g., HIV-infected patients) who have TB. Criteria for interpretation of the PPD test are outlined in Figure 3.16.

Treatment. All cases of TB must be reported to the local and state health department. Respiratory isolation must be instituted when TB is suspected. For

Consider TB in the differential of FUO.

Don't forget about the extrapulmonary manifestations of TB!

TB is the number one infectious disease killer in the world.

PPD is injected intradermally on the volar surface of the arm. The transverse length of induration is measured at 48–72 hours. BCG vaccination typically renders a patient PPD positive for at least one year. The size of induration that indicates a positive test is as follows:

■ Greater than **5 mm:** HIV or risk factors, close TB contacts, CXR evidence of TB.
■ Greater than **10 mm:** Indigent/homeless, developing nations, IVDU, chronic illness, residents of health and correctional institutions.
■ Greater than **15 mm:** Everyone else.

A **negative reaction** with negative controls implies anergy from immunosuppression, old age, or malnutrition and thus does not rule out TB.

FIGURE 3.16. Purified protein derivative placement.

Urosepsis must be considered in any elderly patient with altered mental status.

active TB, multidrug therapy (usually INH, pyrazinamide, rifampin, and ethambutol) are started. Depending on sensitivity, treatment could include rifampin and INH for nine months or INH and rifampin for six months with pyrazinamide during the first two months. Vitamin B_6 (pyridoxine) is commonly given with INH to prevent the common side effect of peripheral neuritis. The prophylactic treatment for HIV-positive and HIV-negative patients less than 35 years of age who show conversion to a positive PPD (see Figure 3.16 for qualifications) but who have no symptoms of active pulmonary TB include INH therapy for nine months. Many physicians forgo INH prophylaxis in patients more than 35 years old because the risk of INH-induced liver toxicity increases with age.

URINARY TRACT INFECTIONS

UTI bugs—

SEEKS PP
S. saprophyticus
E. coli
Enterobacter
Klebsiella
Serratia
Proteus
Pseudomonas

Urinary tract infections are most commonly caused by ascending infections and occur 30 times more frequently in women than in men (due to a short urethra). UTIs in men are usually due to congenital abnormalities or, in elderly men, prostatic enlargement. Risk factors also include sexual intercourse, diaphragm and/or spermicide use, urinary tract instrumentation (e.g., Foley catheters), DM, and immunosuppression. Common microbial causes are listed in Table 3.26. Signs and symptoms include dysuria, suprapubic pain, nocturia, and increased frequency and urgency. Patients with pyelonephritis can have fever, chills, flank pain, and costovertebral angle (CVA) tenderness. The differential includes cystitis, vaginitis, urethritis, vulvar HSV lesions, allergic/chemical reactions, or, rarely, bladder cancer, mycobacterial infection, or urethral spasm. Workup includes a complete history and a routine UA with micro. Dipstick may reveal positive leukocyte esterase and nitrites, elevated urine pH (if *Proteus* is the offending agent), and hematuria. Micro will show pyuria (> 2–5 WBC/hpf) and, in pyelonephritis, WBC casts. The diagnostic gold standard is > 100,000 colony-forming units of bacteria per milliliter of clean-catch urine; however, urine cultures are reserved for recurrent UTIs, pyelonephritis, complicated UTIs, those in men, pregnant women and those in DM or immunocompromised patients. Table 3.27 summarizes treatment options for UTIs.

Complicated UTI: UTI with a resistant organism or in a functionally, anatomically, or metabolically abnormal urinary tract.

TABLE 3.26. Common Microorganisms in Urinary Tract Infections.

Condition	Common Organisms
Uncomplicated UTI or pyelonephritis	*E. coli* (50–80%), *Staphylococcus saprophyticus* (10–30%), *Klebsiella pneumoniae* (8–10%), and *Proteus mirabilis*
Complicated UTI	*E. coli, Proteus, Klebsiella, Serratia, Pseudomonas,* and enterococci

TABLE 3.27. Treatment of Urinary Tract Infections.

Condition	Treatment Choices
Acute, uncomplicated UTIs	Fluoroquinolone (e.g., Cipro) or TMP/SMX DS × 3 days; cephalexin × 5 days, or Macrobid × 7 days; always treat men for 7 days.
Recurrent UTIs	If related to coitus: TMP/SMX DS × 1 dose, postcoitus. If unpredictable, TMP/SMX, cephalexin, or Macrobid qd.
Acute, uncomplicated pyelonephritis; outpatient	Fluoroquinolone (e.g., Cipro) or amoxicillin/clavulanate × 14 days.
Acute, uncomplicated pyelonephritis; inpatient	IV fluoroquinolone, ampicillin, gentamicin, third-generation cephalosporin until afebrile 24–48 hours and then PO Cipro × 14 days.

Rheumatology

SYSTEMIC LUPUS ERYTHEMATOSUS

Systemic lupus erythematosus (SLE) is an inflammatory autoimmune disorder that primarily strikes younger women of child-bearing age (90%). Black women are at an especially high risk. SLE is a multisystem disease that is characterized by recurrent exacerbations and remissions due to autoantibodies and immune complex deposition. Although the etiology remains obscure, there is a familial concordance and a correlation with HLA types DR2 and DR3. Drugs can cause a drug-induced lupus that resolves when the medication is discontinued.

> **Systemic manifestations of SLE—**
>
> **SOAP BRAIN MD**
> **S**erositis
> **O**ral aphthous ulcers
> **A**rthritis
> **P**hotosensitivity
> **B**lood abnormalities (hemolytic anemia, thrombocytopenia, leukopenia, lymphopenia)
> **R**enal disease
> **A**NA +
> **I**mmunologic abnormalities (+ anti-dsDNA, anti-Sm Ab)
> **N**eurologic abnormalities (lupus cerebritis)
> **M**alar Rash
> **D**iscoid rash

DRUGS THAT CAUSE SLE

- α-interferon
- Hydralazine
- INH
- Methyldopa
- Phenytoin
- Penicillamine
- Procainamide
- Quinidine
- Sulfonamides

 **KEY POINT**

Signs and Symptoms. SLE is characterized by multiple systemic complaints, as outlined in the mnemonic "SOAP BRAIN MD" and in Figure 3.17.

Differential. SLE is often hard to diagnose, as its varying systemic presentations seldom make its diagnosis obvious. In addition to SLE, drug-induced lupus and mixed connective tissue disorder (MCTD) can present with multisystem involvement and autoantibodies; discoid lupus presents with the characteristic skin manifestations without systemic involvement. One must also consider epilepsy, various forms of dermatitis, multiple sclerosis (MS), psychiatric disorders, and hematologic disorders, including idiopathic thrombocytopenic purpura (ITP).

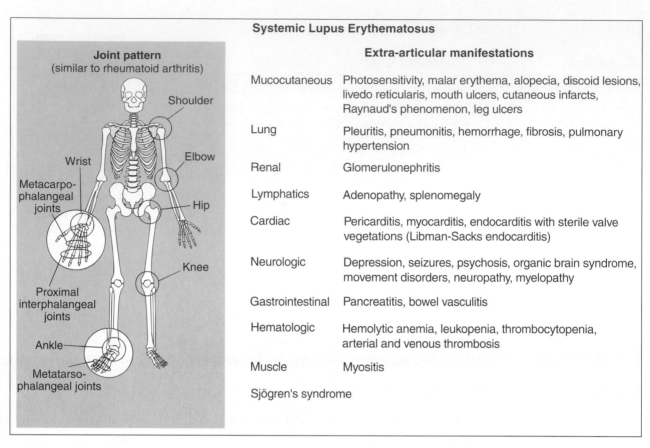

Systemic Lupus Erythematosus

Joint pattern
(similar to rheumatoid arthritis)

Shoulder

Elbow

Wrist

Metacarpo-
phalangeal
joints

Hip

Proximal
interphalangeal
joints

Knee

Ankle

Metatarso-
phalangeal joints

Extra-articular manifestations

Mucocutaneous	Photosensitivity, malar erythema, alopecia, discoid lesions, livedo reticularis, mouth ulcers, cutaneous infarcts, Raynaud's phenomenon, leg ulcers
Lung	Pleuritis, pneumonitis, hemorrhage, fibrosis, pulmonary hypertension
Renal	Glomerulonephritis
Lymphatics	Adenopathy, splenomegaly
Cardiac	Pericarditis, myocarditis, endocarditis with sterile valve vegetations (Libman-Sacks endocarditis)
Neurologic	Depression, seizures, psychosis, organic brain syndrome, movement disorders, neuropathy, myelopathy
Gastrointestinal	Pancreatitis, bowel vasculitis
Hematologic	Hemolytic anemia, leukopenia, thrombocytopenia, arterial and venous thrombosis
Muscle	Myositis
Sjögren's syndrome	

FIGURE 3.17. The many manifestations of SLE. (Reprinted, with permission, from Stobo JD et al. *Principles and Practice of Medicine,* 23rd ed. Stamford, CT: Appleton & Lange, 1996:198.)

Workup. In 1997, the American Rheumatism Association revised the criteria for establishing a diagnosis of SLE. To obtain a diagnosis, the patient must fulfill at least four of the criteria outlined in the "SOAP BRAIN MD" mnemonic. Because of the variable presentation of SLE, however, it might take several years before at least four organ systems are involved and a formal diagnosis can be made. Various antibody tests are perhaps the best screening tool for this disease. Greater than 95% of patients with SLE will have a positive ANA; however, many disorders will also have an abnormal ANA (e.g., scleroderma, chronic liver disease, Epstein-Barr virus, melanoma, ITP, renal dialysis, ovarian cancer, prostate cancer). Anti-dsDNA and anti-Smith antibodies are less common but more specific for making a diagnosis of SLE (see Table 3.28). The presence of antiphospholipid antibody (including lupus anticoagulant and anticardiolipin antibody) increases the risk of stillbirth and abortion in pregnancy. Patients with drug-induced SLE will have the characteristic antihistone antibodies.

Treatment. There is no single treatment for SLE, as treatment depends largely on the systemic manifestations of the disease. Patients are initially treated with NSAIDs, which effectively treat serositis and arthritis. Steroids are used for acute exacerbation; steroids, hydroxychloroquine (Plaquenil), cyclophosphamide, and azathioprine are used in progressive or refractory cases. Plaquenil is especially effective in treating arthritis, skin disease, and fatigue; the cytotoxic

TABLE 3.28. Antibody Tests for Evaluation of SLE.

Test	Sensitivity; Specificity for SLE	Other Disease Associations	Comments
Antinuclear antibody	> 95%; low	Rheumatoid arthritis (RA) (30–50%), discoid lupus, scleroderma (60%), drug-induced lupus (100%), Sjögren's syndrome (80%), miscellaneous inflammatory disorders	Often used as a screening test. A negative test virtually excludes SLE; a positive test, while nonspecific, increases post-test probability. Titer does not correlate with disease activity.
Anti-double-stranded DNA (anti-dsDNA)	60–70%; high	Lupus nephritis, rarely RA, mixed connective tissue disorder (MCID), usually in low titers	The predictive value of a positive test is > 90% for SLE if present in high titers; a decreasing titer may correlate with worsening renal disease. Titer generally correlates with disease activity.
Anti-Smith antibody (anti-Sm)	30–40%; high		SLE-specific. A positive test substantially increases the post-test probability of SLE. Test is rarely indicated.

Reprinted, with permission, from Nicoll D et al. *Pocket Guide to Diagnostic Tests*, 2nd ed. Stamford, CT: Appleton & Lange, 1997:316.

agents (cyclophosphamide and azathioprine) with steroids are effective for lupus nephritis. Pregnant women with prior fetal loss and the presence of antiphospholipid antibodies should receive low-dose heparin. The survival of SLE patients with treatment ranges from 90% to 95% at two years to up to 75% at 20 years; mortality results from end-organ damage and opportunistic infections.

General Medicine

CANCER SCREENING GUIDELINES

Table 3.29 summarizes recommended screening measures.

HIGH-YIELD REFERENCES

CARDIOLOGY

Angina Pectoris, Unstable Angina, and Prinzmetal's (Variant) Angina

ACC/AHA/ACP-ASIM Guidelines for the Management of Patients with Chronic Stable Angina, 1999. Very long, but can review at *http://www.americanheart. org/downloadable/heart/3781_Jun99.pdf*.

TABLE 3.29. Recommended Cancer Screening Measures[a]

Screening Measure	Ages and Intervals
Flexible sigmoidoscopy[b]	q 3–5 years after 50
Fecal occult blood test	q year after 50
Digital rectal examination[b]	q year after 40
Prostate examination[b]	q year after 50
Pap smear	Sexually active or 18, q 1 year; after three normal smears, q 3 years
Pelvic exam	20–40, q 1–3 years; after 40, q year
Endometrial tissue sample[b]	At menopause
Breast self-exam[b]	q month after 20
Breast exam by clinician	20–40, q 3 years; after 40, q year
Mammography	q year after 40–50 (exact timing controversial)
CXR	Not recommended as a screening test

[a]From U.S. Preventative Services Task Force, 1996.
[b]Additional recommendations from the American Cancer Society.
Reprinted, with permission, from Le T et al. *First Aid for the USMLE Step 2*, 3rd ed. New York: McGraw-Hill, 2001:131.

Acute Myocardial Infarction

The GUSTO Investigators. An international randomized trial comparing four thrombolytic strategies for acute myocardial infarction. *NEJM* 1993;329: 673–682. A landmark paper supporting the use of accelerated tPA and heparin in patients with evolving MI. Overall, the combined end point of death or disabling stroke was significantly lower in the accelerated tPA group than in the streptokinase-only groups.

Arrhythmias (i.e., Bradyarrhythmias, Tachyarrhythmias, and Atrial Fibrillation)

ACC/AHA/ESC Guidelines for the Management of Patients with Atrial Fibrillation, 2001. Very long, but can review at: *http://www.americanheart.org/downloadable/heart/222_ja20017993p_1.pdf*.

Benjamin E et al. Impact of atrial fibrillation on the risk of death: the Framingham Heart Study. *Circulation* 1998;98:946–952. A retrospective analysis of the first 40 years of the Framingham Heart Study showing that subjects with AF were significantly more likely than subjects without AF to have cardiovascular disease risk factors and preexisting disease at baseline; AF was associated with a statistically significant increase risk of death (1.5 odds ratio in men; 1.9 odds ratio in women).

Stroke Prevention in Atrial Fibrillation Investigators. Adjusted-dose warfarin versus low-intensity, fixed-dose warfarin plus aspirin for high-risk patients with atrial fibrillation: Stroke Prevention in Atrial Fibrillation III randomised clinical trial. *Lancet* 1996;348:633–638. Landmark study (double-blind randomized controlled trial [RCT]) showing a statistically significant reduction of stroke in high-risk AF patients treated with Coumadin (INR 2.0–3.0) when compared with those treated with aspirin alone.

Congestive Heart Failure

The CONSENSUS Trial Study Group. The effect of enalapril on mortality in severe congestive heart failure: results of the Cooperative North Scandinavian Enalapril Survival Study (CONSENSUS). *NEJM* 1987;30:518–526. A double-blind RCT in which Class IV CHF subjects were given placebo or enalapril; overall reduction in mortality (27%), NYHA classification (symptoms), heart size, and CHF medication requirement in the enalapril group.

The SOLVD Investigators. Effect of enalapril on survival in patients with reduced left ventricular ejection fractions and chronic congestive heart failure. *NEJM* 1991;325:303–310. A landmark trial (double-blind RCT) establishing the role of ACEI in the management of CHF.

Packer M et al. The effect of carvedilol on morbidity and mortality in patients with chronic heart failure. *NEJM* 1996;334:1349–1355. A double-blind RCT with Class II–IV CHF (EF 35%) subjects that demonstrates a reduction in morbidity (65% risk reduction), hospitalization (27% risk reduction), and combined morbidity/hospitalization (38% risk reduction) in mild to moderate CHF.

Packer M et al. Effect of carvedilol on survival in severe chronic heart failure. NEJM 2001;344:1651–1658. Double-blind RCT in which subjects with severe CLTF Class IV with EF < 25% had statistically and combined mortality/ hospitalization when administered carvedilol.

The Digitalis Investigators Group. The effect of digoxin on mortality and morbidity in patients with heart failure. *NEJM* 1997;336:525–533. A double-blind RCT demonstrating decreased morbidity in CHF patients treated with digoxin but no significant change in mortality.

Pitt B et al, for the Randomized Aldactone Workup Study Investigators. The effect of spironolactone on morbidity and mortality in patients with severe heart failure. *NEJM* 1999;341:709–717. A double-blind RCT in which CHF patients treated with spironolactone had a 30% risk reduction in mortality, a 35% reduction in hospitalization, and a significant reduction in symptoms.

ACC/AHA Guidelines for the Workup and Management of Chronic Heart Failure in the Adult. American College of Cardiology and the American Heart Association, 2001. This and other American Heart Association guideline papers can be viewed at *http://www.americanheart.org/presenter.jhtml?iden tifier=9181.*

Hypertension

The sixth report of the Joint National Committee on Prevention, Detection, Workup, and Treatment of High Blood Pressure. *Arch Intern Med* 1997;157:2413–2439. Widely accepted guidelines for the management of hypertension. For the time-impaired, a handy summary is available at *http://www.nhlbi.nih.gov/guidelines/hypertension/*.

PULMONOLOGY

Chronic Obstructive Pulmonary Disease

American Thoracic Society. Standards for the diagnosis and care of patients with chronic obstructive pulmonary disease. *Am J Respir Crit Care Med* 1995;152:S77–S120. A lengthy summary of the current knowledge on pathophysiology and management (pharmacotherapy, home oxygen, and surgery) in COPD patients. Refer to *http://www.thoracic.org/statements/* for other ATS statement articles.

Barnes PJ. Medical progress: chronic obstructive pulmonary disease. *NEJM* 2000; 343:269–280. Review article on types, pathophysiology, and management of COPD.

Pneumonia

Bartlett JG, Mundy LM. Current concepts: community-acquired pneumonia. *NEJM* 1995;333:1618–1624. Outlines common pathogens, signs/symptoms, diagnosis/laboratory tests/radiographic results, and treatment (by subgroup) of community-acquired pneumonia.

Pulmonary Embolism

The PIOPED Investigators. Value of the ventilation/perfusion scan in acute pulmonary embolism: results of the Prospective Investigation of Pulmonary Embolism Diagnosis (PIOPED). *JAMA* 1990;263:2753–2759. A randomized, prospective study to determine sensitivity/specificity of V/Q scans in the diagnosis of PE. It was determined that a history/physical with V/Q scan established/excluded the diagnosis of PE only in the minority of patients with clear, high-probability findings.

GASTROENTEROLOGY

Hepatic Disease (i.e., Cirrhosis and Hepatic Encephalopathy, Acute Hepatitis, Portal Hypertension)

Riordan SM, Williams R. Treatment of hepatic encephalopathy. *NEJM* 1997;337:473–479. A review article of the treatment of hepatic encephalopathy based on the pathophysiological mechanisms causing the disorder. Includes good summary charts of causes and current research on various treatments.

Peptic Ulcer Disease

American Gastroenterological Association. American Gastroenterological Association medical position statement: workup of dyspepsia. *Gastroenterology* 1998;114:579–581. Summarizes differential diagnoses and provides an excellent flow chart on the diagnosis and management of various causes of dyspepsia. *http://www.gastrojournal.org/cgi/reprint/114/3/579.pdf.*

HEMATOLOGY

Neutropenic Fever

Hughes WT et al. 1997 guidelines for the use of antimicrobial agents in neutropenic patients with unexplained fever. *Clin Infect Dis* 1997;25:551–573. Guidelines for determining the causes and treatment of neutropenic fever. Excellent flow charts. Refer to *http://www.idsociety.org/* for management guidelines on various infectious diseases.

ENDOCRINOLOGY

Diabetes Mellitus (Types 1 and 2), Including Diabetic Ketoacidosis

The Diabetes Control and Complications Trial Research Group. The effect of intensive treatment of diabetes on the development and progression of long-term complications in insulin-dependent diabetes mellitus. *NEJM* 1993;329:977–986. A landmark article in which type 1 DM patients with absent or mild retinopathy at baseline were randomized to intensive or conventional blood glucose management. A statistically significant reduction in the appearance or progression of retinopathy, nephropathy, and neuropathy was demonstrated.

Florence JA, Yeager BF. Treatment of type 2 diabetes mellitus. *Am Fam Physician* 1999;59:2835–2844. A review of pharmacologic treatment regimens for type 2 DM. *http://www.aafp.org/afp/990515ap/2835.html.*

The Expert Committee on the Diagnosis and Classification of Diabetes Mellitus. Report of the Expert Committee on the Diagnosis and Classification of Diabetes Mellitus. *Diabetes Care* 2002;25:S5–S20. The most recent guidelines on the types, pathophysiology, and diagnostic tests for DM.

Hyperlipidemias

Randomized trial of cholesterol lowering in 4444 patients with coronary heart disease: the Scandinavian Simvastatin Survival Study (4S). *Lancet* 1994;344:1383–1389. The relative risk of death and a major coronary event in the simvastatin group were decreased in patients with angina or history of MI (0.70 and 0.66, respectively).

Executive summary of the third report of the National Cholesterol Education Program (NCEP) Expert Panel on Detection, Workup, and Treatment of High Blood Cholesterol in Adults (Adult Treatment Panel III), *JAMA* 2001;285:2486–2509. The current guidelines for management of hypercholesterolemia.

THYROID DISORDERS

Singer PA et al. Treatment guidelines for patients with hyperthyroidism and hypothyroidism. *JAMA* 1995;273:808–812. American Thyroid Association standards for the diagnosis and treatment of hyper- and hypothyroidism.

INFECTIOUS DISEASE

HIV and AIDS

1999 USPHS/IDSA guidelines for the prevention of opportunistic infections in persons infected with HIV: part I. Prevention of exposure. *Am Fam Physician* 2000;61:163–174. A three-part series on the prevention and treatment of opportunistic infections in HIV patients. *http://www.aafp.org/afp/20000101/163.html*.

1999 USPHS/IDSA guidelines for the prevention of opportunistic infections in persons infected with HIV: part II. Prevention of the first episode of disease. U.S. Department of Health and Human Services, Public Health Service, Centers for Disease Control and Prevention. U.S. Public Health Service/Infectious Diseases Society of America. *Am Fam Physician* 2000;61:441–442, 445–449, 453–454 passim. *http://www.aafp.org/afp/20000115/441.html*.

1999 USPHS/IDSA guidelines for the prevention of opportunistic infections in persons infected with HIV: part III. Prevention of disease recurrence. United States Public Health Service/Infectious Diseases Society of America. *Am Fam Physician* 2000;61:771–778, 780, 785. *http://www.aafp.org/afp/20000201/771.html*.

Kovacs JA, Masur H. Prophylaxis against opportunistic infections in patients with human immunodeficiency virus infection. *NEJM* 2000;342:1416–1429. A review article that includes opportunistic infections by CD4+ count deficiencies, prophylactic regimens, and current standards for discontinuation of medication for various HIV-associated opportunistic infections.

Tuberculosis

Small PM, Fujiwara PA. Management of tuberculosis in the United States. *NEJM* 2001;345:189–200. An excellent review article of treatment of TB, including treatment in drug-resistant and HIV-associated cases. Also provides a summary of tuberculin skin reactions and patient compliance issues.

Urinary Tract Infections

Stamm WE, Hooton TM. Management of urinary tract infections in adults. *NEJM* 1993;329:1328–1334. A review article that outlines causes and treatment of UTIs based on subtype.

GENERAL MEDICINE

Cancer Screening

Gates TJ. Screening for cancer: evaluating the evidence. *Am Fam Physician* 2001;63:513–522. Rates the evidence on various cancer screening tests. Lengthy but comprehensive. *http://www.aafp.org/afp/ 20010201/513.html.*

TOP-RATED BOOKS

Handbook/Pocketbook

Practical Guide to the Care of the Medical Patient $38.95
Ferri

Mosby, 2001, 5th edition, 1095 pages, ISBN 0323012841

A well-organized and easy-to-read pocketbook for common diseases, written at an appropriate level for medical students. Includes a discussion of etiology, differentials, diagnostic approach, laboratory interpretation, and management. Excellent tables and algorithms are available for the wards. Outline form focuses on enhancing readers' understanding of disease processes and their evaluation. Some treatment sections are better covered in more specialized handbooks.

Saint-Frances Guide to Inpatient Medicine $25.95
Saint

Lippincott Williams & Wilkins, 1997, 1st edition, 533 pages, ISBN 0683075470

An excellent, cheap, and concise pocketbook emphasizing the development of a basic, organized approach toward many common diseases. Makes good use of tables and charts, and devotes a substantial portion of its text to medical mnemonics. However, cannot be used as a primary resource because it lacks extensive discussion of pathophysiology, diagnostic evaluation, management, and treatment. Best used as prerotation reading, as it gives a good overview of differential diagnosis and simplifies the approach toward complex medical issues. Small size makes it easy to carry around. Needs updating.

Saint-Frances Guide to Outpatient Medicine $25.95
Saint

Lippincott Williams & Wilkins, 1999, 2nd edition, 713 pages, ISBN 0781726123

Like its inpatient counterpart, this pocketbook contains numerous medical mnemonics and useful algorithms applicable to an office-care environment. The last part of each section provides useful recommendations on follow-up, which is significant for outpatient medicine. Its portability makes this text an excellent supplement to a more thorough and detailed textbook.

The Washington Manual of Medical Therapeutics $39.95
Ahya

Lippincott Williams & Wilkins, 2001, 30th edition, 697 pages, ISBN 0781723590

An excellent handbook outlining the pathophysiology and diagnosis of common diseases. Contains highly detailed descriptions of various therapeutic options. Aimed toward medical residents, but highly useful for medical students and especially subinterns. Tight fit in most coat pockets. Contains references for the retrieval of primary sources.

Current Clinical Strategies: Medicine $14.95

Chan

Current Clinical Strategies, 2000/2001 edition, 112 pages, ISBN 1881528839

A compilation of admission orders for commonly encountered diseases, including detailed pharmacologic treatment options. This inexpensive pocketbook is especially useful for those doing internal medicine subinternships. A quick reference for management on the wards.

 ### Harrison's Manual of Medicine $39.95

Braunwald

McGraw-Hill, 2001, 15th edition, 1021 pages, ISBN 0071373772

"A baby" pocket version of the parent book, this manual focuses on commonly encountered diseases, providing a wealth of information on pathophysiology, clinical manifestations, and therapeutics. Useful for quick reading on established diagnoses, although dense, large blocks of text make it difficult to skim. Not particularly practical for day-to-day wards problems, as it lacks thorough explanations of the approach toward diagnosis and management. Great as a pocket reference book with which to review diseases that you have encountered or are thinking about on your differential.

TOP-RATED BOOKS

 ### Internal Medicine on Call $29.95

Haist

McGraw-Hill, 1997, 2nd edition, 593 pages, ISBN 0838540562

A quick-reference guidebook to a step-by-step approach toward most commonly encountered medical "on-call" problems. Includes sections on laboratory interpretation, procedures, fluids and electrolytes, ventilator management, and commonly used drugs. Would benefit from more diagrams and tables.

 ### Pocket Companion to Cecil Textbook of Medicine $49.95

Goldman

W. B. Saunders, 2001, 21st edition, 856 pages, ISBN 0721689728

A compact pocket version of the parent book, this text is similar in scope to *Harrison's Manual of Medicine,* succinctly summarizing key points of pathophysiology, diagnosis, and treatment. More information is presented in table and algorithm format than in *Harrison's Manual,* so personal preference will dictate which book is better for you. Refer to other pocketbooks for more detailed management discussions applicable to wards work.

Handbook/Pocketbook

 ### Pocket Medicine $27.95

Sabatine

Lippincott Williams & Wilkins, 1999, 1st edition, 225 pages, ISBN 0781716407

A small pocketbook with great overviews of most diseases along with the latest management. Offers up-to-date references to primary literature after each subject. Also includes handy tables and charts, although the small print may be a drawback. Extra space on each page lends itself to note taking, and personal note cards may be easily added to the ring-bound pocketbook. Limited in detail owing to its size and scope. Compare to *Practical Guide to the Care of the Medical Patient* and *Washington Manual of Medical Therapeutics.*

B **Essentials of Diagnosis and Treatment** $34.95

Tierney

McGraw-Hill, 2001, 2nd edition, 525 pages, ISBN 007137826X

An abridged version of *Current Medical Diagnosis & Treatment* that provides a quick reference for wards and outpatient medicine, organized into bulleted lists containing the essentials of diagnosis, differentials, and treatment. Each medical disorder has its own dedicated page, enlightening clinical pearl, and general primary reference with the primary goal of highlighting crucial points of each disease. Detailed discussions of pathophysiology, diagnosis, and management are beyond the scope of this book, limiting its usefulness on the wards. Consider as a quick-review supplement to its parent book or another textbook.

C **The Portable Internist** $41.95

Zollo

Hanley & Belfus, 1995, 1st edition, 704 pages, ISBN 1560530669

Broad but superficial coverage of various disease processes. Good for quick reading but not as a primary reference source. Given its dimensions (6" × 9"), it is not as portable as the name implies. Has not been updated for several years.

B **Tarascon Internal Medicine & Critical Care Pocketbook** $11.95

Lederman

Tarascon Publishing, 2000, 2nd edition, 191 pages, ISBN 1882742206

A small, cheap, pocket-sized book containing a great deal of information. Excellent tables, graphs, and algorithms present the diagnostic workup and treatment of common emergency problems encountered in internal medicine. A section at the end is dedicated to a description of commonly used drugs in the critical care setting. Occasionally too complex, as information is presented in a highly technical manner with little discussion; geared more toward those with a prior knowledge of the highlighted diseases. Useful for subinterns during their ICU rotations.

Color Atlas and Text of Clinical Medicine $52.00
Forbes

Mosby, 1997, 2nd edition, 534 pages, ISBN 0723421986

A sizable softcover text that gives a broad overview of medicine in an excellent and readable format. Although it offers great figures and tables, its strength lies in its more than 1500 color photos. Excellent illustrations include physical signs of disease, radiographic images, and pathology slides. Not meant for in-depth review, but excellent as an introductory clinical text and as a visual encyclopedia. An excellent investment and supplement to more traditional reference textbooks.

Cecil Essentials of Medicine $49.95
Andreoli

W.B. Saunders, 2000, 5th edition, 975 pages, ISBN 0721681794

A great condensed version of the parent book. Offers clear, detailed explanations of pathophysiology, but not as useful as a treatment reference or for differential diagnosis. More for reference than for practical wards work. Contains many great tables and charts. Not portable.

First Aid for the Medicine Clerkship $29.95
Stead

McGraw-Hill, 2001, 1st edition, 406 pages, ISBN 0071364218

A highly comprehensive overview of pertinent topics in internal medicine, written in outline format and intended for NBME shelf and USMLE Step 2 exam study. Covers essential high-yield information in a succinct, well-written manner. "Exam tips" and "ward tips" included in the margins are too numerous, detracting from their overall utility. Few figures and photographs provided. Short section at end mentions some general Websites, extracurricular activities, and scholarships pertaining to internal medicine. Overall, an excellent review of the broad field of internal medicine. Publication not related to the authors of *First Aid for the Wards*.

Outpatient Medicine $63.95
Fihn

W.B. Saunders, 1998, 2nd edition, 774 pages, ISBN 0721662579

Efficiently summarizes common problems encountered in outpatient medicine. Each section can be read as a five-minute rapid overview of prevention, presentation, clinical approach, treatment, and follow-up. Excellent cross-referencing is provided. Individualized comments are provided for primary references at the end of each section. A good quick reference for outpatient adult medicine.

TOP-RATED BOOKS

Review/Mini-Reference

A⁻ **Underground Clinical Vignettes: Internal Medicine, Vol. 1** $24.95

Bhushan

Blackwell Science, 2002, 2nd edition, 56 pages, ISBN 0632045639

A well-organized review of clinical vignettes commonly encountered on NBME shelf and USMLE Step 2 exams. Includes a focused, high-yield discussion of pathogenesis, epidemiology, management, and complications. Black-and-white images are included where relevant. Also contains several "mini-cases" in which only key facts related to each disease are presented. An entertaining, and easy-to-use supplement for studying during your clinical rotation. A color atlas supplement comes with the purchase of the full set of *Underground Clinical Vignettes*.

 A⁻ **Underground Clinical Vignettes: Internal Medicine, Vol. 2** $24.95

Bhushan

Blackwell Science, 2002, 2nd edition, 58 pages, ISBN 0632045655

See above review of *Underground Clinical Vignettes: Internal Medicine, Vol. 1*.

 B⁺ **Blueprints in Medicine** $34.95

Young

Blackwell Science, 2000, 2nd edition, 354 pages, ISBN 0632044845

A good basic review that students can read early in the rotation to learn the fundamentals of internal medicine. Easy to read, with good tables and charts to illustrate key points. Although some students feel it is too simplistic and not comprehensive enough for the NBME shelf exam, it may be adequate for the USMLE Step 2. Compare with *NMS Medicine*. Consider using as a supplement to textbooks or for more advanced review.

 B⁺ **Common Medical Diagnosis: An Algorithmic Approach** $39.95

Healey

W.B. Saunders, 2000, 3rd edition, 235 pages, ISBN 0721677320

An interesting book dedicated solely to algorithms; organized by body system and presenting sign. Guides you from the differential through the appropriate clinical workup to a more definitive diagnosis. Algorithms are easy to follow and include commentaries on the pathophysiology underlying the diagnostic approach; helping you organize your approach to medical problems. Only the "bread-and-butter" medical problems are covered, requiring you to look in other books for uncommon conditions, but overall a good resource for the seasoned medical student.

 B⁺ **Guide to Internal Medicine** $32.00

Paauw

Mosby, 1999, 1st edition, 302 pages, ISBN 0323009212

Designed specifically for medical students beginning their internal medicine clerkships. Divided into sections by basic skills necessary for the clerkship, common symptoms, and common diseases. Covers practical core knowledge of common medical conditions that all students should have mastered by the end of their rotation. Basic questions and answers help guide the transition to clinical thinking. Too over simplified for any long-term value, but a good, concise overview of internal medicine while on the clerkship.

Kelley's Essentials of Internal Medicine $49.95

Humes

Lippincott Williams & Wilkins, 2001, 2nd edition, 920 pages, ISBN 0781719372

A condensed version of *Kelley's Textbook*, written at the medical student level with the basics for patient workup and diagnosis. Offers good tables and algorithms for a problem- or symptom-based approach to evaluation and differential diagnosis. Slightly less detailed than *Cecils' Essentials*.

 NMS Medicine $32.00

Myers

Lippincott Williams & Wilkins, 2000, 4th edition, 776 pages, ISBN 078172144X

Organized by system with easy-to-read chapters in outline form. Includes questions at the end of each chapter to solidify concepts just learned and a comprehensive exam at the end. Geared toward NBME shelf exam and USMLE Step 2 study, but can be used to review topics on wards. Few diagrams, tables, and illustrations; not always up to date. Thorough and highly detailed, although its inclusion of some esoteric information may make it difficult to find the essentials.

 Principles and Practice of Medicine $54.95

Stobo

McGraw-Hill, 1996, 23rd edition, 1046 pages, ISBN 038579639

Organized by organ system, this text gives a useful "how-to-approach" discussion for each disease process and a summary of key points at the end of each chapter. The level of detail is moderate and manageable, placing this text in between a primary reference and a pocketbook. New edition is expected in January 2004.

B **Internal Medicine Pearls** $45.00

Heffner

Lippincott Williams & Wilkins, 2000, 2nd edition, 275 pages, ISBN 1560534044

Detailed clinical vignettes with laboratory and radiographic findings, followed by a discussion of clinically important "pearls." Questions focus on clinical decision making and management. Only selected topics are covered, so it is not comprehensive, and discussions may be too detailed for review purposes. A good, clinically focused supplement.

B **Medical Secrets** $39.95

Zollo

Hanley & Belfus, 2001, 3rd edition, 564 pages, ISBN 1560534761

An interesting but dense compilation of useful and clinically relevant information presented in a question-and-answer format. Designed for surviving wards pimping sessions, although one is inevitably never asked the majority of these questions. Excellent tables are good for quick reviews. May not be a prudent buy if one does not like the format.

B   Medicine $36.00

Fishman

Lippincott Williams & Wilkins, 1996, 4th edition, 654 pages, ISBN 0397514646

A highly readable and approachable text organized by body system. Sometimes simplistic and lacking in detail. Makes good use of tables, but includes few illustrations. Not a replacement for a medicine reference book, but adequately presents the basics.

B   Outpatient Medicine Recall $29.95

Franko

Lippincott Williams & Wilkins, 1998, 1st edition, 275 pages, ISBN 0683180185

A small, easy-to-carry book with a question-and-answer format typical of the *Recall* series, with a focus on outpatient management. Well-written material is good for self-testing but is neither as concise nor as comprehensive as other resources. No images or diagrams are provided.

B⁻   Medicine Recall $28.00

Bergin

Lippincott Williams & Wilkins, 1997, 1st edition, 928 pages, ISBN 0683180983

A good but not-so-portable book for rapid review and answering pimp questions. Follows the standard *Recall* series question-and-answer format of high-yield information, organized by medical specialty. Requires a significant time commitment to complete. No images are provided, and some information is incorrect or out of date. Not as useful on the wards as its counterpart, *Surgical Recall*. Useful as a supplement to other resources.

B⁻   Most Commons in Medicine $26.95

Goljan

W. B. Saunders, 2000, 1st edition, 857 pages, ISBN 0721687598

Breaks information down into several tables of the most common causes, clinical findings, complications, and treatment options of a wide range of medical disorders. Not designed for primary learning, but more for quick review on the wards when one has spare time. Explanations given for answers are short and limited, if presented at all. Decent preparation for wards pimp questions.

B⁻   Pathophysiology of Disease: An Introduction to Clinical Medicine $44.95

McPhee

McGraw-Hill, 1999, 3rd edition, 662 pages, ISBN 0838581609

A concise, interdisciplinary reference text of the pathophysiology of common diseases, organized by system. Offers excellent explanations of disease processes. Not designed for wards or for dealing with treatment and management issues, but useful as an adjunct to a more traditional textbook. Some students find it more appropriate for pathophysiology classes during preclinical years.

Current Medical Diagnosis & Treatment 2002 $54.95

Tierney

McGraw-Hill, 2002, 41st edition, 1880 pages, ISBN 0071390065

A clinically oriented reference that is concise yet detailed and very readable for medical students compared to other texts. Well organized with excellent descriptions of pathophysiology, clinical findings, and treatment. The beginning of each section offers the essentials of diagnosis. Revised annually, thus offering useful tables and up-to-date references. Strong coverage of ambulatory care relative to more conventional textbooks.

 ## Harrison's Principles of Internal Medicine $125.00

Braunwald

McGraw-Hill, 2001, 15th edition, 2629 pages, ISBN 0070072728

An excellent, comprehensive reference considered by many to be the "gold standard" of internal medicine textbooks. Excellent use of tables, graphs, illustrations, and radiographs. Not for quick reference, but rather for in-depth home reading on specific topics. Incredibly detailed and can be overwhelming at times. Requires serious concentration and reading time, but will provide some of the most thorough reviews of disease processes that you will ever find. A great reference for those considering internal medicine as a career. Available as a single- or double-volume text.

 ## Cecil Textbook of Medicine $110.00

Goldman

W. B. Saunders, 2000, 21st edition, 2308 pages, ISBN 072167996X

One of the classic textbooks of medicine. Comparable to and easier reading than *Harrison's*, but not as comprehensive or detailed. Great tables, charts, and index organization. Available as a single- or double-volume text.

 ## The Merck Manual of Diagnosis & Therapy $35.00

Beers

Merck, 1999, 17th edition, 2833 pages, ISBN 0911910107

Offers clear discussions of a wide variety of diseases, but with limited tables, charts, and illustrations. Well organized, comprehensive, and well indexed. May be used as a reference book, but not as extensive as *Harrison's*. Useful as an adjunctive, quick home-reference textbook.

Kelley's Textbook of Internal Medicine $115.00

Hume

Lippincott Williams & Wilkins, 2000, 4th edition, 3254 pages, ISBN 0781717876

Offers well-organized, straightforward discussions of pathophysiology, clinical findings, diagnosis, and management. Not yet on the same level as *Harrison's*, but subsequent editions have improved. The recent edition places more emphasis on evidence-based medicine with specialized "clinical decision guides" based on the most recent research.

TOP-RATED BOOKS

Textbook/Reference

B⁺ **Textbook of Internal Medicine** $125.00

Stein

McGraw-Hill, 1998, 5th edition, 2515 pages, ISBN 0815186983

A comprehensive reference book that is not at the same level of detail as the previously mentioned textbooks but it is more approachable and friendly. Offers good explanations of pathophysiology with good sections on diagnostic evaluation. A slightly older reference than the other textbooks.

B⁻ **Ferri's Clinical Advisor: Instant Diagnosis and Treatment** $59.95

Ferri

Mosby, 2001/2002 edition, 1568 pages, ISBN 0323013007

A large, annually revised text divided into brief discussions of medical disorders, differential diagnosis of signs and symptoms, clinical algorithms, laboratory interpretation, and preventive guidelines. Quick, easy-to-read bulleted lists and tables are provided on every page. Provides easy access to high-yield information in user-friendly format. Differential lists can be hefty, and some sections have minimal primary references. Some algorithms are over simplified and lack descriptions of the clinical thought process. Refer to other textbooks for in-depth evaluation of disease.

CHAPTER 4

Neurology

Ward Tips
High-Yield Topics
High-Yield References
Top-Rated Books

"Where's the lesion?"

Welcome to your neurology rotation! In the next few weeks, you will focus on the function and dysfunction of the nervous system. In this highly academic and scientific field, you will discover one of the things neurologists love to do: talk, talk, and talk about neurology. So get ready for lengthy rounds in which you'll discuss detailed differentials, neuroscience, and the latest research while simultaneously attempting to answer the ever-present question, "Where's the lesion?" Naturally, you won't be expected to learn all of neurology in a few weeks—so, as in many other rotations, your questions will be more important than your answers. The more interested you are, the better you'll do in the neurology rotation and the more you'll get out of it.

WHAT IS THE ROTATION LIKE?

Neurology rotations differ notably from site to site, so the first thing to do is find out how your responsibilities will be divided between inpatient wards, outpatient clinics, consult-liaison, and neurosurgery. Inpatient neurology tends to be like medicine but is typically less demanding. Student responsibilities center on admission history and physicals (H&Ps), working with the residents on acute management, developing differential diagnoses, and presenting to the team. Day-to-day activities include following labs and neuro exams, writing notes, and playing a supportive role in management. The workload tends to depend on the number of students per team, the presence of interns, the number of admissions, and the inpatient census. Don't hesitate to ask your residents/attendings on the first day: Who evaluates me? What are my responsibilities? Whom can I ask for help? What is the call schedule, and is it home call or in-house?

One of your primary goals during this rotation should be to learn how to conduct and present a complete screening neurologic exam. In addition, you should plan to read about your patients and understand the neuroanatomy, pathophysiology, and treatment involved. *Always* try to trace the neuroanatomic pathways that can cause your patient's symptoms so that you can localize the lesion.

The patient population in neurology can be highly variable from one hospital to another. Patients tend to be admitted for ischemic strokes and hemorrhages, status epilepticus, meningitis and encephalitis, Guillain-Barré syndrome (GBS), myasthenic crises, and acute changes in mental status of unknown etiology, to name but a few. Trauma and tumor patients are often managed by neurosurgery. Outpatient clinics are a great place to see a spectrum of common and uncommon nonacute diseases, such as peripheral neuropathies, multiple sclerosis (MS), migraine, and movement disorders. If you have a particular area of interest, such as neuromuscular disorders, you may want to find out if you can spend a few afternoons each week seeing patients in clinic and observing electrophysiologic testing. In general, you are encouraged to seek out the variety of interesting experiences neurology offers. Your residents and attendings will likely be impressed by your initiative, and you will benefit from the experience.

WHO ARE THE PLAYERS?

Team Neuro often works like a medicine team, with a senior resident (R3 or R4) and at least one junior resident (R2). If there are interns, they tend to be from medicine or psychiatry; if there are no interns, the junior residents may function as "resi-terns." There may also be fourth-year medical students who serve as subinterns and a handful of third-years. In addition, there is usually one ward attending, and there may be private attendings, subspecialty attendings (such as neurovascular or epilepsy), and various fellows. As a result, you may end up presenting patients to a number of different attendings and teams. Other important players include the nursing staff, who among other things are trained to do neuro exams (ICU) and to report on seizures; the social worker, who is an indispensable resource on psychosocial issues and discharge planning; the pharmacist; and the technicians (who do EEGs, blood work, etc.).

HOW IS THE DAY SET UP?

A typical day might consist of the following, although the precise schedule may vary widely by institution:

7:30–8:00 AM	Prerounds
8:00–8:45 AM	Team work rounds
9:00–10:30 AM	Attending rounds
11:00 AM–12:00 NOON	Subspecialty rounds
1:30–4:30 PM	Clinic
5:00 PM–?	Go home (once you've finished your notes, checked labs, etc.)

Call days vary depending on how busy the service is, how many patients you are expected to carry, and how many admits are scheduled. When you are on call, you should find out who the admitting resident is. Often, the consult resident will screen patients in the ER, decide whom to admit, and write the initial orders; you may want to ask this resident to page you so that you can see each patient's initial presentation and take part in formulating the differential diagnosis. This is particularly important in patients with rapidly changing neuro exams.

Conferences can be long, overly theoretical, and difficult to follow. Don't be afraid to ask questions or to ask your residents to clarify points you didn't understand. If most of the conferences are over your head and you feel you aren't learning the basics, consider self-study using a basic clinical neurology handbook (see Top-Rated Books). Ask your resident or attending if he or she would be willing to improvise a few lectures on topics such as "Management of Acute Stroke," "Workup of Altered Mental Status," etc. Depending on the hospital, there may also be neuroradiology conferences to review films on the interesting patients on your team. The more CTs and MRIs you look at, the more familiar you will become with neuroanatomy. Anatomic localization is key to the formulation of meaningful differentials.

Review your neuroanatomy and neuropathophysiology.

HOW DO I DO WELL IN THIS ROTATION?

Doing well in neurology is no different from any other rotation: Be prompt and courteous, take good care of your patients, try to know them better than anyone else, read about their diseases, ask questions, and demonstrate your lifelong interest in the subject. Attendings and fellows love to teach students who are interested, so focus on the basics, reviewing neuroanatomy and studying disease presentation, workup, and treatment. You shouldn't be expected to understand obscure diseases or to track down unintelligible articles (unless your patient happens to have a rare and interesting condition). However, if you find yourself researching a case out of genuine interest, your residents and fellow students might appreciate a report or article that you find. At the very least, your residents will notice your effort and, quite possibly, find the information useful and decide to add the article to their review files (a rare honor indeed). It is always appropriate to try to educate yourself and the other medical students on your team about something interesting, as long as you are not pompous or condescending about it. You may also want to develop a list of course objectives that fit your future aspirations—perhaps focusing on the execution of the neuro exam and on a basic understanding of the common neurologic diseases.

KEY NOTES

Neurology admission notes are like medicine notes with a few key distinctions:

- Indicate the handedness of the patient in ID (e.g., "46 y.o. RH [right-handed] male").
- Take a full medical history as well as a neurologic history, including a history of seizures, cerebrovascular accidents (CVAs), transient ischemic attacks (TIAs), diabetes mellitus (DM), MIs, and other indicators of peripheral vascular disease.
- Remember to note the patient's risk factors, substance use, family history, and social situation.
- Don't forget to record the complete physical exam, noting vital signs, cardiac exam, jaundice, neck stiffness, and so on.
- When you are documenting the neuro exam, remember that the admission H&P should include the full exam; progress notes can be brief. An example of a brief physical/neuro exam with commonly used abbreviations is shown on the following page.
- Don't forget to report imaging studies and lumbar puncture (LP) results.
- The assessment is a good place to organize and summarize: Include the important symptoms and findings; localize the lesions to an anatomic location; and, finally, give an organized differential diagnosis by likelihood.

Sample Neurology Physical Exam

Gen: Elderly Caucasian male in mild discomfort, moaning

VS: T 37.2 P 59 BP 167/89 RR 18 Sat 98% RA

HEENT: NCAT, sclera anicteric

Neck: stiff neck + Brudzinksi + meningismus

Lungs: CTAB

Cardiac: RRR, no m/r/g

Abd: Obese, soft, NTND, NABS × 4 quadrants, no HSM, no masses

Ext: No c/c/e

MSE: A & O × 3

> Normal repetition, naming

> Follows commands

> 7-digit span, able to attend and concentrate

> Memory: 3/3 registration, 0/3 → 2/3 with prompts at 5 minutes

CN: VFFTC, PERRL, 3 → 2 bilaterally

> Fundi normal, no papilledema, exudates, hemorrhages

> EOMI without nystagmus or diplopia

> Face symmetric, nasolabial folds appear equal bilaterally

> Tongue and palate midline, normal tongue motion, no dysarthria

Motor: Strength 4/5 throughout LUE and LLE, 5/5 RUE and RLE

> LUE spasticity

> Normal bulk/tone throughout without tremor or fasciculations

Sensory: Grossly intact to light touch and pinprick throughout bilateral UE and LE

Coordination: RAM: slow with LUE, normal with RUE

> Normal finger-to-nose and heel-to-shin

> No dysmetria

> Negative Romberg

Gait: Stable, normal tandem, cannot walk on heels or tiptoes

Reflexes:

A&O × 3 = Alert and oriented to person, place, and date

c/c/e = Clubbing, cyanosis, edema

CTAB = Clear to auscultation bilaterally

EOMI = Extraocular movement intact

HSM = Hepatosplenomegaly

LE = Lower extremity

LLE = Left lower extremity

LUE = Left upper extremity

m/r/g = Murmurs, rubs, gallops

MSE = Mental status examination

NABS = Normoactive bowel sounds

NCAT = Normocephalic

NTND = Nontender, nondistended

PERRL – Pupils equal, round, and reactive to light

RAM = Rapid alternating movements

RLE = Right lower extremity

RRR = Regular rate and rhythm

RUE = Right upper extremity

UE = Upper extremities

VFFTC = Visual fields full to confrontation

Always rule out increased intracranial pressure or focal neurologic deficit before attempting an LP.

KEY PROCEDURES

The main procedure in inpatient neurology is the LP, known to your patients as the dreaded "spinal tap." Make sure your resident knows that you are interested in doing LPs; it's a good chance to practice. Check *Clinical Neurology, Clinician's Pocket Reference,* Ferri's *Care of the Medical Patient,* or similar guides for a description of the procedure. Contraindications include suspected intracranial mass lesion, local infection, spinal cord mass, or coagulopathy. Remember, the patient must give informed consent (although this is not always possible in cases with altered mental status), and you must write a procedure note documenting both the indications for the LP and a summary of the procedure (see Chapter 1 for a sample procedure note). You should also find a good and enthusiastic teacher and ask for plenty of supervision early on. Attempting a difficult LP alone can be a nightmare both for you and for the patient.

WHAT DO I CARRY IN MY POCKETS?

Checklist
- ❑ Stethoscope
- ❑ Ophthalmoscope (optional)
- ❑ Eye chart
- ❑ Tuning fork (512 Hz for testing hearing, 256 Hz for vibration testing)
- ❑ Penlight
- ❑ Reflex hammer (the larger the better)
- ❑ Pins (for testing pain sensation; do not reuse them)
- ❑ Cotton swabs or clean tissues (for corneal reflex) and tongue blades

With the items listed above, you will be well equipped to perform a full neuro exam. Keep these items within reach on attending rounds; providing your residents or attendings with such implements is a common courtesy.

HIGH-YIELD TOPICS

ROTATION OBJECTIVES

Probably the most important things to learn in your neurology rotation are the screening and complete neurologic exams as well as the workup and management of common neurologic problems, such as headache, seizure, low back pain, and stroke. You should focus on the history, physical exam, and studies; on the development of differentials; and on the recognition of emergency conditions. This is also a good time to learn about the indications for and interpretation of investigational studies, especially CT, MRI, LP, and, perhaps, EEG, electromyographic (EMG), and nerve conduction studies.

The following is a list of topics that you should review during this rotation. Topics in italics are discussed in greater detail in this chapter.

The Complete Neurologic Exam

Screening Exam
- *For mental status*
- *For cranial nerves*
- *For motor and coordination*
- *For sensation*

Imaging Basics
- *Computed tomography*
- *Magnetic resonance imaging*
- *Contrast*

Lumbar Puncture Results
- *CSF profiles*

Management of Intracranial Pressure

Aphasias
- *Broca's aphasia*
- *Wernicke's aphasia*
- *Transcortical aphasias*
- *Conduction aphasia*
- *Global aphasia*

Coma
- *Anatomic and metabolic etiologies*
- *Assessing a comatose patient (use of Glasgow Coma Scale)*
- *Primitive brain stem reflexes*
- *Workup and treatment of comatose patients*
- *Coma, persistent vegetative state, and locked-in syndrome*

Delirium and Dementia
- *Delirium vs. dementia*
- *Common and treatable causes of delirium*
- Wernicke's encephalopathy
- Delirium tremens
- *Causes of dementia*
- *Alzheimer's disease*

Dysequilibrium
- *Central vs. peripheral dysequilibrium*
- *Common etiologies*
- Nystagmus

Headache
- *Migraine*
- *Cluster*

- *Tension*
- Subarachnoid hemorrhage (see Intracranial hemorrhages)
- Temporal arteritis
- Intracranial tumor (see Intracranial neoplasms)
- Subdural hematoma (see Intracranial hemorrhages)

Infections
- Meningitis: bacterial and viral (see Pediatrics, Chapter 6)
- HIV infection (both primary and opportunistic)
- Tuberculosis and Herpes Simplex Virus infection
- Encephalitis and cerebral abscess
- Polio and postpolio syndrome

Intracranial Hemorrhages
- *Subarachnoid*
- *Epidural hematoma*
- *Subdural*
- *Intraparenchymal*

Intracranial Neoplasms
- Primary brain tumors
- Metastatic brain tumors
- Presentation of brain tumors
- Tumors in children and adults

Low Back Pain, Spinal Cord Injuries
- Cord lesions, cord compression, and common myelopathies
- Differential diagnosis, workup, and protocol
- Cervical spine injury

Movement Disorders
- *Hyperkinetic vs. hypokinetic disorders*
- *Parkinson's disease*
- *Huntington's disease*
- *Multiple sclerosis*
- Wilson's disease

Seizures
- *Partial*
- *Generalized*
- *Absence (petit mal)*
- *Tonic-clonic (grand mal)*
- *Status epilepticus*

Stroke

- *Clinical features*
- *Risk factors and preventive therapies*
- *Approach to workup, treatment, and management*

Weakness

- *Upper motor neuron vs. lower motor neuron weakness*
- *Differential diagnosis classified by anatomic localization*
- *Carpal tunnel syndrome*
- *Guillain-Barré syndrome*
- *Myasthenia gravis*

The Complete Neurologic Exam

Learning to do a complete neurologic exam is one of the most important objectives of your rotation. Don't expect to master it in a few weeks, however; instead, spend time creating a systematic approach to the exam and learning to feel comfortable with its components. Perhaps the best advice is to carefully observe the exams (and notes) of your residents and attendings, taking note of how (and why) they chose to abbreviate or focus their exams. Also pay attention to which specific neurologic exams help them find subtle deficits. Tables 4.1 through 4.4 provide information for a complete exam; shown below is the abbreviated version. Good luck!

Create a systematic approach!

SCREENING EXAM FOR MENTAL STATUS

A screening for mental status exam should include the following (see Table 4.1):

1. Assess the patient's level of consciousness and orientation (to person, place, date, and time).
2. Assess the patient's attention. Can the patient attend to commands? Can he or she concentrate on giving a history? If not, check a digit span or the A-test (the former is a better test). The digit span consists of determining how many digits the patient can repeat (five to seven is normal). In the A-test, you recite a series of letters and ask the patient to raise his or her hand each time the letter "A" is heard.
3. Pay attention to the patient's use of language and comprehension of your requests during the exam. Ask if the patient knows what's going on with his or her care and condition. Check repetition and naming (a sensitive test of aphasia).
4. Finally, check memory and higher cognitive function. Ask the patient how he or she got to the hospital. What tests were done today? Ask the patient to recall three items after five minutes. Who is the president? What are some current events? Test abstraction. What does it mean when you say, "Two heads are better than one"?

TABLE 4.1. Mental Status Exam.

What You're Testing	What You're Looking For	What You're Doing
Level of consciousness[a]	Alertness	Observe (eyes open? drowsy looking?).
	Orientation	Can patient answer: What's your name? What is the day of week, date, month, year? Where are you? What floor?
	Response to voice	Call patient's name; ask to open eyes.
	Response to pain	Try sternal rub, pinching extremities, and watch response for purposefulness.
Attention[a]	Ability to focus on a task	Ask patient to repeat digit spans (e.g., "02139") or use the A-test (described above).
Language	Comprehension of spoken word	Ask patient to close eyes, show three fingers, and touch right ear with left thumb.
	Comprehension of written word	Hold up card reading "Close your eyes."
	Repetition of phrases	Have patient repeat, "No ifs, ands, or buts" or "Around the rugged rock the ragged rascal ran," and write "Today is a sunny day."
	Fluency of speech	Is it intelligible, fluent, grammatical? Can patient write a complete sentence?
	Naming	Try pointing to watch and parts to elicit "watch, band, crystal."
Concentration	Ability to maintain focus	Have patient serially subtract 7 from 100 (or 3 from 20) or spell "world" backwards.
Mood, insight, thought process and content	Look for signs of depression, other psychiatric disturbance, denial	Ask patient, "How are your spirits?" "Do you know why you are here in the hospital?"
Memory	Registration	List three words (e.g., "apple, England, and John Lennon)" and ask patient to repeat.
	Short term	Three minutes later, ask patient to recall three items. Offer prompts if patient is unable to do so (such as "a kind of fruit," "a country in Europe," "the best Beatle"); can also try current events.
	Long term	Ask for birthdate, Social Security Number, history.
Higher cognitive function	Fund of knowledge	Ask for names of current/past presidents.
	Calculations	Try simple addition and division (how many quarters in $2.50), subtraction (making change from $5.00 for $1.39).
	Abstractions	Ask patient to interpret a proverb such as "A rolling stone gathers no moss." Be aware of cultural differences.
	Constructions	Ask patient to copy sketches (square, cube) and to draw a clock (analog).

[a]If level of consciousness and attention are abnormal, the other components of the exam are more difficult to interpret.

SCREENING EXAM FOR CRANIAL NERVES

A screening for cranial nerves exam should include the following (see Table 4.2):

1. Focus on the eyes: check acuity, visual fields (by confrontation), pupillary size/shape/constriction to light and accommodation, and extraocular movements. Ask about diplopia. Don't leave out the funduscopic exam.
2. Check light touch and temperature sensation in the face using the "cold" tuning fork. Check corneal reflexes if the patient has a depressed level of consciousness. Intact corneal reflexes will tell you that both cranial nerves (CN) V and VII are intact.
3. Check the face for asymmetries. Check the symmetric movement of the facial muscles. Determine if any facial weakness is central (only the lower half of the face is affected) or peripheral (one entire half of the face is affected).
4. Determine if there are gross differences in hearing between the ears. Check for vestibular dysfunction by inspecting gait and doing a Romberg test.
5. Listen to the voice for hoarseness and dysarthria.
6. Determine if the tongue and uvula are midline.

SCREENING EXAM FOR MOTOR NERVES

A screening for motor nerves exam should include the following (see Table 4.3, 4.4, and 4.5):

1. Observe! Does the patient have atrophy, abnormal movements or postures, or a tendency to favor one side of the body over the other? Are there localizing findings?
2. Check tone in all four extremities.
3. Check strength throughout major muscle groups in the upper and lower extremities using the standardized grading scale (see Table 4.4). Note asymmetries between right and left extremities or between proximal and distal muscle groups.
4. Check the strength of finger extension, index finger abduction, and big toe dorsiflexion and plantar flexion to look for subtle distal weakness.
5. Check pronator drift by asking the patient to extend both arms with palms up and eyes closed. Weakness manifests as pronation or downward drift.
6. Check rapid hand movements such as quickly tapping the index finger on the thumb for weakness or loss of coordination. Also check rapid foot tapping.
7. Check DTRs (biceps, triceps, brachioradialis, patellar, ankle) and plantar responses (see Table 4.5 for grading scale).
8. Check for functional weakness of gait with heel and toe walking. Assess tandem and casual gait.

TABLE 4.2. Cranial Nerve Exam.

What You're Testing	What You're Looking For	What You're Doing
Olfactory nerve	Ability to discern smells	Usually omitted—can check with coffee, ammonia, orange or lemon extract.
Optic nerve	Visual acuity	Use Snellen eye chart.
	Visual fields	Test by confrontation if patient cooperates, or estimate by visual threat otherwise.
	Ocular fundi (funduscopic exam)	Look for papilledema, retinal/subhyaloid hemorrhages, retinopathy, and/or optic atrophy.
Oculomotor nerve	Pupillary function	Check baseline size, shape, and symmetry; direct and consensual constriction (using penlight); and accommodation.
	Function of levator palpebrae	Check for elevation of eyelid and ptosis.
	Function of superior rectus	Extraocular muscles (EOM) (elevate gaze).
	Function of inferior rectus	EOM (depress gaze).
	Function of inferior oblique	EOM (elevate adducted eye).
Trochlear nerve	Function of superior oblique	EOM (depress adducted eye).
Abducens nerve	Function of lateral rectus	EOM (abduction).
	Assessment of EOMs	Ask patient to follow target in H shape, looking for full movement and coordination.
Trigeminal nerve	Motor: temporal, masseter muscles	Palpate muscles as patient clenches teeth.
	Sensory: V1, V2, V3	Check sensation to forehead, cheek, and jaw.
	Reflex: corneal blink	Touch cornea with cotton thread or tissue.
Facial nerve	Motor to facial muscles (also checked in motor response to the corneal reflex)	Check raised eyebrows, tightly squinted eyes, smile, and puffed-out cheeks, looking for asymmetries.
Vestibulocochlear nerve	Auditory function	Grossly test hearing by rubbing fingers together by each ear or scratching pillow. Also consider doing Weber and Rinne's tests
	Vestibular function	Check for nystagmus, h/o vertigo.
Glossopharyngeal nerve	Sensory: palate, pharynx	Check gag reflex (stroke back of throat).
Vagus nerve	Motor: palate, pharynx, vocal cords	Check voice for hoarseness, articulation; check palatal elevation, uvular position, gag reflex.
Spinal accessory nerve	Motor: trapezius	Have patient shrug shoulders with resistance.
	Motor: sternocleidomastoid (SCM)	Have patient check SCM strength.
Hypoglossal nerve	Motor: tongue	Look at tongue in mouth for position, atrophy, and fasciculations; have patient protrude tongue and move side to side (check for asymmetry).

TABLE 4.3. Motor Nerve Exam.

What You're Testing	What You're Looking For	What You're Doing
Appearance	Bulk (atrophy, hypertrophy), fasciculations, spasms, spontaneous motion.	Observing.
Tone	Resistance to passive motion.	Check wrists, elbows, ankles, knees; remind patient to relax, shake gently, move evenly through range of motion, then move abruptly (note pattern of resistance).
Descriptions of tone	Rigidity: Increased in full range of motion, not dependent on rate or location; may be constant (lead-pipe rigidity) or ratchety (cogwheel rigidity). Spasticity: Tone increased most in arm flexors and leg extensors, increases as rate of motion increases, more noted at initiation of motion than continuation. Flaccidity: Decreased tone, joints tend to flop and hyperextend like a rag doll. Paratonia: Changes in tone over time/position caused by an inability to relax.	
Strength	Discover pattern of weakness (or absence of weakness). Explore extent of weakness and elucidate possible etiologies.	History (weakness, clumsiness). Screening exam (see below). Focused motor exam based on information given in history and screen. Also use functional testing (see entry on *gait* below). Examination tips: Give patient mechanical advantage (start with joint in midposition) and apply force to overcome patient's strength, not to match it. Palpate muscle belly during exam.
Reflexes	Deep tendon reflexes (jaw, biceps, brachioradialis, triceps, finger flexors, patellar, thigh adductors, ankle jerk) Superficial reflexes (abdominal, cremasteric). Pathological reflexes (Babinski, frontal release).	Ask patient to relax, position limbs, alternate from side to side for comparison. Watch for clonus, and record briskness (0 = areflexia, 1 = weak reflex, 2 = normal, 3 = "spread" of reflex to other muscle groups, 4 = clonus). Pay attention to symmetry! For Babinski (plantar response), stroke the lateral plantar surface of the foot with a key; look for direction of big toe motion (dorsiflexion = Babinski sign).

TABLE 4.3 (continued). Motor Nerve Exam.

What You're Testing	What You're Looking For	What You're Doing
Coordination	Point-to-point testing.	Finger-to-nose (upper): Have patient touch his nose, then your finger, repeat. Heel-to-shin (lower): Have patient run heel up and down opposite shin from knee to foot.
	Rapid movements (strength and coordination).	Index finger tapping on thumb, foot tapping on the ground or on your palm.
Gait	Normal gait. Important for testing power of the lower extremities; functional testing is more sensitive than manual testing.	Is gait balanced and coordinated with feet no wider than shoulders and arms swinging?
	Test for ataxia (tandem gait).	Can patient walk in a line heel-to-toe?
	Test for distal weakness.	Have patient walk on toes (plantar flexion) and on heels (dorsiflexion of ankles).
	Test for proximal weakness.	Have patient hop on one foot or try a knee bend (standing on one foot). Can patient get out of chair without using arms?

TABLE 4.4. Muscle Strength Grading.

Score	Strength
0	No movement
1	Flicker of contraction
2	Full range of motion with gravity eliminated
3	Full range of motion against gravity
4	Full range of motion against gravity and some resistance
5	Full power

TABLE 4.5. Deep Tendon Reflex Grading.

Score	Reflex
0	Absent
1	Hypoactive
2	Normal
3	Hyperactive with spread across a joint
4	Hyperactive with clonus

SCREENING EXAM FOR SENSATION (TABLE 4.6)

1. Check pain (or temperature) sensation in the hands and feet.
2. Check vibration (or joint position sense) in the hands and feet.
3. Check light touch on arms and legs, looking for asymmetry.

Be familiar with dermatomal patterns.

Imaging Basics

After you have conducted a complete neurologic exam, you should theoretically be able to localize a lesion in the nervous system. However, modern neurology increasingly relies on imaging for confirmation and diagnostic purposes. You will thus be a step ahead if you are familiar with the basic imaging modalities used in neurology before you start your rotation. But remember, nothing can replace a complete neurologic exam!

The two modalities used most in neurology are CT and MRI (see Figure 4.1). Both modalities have their advantages and disadvantages, and each is indicated under different circumstances. Always identify what type of image you are looking at before trying to interpret it; otherwise, you may run into some trouble.

TABLE 4.6. Sensory Exam.

What You're Testing	What You're Looking For	What You're Doing
Sensory Modalities—Seeking to identify a pattern of sensory loss/disruption		
Pain	Ability/inability to identify "sharp"	Pricking with a safety pin or a Q-tip stick broken in half.
Temperature	Ability/inability to identify "cold"	Touching with cool tuning fork.
Vibration	Ability/inability to identify "buzz"	Buzzing tuning fork touched to bone and joint.
Joint position sense	Ability to sense direction of motion	Moving patient's finger or toe up or down.
		Romberg test: Stand with feet together and eyes closed for 10 seconds. If patient is okay with eyes open but not closed, test is positive.
Light touch	Ability/inability to identify touch	Lightly touch patient with finger or cotton.
Higher Sensory Function—Deficits in the discriminative sensations, testing cortical/peripheral		
Graphesthesia	Ability to recognize object by feeling	Ask patient to identify object in hand without seeing it, such as a paper clip, or to identify heads/tails of a coin.
Point localization	Ability to localize sensory input	Quickly touch patient, then ask to identify location.
Extinction	Ability to recognize dual, bilateral stimuli	Touch same areas bilaterally and ask patient to identify location of stimulus.

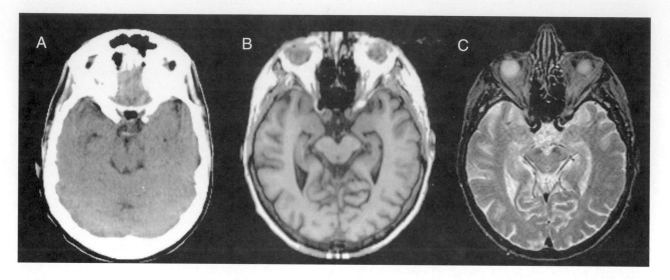

FIGURE 4.1. The three major types of brain images you can expect to see on your neurology rotation are (A) CT, (B) T1 MRI, and (C) T2 MRI. (Images courtesy of the UCLA Laboratory of Neuroimaging.)

COMPUTED TOMOGRAPHY

CT scans are basically three-dimensional x-rays. The images show high-attenuation (white) bony structures surrounding the brain and often show a darker (low attenuation) cortical ribbon surrounding the white matter; cerebrospinal fluid (CSF) appears black. CT image quality is generally considered inferior to MRI. Even so, there are specific circumstances in which CT is far more useful than MRI, including the following:

- **Suspected skull fracture:** Because CT uses x-rays for imaging, bone abnormalities are easily discerned. Bone cannot be imaged using MRI.
- **Suspected intracranial bleeds:** Acute bleeds appear white on CT scans within 20 minutes of their onset. CT is especially useful in suspected subarachnoid bleeds (e.g., ruptured aneurysms), looking for blood around the cerebral peduncles. Blood takes hours to appear on MRI.
- **Trauma:** CT is safer than MRI in a trauma setting, when a patient may have metallic implants, fragments, or pacemakers in the body. In addition, when time is of the essence, CT is preferable to MRI.
- **Monitoring hydrocephalus:** The ventricles are relatively large structures. Therefore, the monitoring of increased ventricle size (hydrocephalus) does not require high-resolution imaging. The cheaper and faster imaging modality (CT) is thus preferred.

MAGNETIC RESONANCE IMAGING

MRI uses a combination of magnetic field and radio-frequency (RF) waves to produce images. Different timing sequences and RF waves can be used to produce different types of MRI images. You should know the two major types of MRI: T1 and T2. However, don't worry about what T1 and T2 mean from a physics perspective. Instead, be able to recognize both types and know what each can tell you about the brain.

- **T1:** T1 images look like what you expect the brain to look like: Gray matter is darker, white matter is lighter, and CSF is clear (i.e., it does not produce any signal). Remember, bone does not produce an MRI signal. In general, T1 images are used for studying the anatomy of the brain. Pathology may also be appreciated in these images as lighter or darker areas, but such areas will not be very pronounced. Also, the spatial extent of pathology is often underestimated by T1 imaging. Gadolinium enhancement can be used to increase resolution of certain pathological processes.
- **T2:** T2 images are almost the inverse of T1: Gray matter is lighter, white matter is darker, and CSF appears white. Unlike T1 images, pathology in T2 images will stand out (as bright white). Pathology appears white owing to edema and water accumulation in the area of pathology. Note that both edema and CSF have a large water component, and therefore both appear white. T2 is study of choice for identifying pathology.

Diffusion-weighted imaging (DWI) is a specific T2 sequence with which you should be familiar. DWI is used in suspected cases of acute stroke to determine if an ischemic event is occurring in the brain. As expected, the ischemic area appears white. DWI is especially useful because it reveals ischemic areas within minutes of onset.

CONTRAST

CT and MRI studies will often be ordered with contrast. Adding contrast to a study will tell you whether the blood-brain barrier (BBB) has been compromised. If the BBB is interrupted, contrast will "leak" into the brain and enhance the signal from that region. This tells the clinician about the severity of the condition and can increase the resolution of a study. Iodinated contrast agents are used for CT contrast and gadolinium is used for MRI contrast.

Lumbar Puncture Results

One of the unique procedures and laboratory results you may encounter in your neurology rotation is the LP. As you read through this chapter, you will notice that in many cases an LP may be ordered to narrow the differential. It will be important for you to be able to recognize CSF patterns in order to discern different disease processes. Table 4.7 provides CSF profiles for different neurologic diseases you may encounter.

TABLE 4.7. CSF Profiles.

	RBC (per mm^3)	WBC (per mm^3)	Glucose (mg/dL)	Protein (mg/dL)	Opening Pressure (cmH$_2$O)	Appearance	Gamma Globulin (% protein)
Normal	< 10	< 5	~2/3 of serum	15–45	10–20	Clear	3–12
Bacterial meningitis	↔	↑ (PMN)	↓	↑	↑	Cloudy	↔ or ↑
Viral meningitis	↔	↑ (mono)	↔	↔ or ↑	↔ or ↑	Most often clear	↔ or ↑
Subarachnoid hemorrhage	↑↑	↑	↔	↑	↔ or ↑	Yellow/Red	↔ or ↑
GBS	↔	↔	↔ or ↑	↑↑	↔	Clear or yellow (high protein)	↔
Multiple sclerosis	↔	↔ or ↑	↔	↔	↔	Clear	↑↑
Pseudotumor cerebri	↔	↔	↔	↔	↑↑↑	Clear	↔

Aphasias

Aphasia is a general term used to describe language disorders. There are eight main types of aphasias, so it is important to determine the type your patient has. The two principal aphasias with which you should be familiar are Broca's and Wernicke's (Figure 4.2). An overview of the different aphasias is presented in Table 4.8.

Aphasias generally result from insults (strokes, tumors, abscesses, etc.) to the language centers in the "dominant hemisphere." The left hemisphere is dominant in 90% of right-handed people and in 50% of left-handed people. In order to fully characterize an aphasia, you must assess the patient's language abilities in three domains: production, comprehension, and repetition. Reading and writing are other aspects of language you may want to evaluate.

BROCA'S APHASIA

*Broca's is **B**roken speech.*

Broca's aphasia is an expressive aphasia; it is a disorder of language production and repetition without a deficit in comprehension. Features include the following:

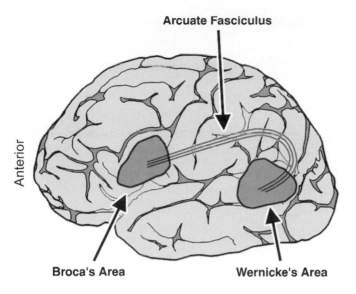

Arcuate Fasciculus

Broca's Area

Wernicke's Area

Anterior

FIGURE 4.2. Broca's and Wernicke's areas are the two major language centers in the brain. The arcuate fasciculus connects these two areas. Injury to the arcuate fasciculus results in language repetition errors.

TABLE 4.8. Summary of Aphasias.

Aphasia	Fluency	Compre-hension	Repetition	Naming	Reading	Writing	Lesion Localization
Broca's	↓	Normal	↓	↓	↓	↓	Posterior inferior frontal gyrus
Wernicke's	Normal	↓	↓	↓	↓	↓	Posterior superior temporal lobe
Conduction	Normal	Normal	↓	↓	Normal	↓	Arcuate fasciculus
Global	↓	↓	↓	↓	↓	↓	Large portion of left hemisphere
Transcortical motor	↓	Normal	Normal	Mildly ↓	Normal	↓	Anterior/ middle border zone
Transcortical sensory	Normal	↓	Normal	↓	↓	↓	Posterior/ middle border zone

- Speech is nonfluent, with decreased rate, short phrase length, and impaired articulation.
- Repetition is impaired.
- Comprehension is intact. Patients are noticeably frustrated with their speech because they are aware of their deficit.
- Associated features include arm and face hemiparesis, hemisensory loss, and apraxia of oral muscles due to the proximity of Broca's area (posterior inferior frontal gyrus) to the motor and sensory strips (the pre- and postcentral gyri, respectively).
- The lesion is often secondary to a superior middle cerebral artery (MCA) stroke.

Treatment. In addition to treating the underlying pathology, speech therapy is indicated.

WERNICKE'S APHASIA

*Wernicke's is **Wordy** but makes no sense.*

Wernicke's aphasia is a receptive aphasia; it is a disorder of language comprehension and repetition without a deficit in language production. Its features include the following:

- Speech is fluent but empty of meaning.
- Comprehension, naming, and repetition are impaired, with frequent use of marked neologisms (made up words) and paraphasic errors (word substitutions).
- No notable hemiparesis or dysarthria is present.
- Patients are often unaware of their deficit because they lack comprehension.
- The lesion is often in the left posterior superior temporal lobe perisylvian) secondary to left inferior MCA stroke.

Treatment. In addition to treatment of the underlying etiology, speech therapy is indicated, although it is not as successful as is the case for Broca's aphasia.

TRANSCORTICAL APHASIAS

Transcortical motor aphasia and transcortical sensory aphasia are marked by impaired language motor output (production deficit) and impaired language "sensation" (comprehension deficit), respectively. Both are distinct from Broca's and Wernicke's aphasias in that repetition remains intact.

CONDUCTION APHASIA

A conduction aphasia is a subtle aphasia that can be easily missed because both language production and comprehension remain intact, but language repetition is impaired.

GLOBAL APHASIA

A global aphasia is, as the name implies, a global deficit of language production, comprehension, and repetition. It is the most serious and devastating of all the aphasias and is associated with the most widespread insult to the brain. It also carries the worst prognosis.

Coma

Coma is a profound suppression of responses to external and internal stimuli. Coma can be caused either by catastrophic structural injury to the CNS or by diffuse metabolic dysfunction that severely depresses consciousness.

The severity of coma is measured by the Glasgow Coma Scale (GCS), which consists of three parts: motor responses, verbal responses, and eye opening (see Table 4.9). The initial GCS score is a very good predictor of coma outcomes; those with a GCS of 3 or 4 have approximately 95% mortality at one month. Remember, however, that coma etiology is the best predictor of coma outcomes (see below). While coma secondary to drug overdose is associated with 5–10% mortality, coma secondary to anoxia carries a 90% mortality. Another factor that influences outcome is patient age: The younger the patient, the better the prognosis.

Determining coma etiology is critical in that it is the best predictor of outcomes.

Etiology. Insults that lead to coma must be (1) bilateral hemispheric insults, (2) bilateral thalamic insults, or (3) brain stem/reticular activating system insults. It is important to detect supratentorial processes in order to prevent potential herniation and compression of the midbrain and brain stem. Supratentorial processes include hemorrhage (epidural, subdural, or intraparenchymal), infarction, abscesses, and tumors. Infratentorial lesions include hemorrhages of the pons, cerebellum, or posterior fossa; vertebrobasilar strokes; and tumors of the brain stem or cerebellum. Infratentorial masses require prompt evacuation due to impending compression of and damage to the brain stem.

Other diffuse processes that depress consciousness are endogenous disturbances in electrolyte, endocrine, or metabolic function; exogenous toxins

TABLE 4.9. Glasgow Coma Scale.

Verbal Response (5 points)		Eye Opening (4 points)		Motor Response (6 points)	
Oriented	5	Spontaneous	4	Follows commands	6
Confused	4	To voice	3	Localizes	5
Inappropriate words	3	To painful stimulus	2	Withdraws	4
Incomprehensible	2	No eye opening	1	Flexion (decorticate)	3
No response	1			Extension (decerebrate)	2
				No response	1

such as medications, ethanol, and other drugs; infectious or inflammatory disease; subarachnoid blood; and generalized seizure activity or postictal states.

Collateral history may be key to understanding coma etiology. In the history, the temporal progression from alert to comatose yields valuable information. Onset may be sudden, as in brain stem infarctions or subarachnoid hemorrhage (SAH); initially focal but rapidly progressive, as in intracerebral hemorrhage; or subacute, as in tumor, abscess, or subdural hematoma. Structural lesions may initially present with focal neurologic deficits. Diffuse processes such as metabolic or drug intoxication are more likely to present without focal signs.

Differential. Patients with an apparent decrease in level of consciousness may actually be awake. This may be the case with patients who are catatonic, hysterical, "locked in," or in a persistent vegetative state. Locked-in patients are awake and alert but are unable to move anything but their eyes and eyelids. Locked-in states are associated with central pontine myelinolysis, brain stem stroke, and advanced amyotrophic lateral sclerosis (ALS). A patient in a persistent vegetative state appears to have normal wake-sleep cycles but is completely unaware of self or the environment. The most common causes are trauma with diffuse cortical injury or hypoxic ischemic injury.

Reactive pupils in a patient with absent oculocephalic reflexes cannot be truly localized and point to a toxic/metabolic insult.

Workup. The evaluation of the comatose patient initially involves careful history and examination. Further evaluation requires testing of primitive brain stem reflexes, including pupillary light reflex, corneal reflex, oculocephalic reflex, and hot/cold calorics. Absence or asymmetry of reflexes can help localize the lesion and elucidate coma etiology. For example, reactive pupils in a patient with absent oculocephalic reflexes cannot be truly localized and point to a toxic/metabolic insult.

A normal pupillary light reflex is said to occur when the pupils constrict symmetrically to light shone into either eye. A normal corneal reflex occurs when both eyes blink in response to corneal irritation (usually with a Q-tip or a cotton swab). A normal oculocephalic reflex (or "doll's eye" reflex) occurs when the eyes consistently look forward with lateral head rotation such that they move in the direction opposite to head motion. Finally, the normal response to cold-water infusion in an ear is to induce nystagmus in the opposite direction (fast-phase opposite). Note that nystagmus is always described in the direction of the fast phase. To help you remember the normal caloric response, remember the mnemonic "COWS." Also look closely at the size of the pupils. Are they symmetric? A "blown pupil" may be a sign of ipsilateral uncal herniation.

Normal eye deviations to caloric stimulation—

COWS
Cold
Opposite
Warm
Same

Respiratory patterns should also be noted. Patterns include:

- **Cheyne-Stokes:** A crescendo-decrescendo pattern due to bilateral hemisphere dysfunction.
- **Central neurogenic hyperventilation:** Rapid deep breathing due to mesencephalon damage.

- **Apneustic breathing:** Prolonged inspiration with subsequent apnea due to pontine dysfunction.
- **Ataxic breathing:** Irregular breathing due to medullary dysfunction.

Treatment. Treatment consists of the following measures:

1. **Stabilize the patient:** Attend to **ABCs: A**irway, **B**reathing, and **C**irculation.
2. **Reverse the reversible:** Administer **DON'T: D**extrose, **O**xygen, **N**aloxone, and **T**hiamine.
3. **Localize the lesion:** This requires that structural and diffuse processes be differentiated.
   - Labs should be sent to check glucose and electrolytes. In addition, a toxicology screen (for alcohol, drugs of abuse), liver function tests (LFTs), blood urea nitrogen (BUN), creatinine, prothrombin time/partial thromboplastin time (PT/PTT), CBC, arterial blood gases (ABGs), blood cultures (if sepsis is suspected), and an LP (if CNS infection is suspected) should be ordered.
   - A CT scan is indicated, particularly if a structural lesion, trauma, or SAH is suspected.
   - The physical exam should check for vital signs, trauma, nuchal rigidity, and funduscopic changes.
4. **Prevent further damage:** This requires recognition of the progressive and/or treatable etiologies of coma. A few things to look for include the following:
   - Signs of herniation can be managed by decreasing intracranial pressure and/or surgical decompression. It is important to detect supratentorial processes early on and to follow neurologic changes vigilantly.
   - Signs of meningitis include fever and nuchal rigidity; patients with possible meningitis should receive IV antibiotics immediately and an LP within four hours.
   - Signs of SAH warrant emergent CT and LP.
   - Seizure activity should be considered and treated if verified by clinical findings or EEG.
   - Trauma may suggest cervical spine injury and may warrant cervical x-rays and/or a CT.

After the emergent conditions listed above have been attended to or excluded, management can shift to the treatment of metabolic disturbances and further investigation, if indicated, by ECG, CXR, toxicology screens, and EEG.

Delirium and Dementia

Differentiating between delirium and dementia can be challenging. Although both conditions reflect a so-called altered mental status (AMS) and a global decrease in cognition, delirium and dementia differ in terms of their etiologies, their time course, and the cognitive domains affected. Delirium and dementia are compared in tabular format in Table 4.10.

DELIRIUM

Delirium is an acute change in mental status that is usually most pronounced in the domains of attention, concentration, orientation, and perception. Symptoms may include hallucinations, delusions, and persecutory thoughts. Delirium often has a waxing and waning course. The elderly are at particular risk for delirium secondary to medical illness, polypharmacy, and preexisting dementia. Urinary tract infection (UTI) and pneumonia are among the most common causes of delirium in the elderly. Other predisposing factors include unfamiliar surroundings, sleep deprivation, sensory deprivation, or sensory overload. Delirium is associated with a 40% one-year mortality rate.

Etiologies. Delirium may have multiple etiologies. A mnemonic with which to remember the major etiologies is "MOVE STUPID." Remember, however, that any medical condition can cause delirium in a susceptible patient. The more common etiologies are provided in Table 4.11.

Workup. The most important part of a delirium workup is a thorough history of the days leading up to the episode, including the presence of fevers, chills, nausea, vomiting, bowel movements, nutrition, drugs (including prescription and alcohol), and recent illnesses. Pay particular attention to signs of infection or dehydration. Consider chronic medical conditions that may make the patient more susceptible to delirium (including dementia!).

The examination should pay close attention to vital signs and to the complete neurologic exam. Labs must include electrolytes (including calcium), CBC

> **Causes of delirium—**
>
> **MOVE STUPID**
> **M**etabolic
> **O**xygen
> **V**ascular
> **E**ndocrine/
>   **E**lectrolytes
> **S**eizures
> **T**umor/**T**rauma/
>   **T**emperature
> **U**remia
> **P**sychogenic
> **I**nfection/
>   **I**ntoxication
> **D**rugs/
>   **D**egenerative
>   diseases

TABLE 4.10. Differentiating Dementia.

	Dementia	Delirium
Hallmark feature	Memory loss	Fluctuating orientation
Level of arousal	Normal	Stupor or agitation
Development	Slow and insidious	Rapid
Reversibility	Often irreversible	Frequently reversible
Other comments		Brain damage predisposes
		Most common in children and elderly
		Course fluctuates; duration brief

TABLE 4.11. Common Causes of Delirium.	
Type of Insult	**Example**
Metabolic	Hepatic encephalopathy
	Thiamine deficiency
	Hypoglycemia
Oxygen	Hypoxia/hypercarbia
Vascular	MI
	Anemia
Endocrine/Electrolytes	Hyponatremia
	Hypercalcemia
	Fluid imbalance
	Hyper-hypothyroidism
Seizures	Ictal
	Postictal
Tumor/Trauma/Temperature	
Uremia	
Psychogenic	
Infection	UTI
	Pneumonia
	Meningitis
	Sepsis
Intoxication	Alcohol
	Benzodiazepines
	Carbon monoxide
	Barbiturates
	Hallucinogens
	Opioids
Drugs/Degenerative diseases	

with differential (to rule out infection), and urinalysis (UA, to rule out UTI). Labs to consider include ABGs (to rule out hypoxia), ECG (to rule out MI), CXR (to rule out TB, CHF, etc.), urine toxicology, LFTs (to rule out hepatic encephalopathy), thyroid function tests (TFTs), EEG (to rule out seizures), rapid plasma reagin (RPR) or VDRL, LP (to rule out meningitis), and serum B_{12} and folate (to rule out vitamin deficiencies and malnutrition). CT and MRI should be performed (1) if head trauma or CNS pathology is suspected *after* lab work is done and is found to be noncontributory to a medical diagnosis, or (2) if there is a high index of suspicion of CNS pathology.

Treatment. Always treat the underlying cause of delirium. Normalize fluid and electrolyte status, and provide an appropriate sensory environment (windows and light). In addition, use nonsedating antipsychotics (e.g., haloperidol) for agitation but not in alcohol withdrawal; avoid benzodiazepines for sedation, as they will worsen most patients' symptoms (except in the setting of alcohol withdrawal, when benzodiazepines are clearly indicated).

DEMENTIA

Dementia represents a chronic, progressive, global decline in multiple cognitive areas. All dementia patients have a disturbance in memory (amnesia) that affects both short- and long-term memory. Other cognitive deficits include aphasia (language disturbance), apraxia (inability to execute commands), agnosia (disruption of recognition), and disturbances in executive function (e.g., abstraction).

Etiology. The most common etiology of dementia is Alzheimer's disease (AD), which accounts for 70–80% of cases. A useful mnemonic for etiologies is "DEMENTIAS." Be careful not to mistake inattentiveness for a cognitive decline.

Workup. The standard initial workup includes CBC, electrolytes (including calcium), glucose, BUN/creatinine, LFTs, TFTs, B_{12} levels, and RPR or VDRL. Neuroimaging (CT or MRI) is also indicated at some point to identify specific patterns of brain atrophy consistent with a particular etiology. Other tests to consider, although not indicated in all patients, include LP, erythrocyte sedimentation rate (ESR), folate, HIV, CXR, UA, 24-hour urine for heavy metals, and urine toxicology.

Treatment. Treatment is etiology specific. In general, measures should be taken to reduce further insult to the brain by avoiding toxic agents, normalizing diets, and treating any underlying disease that may be exacerbating the dementia. Many believe that therapies designed specifically for AD, including antioxidants (vitamin E and selegiline) and cholinesterase inhibitors (donepezil [Aricept], galantamine) may benefit other dementia victims. Avoid benzodiazepines, as they will often exacerbate disinhibition and confusion. The newer atypical antipsychotics (e.g., risperidone) are safer to use for agitation. It is also important to treat any associated depression.

ALZHEIMER'S DISEASE

Alzheimer's Disease is the most common cause of dementia, and age is the most important risk factor. Other risk factors include female gender, family history, Down syndrome, and low educational level. Pathology includes neurofibrillary tangles, neuritic plaques with amyloid deposition, amyloid angiopathy, and neuronal loss.

Signs and Symptoms. Amnesia is the first sign of AD and includes inability to acquire new information and difficulty recalling remote memories. Subsequent cognitive deficits include aphasias (word-finding and naming difficulties), acalculia, depression, agitation, and apraxia. Survival is approximately five to ten years from the onset of symptoms. Death is usually secondary to aspiration pneumonia or other infections.

The 5 A's of dementia—

Amnesia
Aphasia
Agnosia
Apraxia
Abstract thought disturbances.

DEMENTIAS—

Degenerative diseases (Parkinson's, Huntington's, Pick's, Lewy body)
Endocrine (thyroid, parathyroid, pituitary-adrenal axis)
Metabolic (alcohol, fluid electrolytes, B_{12}, glucose, hepatic, renal, Wilson's disease)
Exogenous (heavy metals, carbon monoxide, drugs)
Neoplasm
Trauma (subdural hematoma)
Infection (meningitis, encephalitis, abscess, endocarditis, HIV, syphilis, prions, Lyme disease)
Affective disorders (pseudodementia secondary to depression)
Stroke/**S**tructure (multi-infarct [vascular] dementia, ischemia, vasculitis, normal pressure hydrocephalus)

Workup. AD is a clinical diagnosis of exclusion; only on autopsy can it be definitively diagnosed. However, a number of neurobehavioral and neuropsychological tests can be ordered to identify patients' specific cognitive deficits. Neuroimaging, especially positron-emission tomography (PET), is increasingly being used to determine specific patterns of hypometabolism that may be highly sensitive and specific for diagnosing AD.

Treatment. Donepezil (Aricept) is first-line therapy. Vitamin E (α-tocopherol) and selegiline, both of which are antioxidants, have been shown to slow cognitive decline.

Dysequilibrium

It is not uncommon for a patient to present to the ER with complaints of feeling "dizzy." Dizziness is a vague term that may signify a number of phenomena, including light-headedness (as one might feel after standing up rapidly from a reclining position), loss of balance, or vertigo (a spinning sensation). Through the history, determine what the patient actually means by "dizziness." Pay particular attention to the duration of the "dizzy spells" (i.e., seconds vs. minutes vs. hours) and the precipitating events.

Equilibrium is maintained through the input of visual, vestibular, and proprioceptive sensory systems and through processing by the cerebellum and brain stem. Dysequilibrium manifests clinically as vertigo or ataxia (incoordination without weakness of voluntary movement of eyes, speech, gait, trunk, or extremities) and can be localized along this axis. The first step to take is to determine if the process is peripheral (dysfunction of the labyrinthine structure or the vestibular nerve) or central (brain stem or cerebellar processes, such as stroke, tumor, or MS).

The most common cause of peripheral dysequilibrium (responsible for 50% of cases) is benign paroxysmal positional vertigo (BPPV). BPPV is marked by brief spells of vertigo triggered by changes in head position and is caused by loose debris within the posterior canal of the inner ear. Other causes of vertigo that you will be expected to know are Ménière's disease (intermittent vertigo due to dilation and periodic rupture of the endolymphatic compartment of the inner ear) and acoustic neuroma (or vestibular schwannoma).

Signs and Symptoms. Peripheral and central vertigo are compared and further discussed in Tables 4.12 and 4.13. The intrinsic brain stem signs cited in Table 4.12 refer to signs such as ataxia, dysarthria, cranial nerve abnormalities, and motor system dysfunction.

Workup. In the neuro exam, be sure to focus on the patient's stance and gait, checking his or her ability to stand still with eyes closed (Romberg's sign) and to march in place. A patient with a cerebellar lesion will be unable to stand still; a patient with a vestibular lesion will often turn or fall in the ipsilateral direction. Also check for nystagmus, paying close attention to direction and

Vertical nystagmus is pathognomonic for a central lesion.

TABLE 4.12. Central vs. Peripheral Dysequilibrium.

	Peripheral	Central
Vertigo	Often intermittent; severe	Often constant; usually less severe
Nystagmus	Always present; unidirectional, never vertical	May be absent, uni- or bidirectional; may be vertical
Associated findings		
Hearing loss or tinnitus	Often present	Rarely present
Intrinsic brain stem signs	Absent	Often present

character. In addition, test for dysmetria, checking finger-to-nose and heel-to-shin coordination; this should be unimpaired in peripheral processes. Don't ignore the rest of the neuro exam. The general exam should carefully rule out other cranial nerve deficits, motor weakness, orthostasis, cardiac arrhythmia, and ear canal occlusions.

Specific testing includes positional testing with the Dix-Hallpike maneuver for BPPV, in which vertigo is elicited with a change in the patient's head position. This exam may elicit symptoms, produce nystagmus, and provide clear evidence of a peripheral lesion. Adjunctive testing to clarify the issue of peripheral versus central dysequilibrium could include an audiogram, brain stem auditory evoked responses (BAERs), and an electronystagmogram (ENG). An MRI should be done if the patient shows signs of central involvement or if a peripheral disturbance cannot be explained by a benign etiology. Other tests might include assessment of thyroid function, B_{12} level,

TABLE 4.13. Etiologies of Peripheral and Central Dysequilibrium.

Peripheral Vestibular Disorders	Acute Central Ataxias	Chronic Central Ataxias
Benign positional vertigo	Drug intoxication	MS
Ménière's disease	Wernicke's encephalopathy	Cerebellar degeneration
Acute peripheral vestibulopathy	Vertebrobasilar ischemia	Hypothyroidism
Otosclerosis	Vertebrobasilar infarction	Wilson's disease, Creutzfeldt-Jakob disease (CJD)
Cerebellopontine-angle tumor	Inflammatory disorders	Posterior fossa masses
Vestibulopathy/ acoustic neuropathy	Cerebellar hemorrhage	Ataxia-telangiectasia

and CSF for cells and oligoclonal bands (to rule out an infectious etiology and MS, respectively).

Treatment. Reducing the symptoms of vertigo may be achieved medicinally with antihistamines (especially meclizine), anticholinergics such as scopolamine, benzodiazepines, and sympathomimetics; these are appropriate in the treatment of benign conditions such as BPPV and Ménière's disease. BPPV can also be treated using repositioning exercises (e.g., the Dix-Hallpike maneuver), although the condition usually subsides spontaneously in weeks to months. Vestibulotoxic drugs such as quinidine, alcohol, and aspirin should be discontinued. When possible, the underlying disorder, such as thiamine deficiency or hypothyroidism, should be dealt with promptly.

Headache

Headaches afflict up to 90% of adults in the United States and represent one of the most common reasons patients seek medical attention. Primary headache is generally classified into three categories: migraine, tension, and cluster. However, headache may also be the presenting symptom of serious neurologic disease. It should therefore be taken seriously. It is your job to differentiate between benign and life-threatening causes.

Workup. There are four important questions that you should ask with regard to headache:

1. **Is this a new or an old headache?** You should ask if the patient has ever had a headache like this before. Is it qualitatively different from headaches he or she has had in the past? Does the patient describe it as the "worst headache of my life"? Any new, severe headache warrants an emergent workup and probably a CT (for "acute" causes of headaches listed below, especially SAH).

2. **What are the characteristics of the pain?** As with any other body pain, you should characterize the headache in terms of onset, duration, quality, location, and what makes it better or worse. Look for clues to differentiate between the three different categories of primary headaches.

3. **Are there any associated symptoms or a relevant past medical history?** Ask about fever, nausea, vomiting, weight loss, and jaw claudication. Also ask about a present and past medical history of cancer or immune compromise (e.g., HIV), since these factors make serious diagnoses more likely. Family history is also important, since migraines may run in families.

4. **Are there associated neurologic symptoms?** The thorough neurologic history and exam is crucial here to determine if the patient has either positive (paresthesias, visual stigmata) or negative (weakness, numbness, ataxia) symptoms. Make sure to ask the patient about photophobia, dizziness, neck stiffness, and a history of auras. A focal exam needs immediate workup.

Differential. The differential can be divided into the following categories:

- **Acute:** *SAH, hemorrhagic stroke, seizure,* meningitis, acute elevated intracranial pressure (ICP), hypertensive encephalopathy, post-LP (spinal headache), ocular disease (glaucoma, iritis), new migraine headache.
- **Subacute:** Temporal arteritis, *intracranial tumor, subdural hematoma,* pseudotumor cerebri, trigeminal/glossopharyngeal neuralgia, postherpetic neuralgia, hypertension.
- **Chronic/episodic:** *Migraine, cluster headache, tension headache,* sinusitis, dental disease, neck pain.

The "chronic/episodic" causes of headache listed in italics are discussed in more detail in the paragraphs that follow. Other causes of headache listed in italics, including intracranial hemorrhage, stroke, seizure, and intracranial tumors, are discussed in other sections.

MIGRAINE HEADACHE

Migraines afflict up to 18% of women (most commonly beginning before the age of 30) and 6% of men. Migraines tend to run in families, so be sure to ask about family history. The etiology is not fully understood; vascular abnormalities (such as intracranial vasoconstriction and extracranial vasodilation) are perhaps secondary to a disorder of serotonergic neurotransmission. Migraines are often precipitated by identifiable triggers, including the intake of certain foods (e.g., chocolate, caffeine), skipping meals, letdown from stress, menses, oral contraceptive use, and bright light.

Signs and Symptoms. The headache is usually throbbing, lasts between 2 and 20 hours, is often unilateral (although it may also be bilateral or occipital), and is associated with nausea and vomiting, photophobia, and noise sensitivity (see Figure 4.3). "Classic migraines" are preceded by a visual aura in the form of either scintillating scotomas (bright light or flashing lights, often in a zigzag pattern, moving across the visual field) or field cuts. Most migraines, however, are not associated with these symptoms and are considered "common migraines."

Workup. CT with contrast or MRI may be warranted on first presentation, especially if there are focal findings on examination (migraine itself can be associated with transient focal neurologic defects). Remember that subacute blood becomes isodense with brain after 2 to 14 days. MRI may therefore be the image modality of choice depending on history and time course.

Treatment. There are two types of therapy: abortive and prophylactic. Abortive therapy seeks to end the headache once it has started and is most effective when a reliable prodrome can be identified. The earlier abortive therapy is initiated in the course of the migraine, the more effective the therapy will be at blunting the symptoms. Abortive therapy includes aspirin/NSAIDs, sumatriptan and other $5HT_1$ agonists, ergots (partial $5HT_1$ agonists), and,

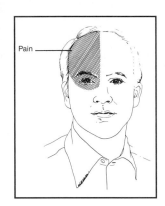

FIGURE 4.3. Pain in migraine headache is most commonly hemicranial. Pain can also be holocephalic, bifrontal, or unilateral frontal. (Reprinted, with permission, from Aminoff MJ et al. *Clinical Neurology,* 3rd ed. Stamford, CT: Appleton & Lange, 1996:91.)

rarely, opiates. For patients with severe and frequent migraines, prophylaxis is indicated, including propranolol (beta blockers), verapamil (calcium-channel blockers), amitriptyline (tricyclic antidepressants [TCAs]), and valproic acid (anticonvulsants). Narcotics should not be used prophylactically. Patients should also be advised to avoid known triggers, have consistent sleep and dietary patterns, and get regular exercise.

CLUSTER HEADACHE

Cluster headaches affect approximately 1% of the population and are seen more often in men than in women. Cluster headaches are much less common than migraines. The average age of onset is 25.

Signs and Symptoms. Cluster headache is a brief, severe, unilateral, periorbital headache lasting 30 minutes to three hours (see Figure 4.4). Attacks tend to occur in clusters (hence the name), affect the same part of the head, and take place at the same time of day (usually at night) and at the same time of the year. Associated symptoms include ipsilateral tearing of the eye and conjunctival injection, Horner's syndrome, and nasal stuffiness. Cluster headache may be precipitated by alcohol intake or vasodilators.

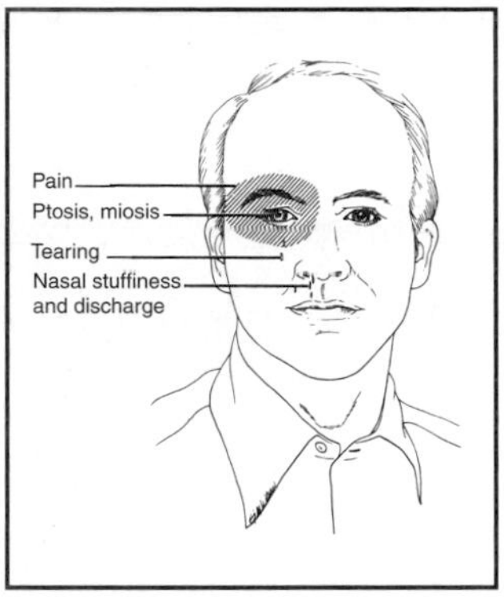

Workup. No workup is necessary if the presentation is classic. However, imaging is often necessary to rule out a more catastrophic cause of this exceptionally painful syndrome (especially with initial presentation).

Treatment. Cluster headache treatment also includes both abortive and prophylactic therapy. Cluster headaches are relieved acutely by 100% oxygen, sumatriptan, ergots, intranasal lidocaine, and corticosteroids. Prophylactic therapy includes calcium-channel blockers, ergots, valproic acid, prednisone, topiramate, and methysergide.

FIGURE 4.4. Distribution of pain in cluster headache. Pain is commonly associated with ipsilateral conjunctival injection, tearing, nasal stuffiness, and Horner's syndrome. (Reprinted, with permission, from Aminoff MJ et al. *Clinical Neurology*, 3rd ed., Stamford, CT: Appleton & Lange, 1996:92.)

TENSION HEADACHE

Tension headaches, which account for 75% of all headaches, are chronic headaches that do not share the specific symptomatology of migraines. Tension headaches are a diagnosis of exclusion, with the diagnosis made once other etiologies have been ruled out.

Signs and Symptoms. Patients complain of a tight, bandlike pain that is exacerbated by noise, bright lights, fatigue, and stress. Patients also report other nonspecific symptoms, such as anxiety, poor concentration, and difficulty sleeping. Headaches are generalized but may be most intense in the occipital or neck region. The surrounding musculature may also be tightly contracted. If a history of nausea and vomiting, photophobia, or family history is elicited, migraine headache is the more likely diagnosis. Many patients appear to have an overlap syndrome with components of both migraine and tension headaches.

Workup. Tension headaches are a diagnosis of exclusion. Other causes of headache must first be considered. There are no focal neurologic signs in tension headache. Headache diaries are helpful in delineating triggers and evaluating treatment trials.

Treatment. Relaxation, massage, hot baths, regular diet, exercise, and avoidance of exacerbating factors may alleviate symptoms. Abortive medications are generally restricted to NSAIDs, although triptans and ergots may be considered. Prophylactic therapy includes TCAs and selective serotonin reuptake inhibitors (SSRIs) as well as calcium-channel blockers and beta blockers. Analgesic overuse should be avoided as this can precipitate an analgesic rebound headache syndrome.

Intracranial Hemorrhages

SUBARACHNOID HEMORRHAGE

Subarachnoid hemorrhage is commonly caused by a ruptured aneurysm (e.g., berry, hypertensive), an arteriovenous malformation (AVM), or trauma to the circle of Willis (often at the MCA). Berry aneurysms are the most common cause and are associated with polycystic kidney disease and coarctation of the aorta (see Figure 4.5). SAH typically occurs at 50 to 60 years of age and has a high mortality rate (35%). Ruptured aneurysms are reported to have a 50% one-month mortality rate.

Signs and Symptoms. SAH is characterized by a sudden-onset, intensely painful headache, often with neck stiffness and other signs of meningeal irri-

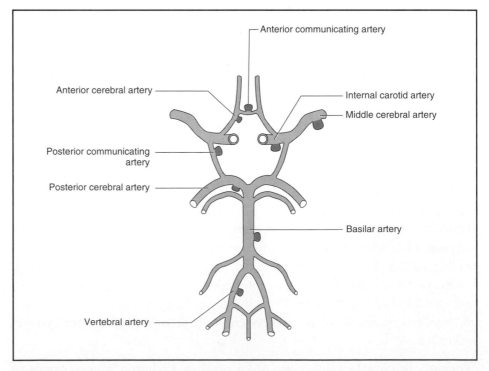

FIGURE 4.5. Frequency distribution of intracranial aneurysms. (Reprinted, with permission, from Aminoff MJ et al. *Clinical Neurology*, 3rd ed., Stamford, CT: Appleton & Lange, 1996:77.)

tation, along with fever, nausea, vomiting, and a fluctuating level of consciousness. SAH may be preceded by "sentinel headaches" in the weeks prior to hemorrhage. Seizure may result from blood irritating the cortex. Third-nerve palsy with pupil involvement is associated with berry aneurysms on the posterior communicating artery. There may be other neurologic deficits or a decreased level of consciousness, or the examination may be normal.

Differential. The differential includes hemorrhagic stroke, trauma, meningitis, and first presentation of migraine headache.

Workup. Workup should include an emergent head CT without contrast, looking for blood in the subarachnoid space, especially around the circle of Willis. Blood appears white on noncontrast CT (see Figure 4.6). If there is a high index of suspicion for SAH but the head CT is negative, obtain an immediate LP to look for red cells (must be in consecutive tubes to rule out traumatic tap), xanthochromia, and elevated ICP. Four-vessel angiography should be performed once SAH has been confirmed to look for an aneurysm.

Treatment. Treatment focuses on preventing rebleeding, which is most likely to occur in the first 48 hours after SAH. Measures include lowering ICP by raising the head of the bed, administering IV fluids and calcium-channel blockers (nimodipine) to prevent vasospasm, treating hypertension, and administering antiseizure medication (phenytoin). Surgical treatment involves open or interventional radiologic clipping or coiling of an aneurysm or AVM.

Complications. The mass effect of a large AVM or aneurysm impinging on brain parenchyma may also cause neurologic deficits. As alluded to above, vasospasm in the first week after SAH is the most common cause of ischemic in-

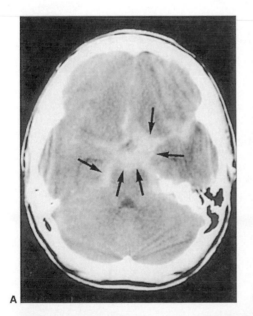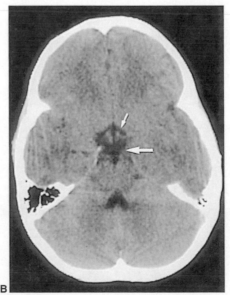

FIGURE 4.6. Head CT scans. (A) Acute SAH. Areas of high density (arrows) represent blood in the subarachnoid space. (B) A normal scan; note the interpeduncular cistern (large arrow) and suprasellar cistern (small arrow). (Reprinted, with permission, from Aminoff MJ et al. *Clinical Neurology,* 3rd ed., Stamford, CT: Appleton & Lange, 1996:78.)

jury to the brain after SAH. Finally, be aware of possible obstructive hydrocephalus secondary to intraventricular blood obstructing CSF drainage or interfering with CSF absorption through the arachnoid granulations.

EPIDURAL HEMATOMA

Epidural hemorrhages are generally traumatic and of arterial origin. They are associated with lateral skull fracture due to blunt trauma with resultant tear of the middle meningeal artery.

Signs and Symptoms. Patients present with a lucid interval ranging from several minutes to hours followed by the onset of headache, progressive obtundation, and hemiparesis. Ultimately, epidural bleeding may lead to a "blown pupil" in which the pupil becomes fixed and dilated; this usually occurs secondary to uncal herniation and compression of CN III.

Workup. CT shows a lens-shaped, convex hyperdensity that is usually limited by the sutures of the cranium where the dura inserts onto the bone (see Figure 4.7). Patients require urgent neurosurgical intervention and intensive monitoring.

Treatment. Treatment consists of emergent neurosurgical evacuation.

A

B

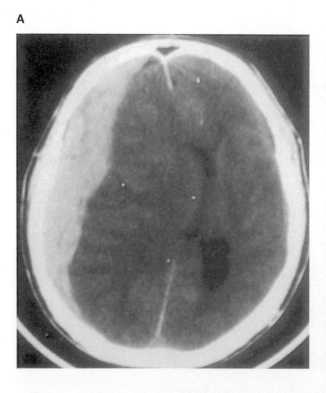 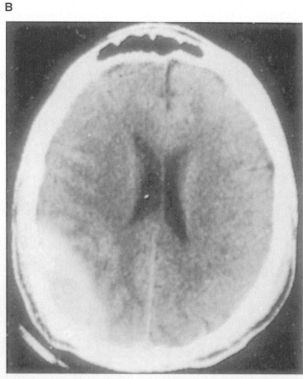

FIGURE 4.7. Head CT scans. (A) Subdural hematoma. Note the crescent shape and the mass effect with midline shift. (B) Epidural hematoma with classic biconvex lens shape. (Reprinted, with permission, from Aminoff MJ et al., *Clinical Neurology*, 3rd ed., Stamford, CT: Appleton & Lange, 1996:296.)

SUBDURAL HEMORRHAGE

Subdural hematoma is typically a result of trauma secondary to rupture of bridging veins from the cortex to the dural sinuses. Subdural hemorrhage is often seen in the elderly and alcoholics, who have significant cortical atrophy that places the bridging veins under tension.

Signs and Symptoms. Signs and symptoms include headache, change in mental status, contralateral hemiparesis, or other focal deficits. Changes can be either subacute or chronic and may present as a new-onset dementia or mental status change. There may be a remote history of a fall.

Workup. CT with and without contrast or MRI demonstrates a crescent-shaped, concave fluid collection, with density depending on the age of the bleed (see Figure 4.7). In some cases, a hematocrit line may be observed where the RBCs have settled down and separated from the plasma.

Treatment. Treatment requires surgical evacuation if the patient is symptomatic; otherwise, just observe. Subdural blood will frequently regress spontaneously.

INTRAPARENCHYMAL HEMORRHAGE

The etiologies of intraparenchymal hemorrhage include hypertension (usually in the basal ganglia), amyloid angiopathy (seen in the elderly), and vascular malformations (AVMs, cavernous hemangiomas). Note that AVMs are more likely to produce an intraparenchymal hemorrhage than an SAH.

Signs and Symptoms. Patients will often present with lethargy and headache. The physical exam may be significant for focal motor or sensory deficits. If a patient presents with hemiparesis or hemianesthesia, a hemorrhagic stroke of the posterior internal capsule should be considered.

Workup. Emergent head CT without contrast reveals an intraparenchymal hemorrhage. Be sure to look for mass effect or edema that may predict herniation.

Treatment. Treatment is similar to that of SAH: Raise the head of the bed, institute seizure prophylaxis, and monitor for and try to prevent ischemic damage secondary to vasospasm. Surgical evacuation may be necessary and lifesaving if a mass effect is observed or if the hemorrhage occurs in the posterior fossa, thereby threatening vital brain stem function.

Intracranial Neoplasms

Intracranial neoplasms may be primary (30%) or metastatic (70%). The most frequently reported primary tumors include meningiomas and glioblastoma multiforme (GBM) in adults and medulloblastomas and astrocytomas in children. Of all primary brain tumors, 40% are benign. Men are more likely than women to have GBM, and women are more likely than men to have meningiomas. In general, benign disease affects those over 65 years old. While two-thirds of primary brain tumors in adults are supratentorial, only one-third are supratentorial in children. Primary tumors rarely spread beyond the CNS. The most common primary neoplasms and their respective presentations and treatments are presented in Table 4.14.

Metastatic tumors to the brain most commonly arise from breast, lung, kidney, and GI tract neoplasms and from melanoma. They most often occur supratentorially, appear at the gray-white junction, and are characterized by rapid growth, invasiveness, necrosis, and neovascularization. When multiple discrete neoplastic nodules appear in the brain simultaneously, metastatic disease should be suspected and a primary source should be sought.

TABLE 4.14. Most Common Primary Neoplasms.

Tumor	Presentation	Treatment
Astrocytoma	Presents with headache and increased ICP May cause unilateral paralysis in CN V-VII and X Slow, protracted course Prognosis much better than that of glioblastoma multiforme	Resection if possible; Radiation
Glioblastoma multiforme (grade IV astrocytoma)	Most common primary brain tumor Often presents with headache and increased ICP Progresses rapidly Poor prognosis (< 1 year from the time of prognosis)	Surgical removal/resection; Radiation and chemotherapy have variable results
Meningioma	Originates from dura mater or arachnoid Good prognosis Incidence increases with age	Surgical resection Radiation for unresectable tumors
Acoustic neuroma (schwannoma)	Presents with ipsilateral hearing loss, tinnitus, vertigo, and signs of cerebellar dysfunction Derived from Schwann cells	Surgical removal
Medulloblastoma	Common in children Arises from fourth ventricle and leads to increased ICP Highly malignant; may seed subarachnoid space	Surgical resection coupled with radiation and chemotherapy
Ependymoma	Common in children May arise from ependyma of a ventricle (commonly the fourth) or the spinal cord; may lead to hydrocephalus	Surgical resection; Radiation

Signs and Symptoms. Symptoms usually develop gradually. Patients often complain of persistent vomiting and headache or focal neurologic deficits. Other common symptoms include personality changes, lethargy, intellectual decline, aphasias, seizures, and mood swings. Only 30% of patients present with headache. When present, headache is typically dull and steady, worse in the morning, associated with nausea and vomiting, and exacerbated by coughing, changing position, or exertion. Symptomatology is due to local growth and resulting mass effect, cerebral edema, ventricular obstruction, and increased ICP.

Workup. Workup should include CT with contrast and MRI with gadolinium to localize and determine the extent of the lesion. Histologic diagnosis may be obtained via CT-guided biopsy or during surgical tumor debulking, although the most likely diagnosis may be evident by tumor morphology and location.

Treatment. Management depends on tumor type. Some types (e.g., benign meningioma) can be observed or cured with resection. Low-grade primary CNS tumors can be cured with resection, radiation therapy, and/or chemotherapy. Other types (e.g., GBM) may be poorly responsive and require palliative care.

Movement Disorders

Movement disorders can be classified as hyperkinetic or hypokinetic, meaning that there is either too much movement or significantly decreased movement. Three commonly seen movement disorders are Parkinson's disease (PD), Huntington's disease (HD), and MS.

PARKINSON'S DISEASE

Parkinsonism is a hypokinetic syndrome characterized by tremor, rigidity, bradykinesia, and abnormal gait and posture (see Figure 4.8). There are many etiologies of parkinsonism that may be indistinguishable clinically. The most common cause of parkinsonism is idiopathic degeneration of the dopaminergic nigrostriatal tract with a resulting imbalance between dopamine and acetylcholine. Idiopathic parkinsonism is called Parkinson's disease (PD). The usual age of onset of PD is about 60. PD has a prevalence of 100–200/100,000 and an annual incidence of roughly 20/100,000. Life expectancy from the time of diagnosis is approximately nine years.

Other insults that decrease dopaminergic activity can lead to parkinsonism, including postencephalitic, toxic (e.g., carbon disulfide, manganese, "designer drugs" such as MPTP), bihemispheric ischemic, traumatic, and iatrogenic (especially neuroleptic) insults.

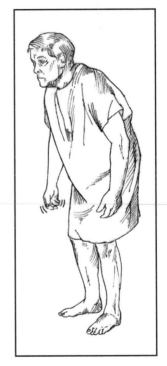

FIGURE 4.8. Patient with parkinsonism in typical flexed posture. Note the masklike facies and resting hand tremor. (Reprinted, with permission, from Aminoff MJ et al *Clinical Neurology*, 3rd ed., Stamford, CT: Appleton & Lange, 1996:220.)

Signs and Symptoms. The "Parkinson's tetrad" consists of the following:

1. Resting tremor (especially coarse "pill-rolling" tremor of the hands, but may affect all extremities, the head, and the trunk) is one of the earliest symptoms.
2. Rigidity is noted as increased resistance to passive range of motion. "Cogwheeling" is a phenomenon attributable to the combined effects of rigidity and tremor.
3. Bradykinesia, which literally means slowed *(brady)* movements *(kinesia)*. Bradykinesia encompasses both slowed movements and difficulty initiating movements. Patient also exhibit a typical shuffling, festinating gait (wide leg stance with short accelerating steps) without arm swing.
4. Postural instability (e.g., stooped posture, impaired righting reflexes, freezing, falls).

Mild dementia (subcortical in etiology) is common as well but typically is not profound. Other telltale signs include masked facies and decreased amplitude of movements (seen in micrographia and hypophonia).

Differential. It is important to consider treatable causes of tremors, psychomotor slowing, and instability, such as depression, normal pressure hydrocephalus, and Wilson's disease. Also consider Parkinson's-plus syndromes, which are distinguished from idiopathic PD by the presence of additional prominent neurologic abnormalities. Syndromes to consider in this context include progressive supranuclear palsy (PSP), cortical-basal ganglionic degeneration (CBGD), and multiple-system atrophy (MSA). Other conditions to include in the differential are CJD, Shy-Drager syndrome, and HD.

Treatment. Treatment for parkinsonism should seek to improve the balance between dopamine and acetylcholine by increasing dopaminergic tone with agonists such as levodopa and bromocriptine; decreasing dopamine-antagonizing neuroleptics; or decreasing acetylcholine with anticholinergic medications (e.g., benztropine [Cogentin]). Amantadine may also be useful as well for tremor, although the mechanism is unknown. Some studies have shown that other dopamine agonists (pramipexole [Mirapex]) can be used as an adjunct to levadopa or as a sole therapy early in the disease. Surgical management may be helpful in intractable cases; pallidotomy has reemerged as a potentially important treatment, as has chronic deep brain stimulation of the subthalamic nucleus.

HUNTINGTON'S DISEASE

Huntington's disease is a hyperkinetic disease and is a rare autosomal-dominant condition involving multiple abnormal CAG triplet repeats on chromosome 4p. The number of repeats can expand from generation to generation, causing earlier expression and more severe disease in subsequent generations through a process known as anticipation. Fewer than 29 CAG repeats are considered normal, while mutant genes generally have greater than 39 repeats (there is a gray area in between). The disease is invariably fatal, with death often occurring within 20 years of diagnosis.

Signs and Symptoms. HD usually presents in patients 30 to 50 years of age with a gradual onset of chorea, altered behavior, and dementia. Early motor symptoms of rigidity and stiffness give way to prominent choreiform activity. Patients are often highly cognizant of these movements and try to incorporate them into their normal movements so as to disguise them. Dementia begins as irritability, moodiness, and antisocial behavior. This develops into schizophreniform illness and depression.

Differential. Tic disorders (including Tourette's syndrome), senile chorea, hemiballismus, Wilson's disease, and PD should be considered in the differential.

Workup. Diagnosis is made on a clinical basis. CT scans and MRI show cerebral atrophy (especially of the striatum, which includes the caudate and putamen). Molecular genetic testing is also available to determine the number of CAG repeats in the gene.

Treatment. There is no cure for HD, and disease progression cannot be halted. However, symptomatic therapy can improve quality of life. Haloperidol can be used for the treatment of psychosis, and reserpine can minimize unwanted movements. Antidepressants can be used to treat depression. Finally, benzodiazepines can be used to treat symptoms of anxiety. Genetic counseling should be offered to offspring with special attention given to the social aspects of the disease.

MULTIPLE SCLEROSIS

Multiple sclerosis is a hypokinetic disease and is an autoimmune demyelinating disorder of the CNS that is most likely T-cell mediated. MS has a female-to-male ratio of 2:1, shows a peak incidence at 20 to 40 years of age, and is thought to have a genetic component. The incidence of MS increases with increased distance from the equator; those who move before the age of 15 inherit the susceptibility of the new geographic location, while those who move after the age of 15 retain the risk that characterizes the geographic area in which they grew up. The prevalence ranges from 50 to 150 per 100,000. These geographic differences have led some to hypothesize that MS may be triggered by a viral infection. The clinical course of MS is variable.

The types of MS, in order of decreasing frequency, are relapsing-remitting, secondary progressive, primary progressive, and progressive-relapsing. The type of MS that is ultimately diagnosed offers the best prognostic indicator. The best prognosis is conferred on those with a relapsing-remitting course with discrete exacerbations, full recovery of function after each episode, and an early age of onset of the initial attack. The Kurtzke five-year rule states that the absence of significant motor or cerebellar dysfunction five years after diagnosis correlates with limited disability at 15 years. Fifteen years after diagnosis, approximately 20% of MS patients have no functional limitation; 70%

are limited or are unable to perform major activities of daily living, and 75% are not employed. Morbidity and mortality are related to the accumulation of physical disabilities due to incomplete recovery from sequential attacks.

Signs and Symptoms. Patients present with neurologic complaints that are separated in time and space and cannot be explained by a single lesion. The most common presentations include limb weakness, visual loss, paresthesias, diplopia, urinary retention, and vertigo. Signs of MS are abundant, since the disease can affect any white-matter region of the CNS. However, one should look in particular for optic pallor or atrophy, medial longitudinal fasciculus lesions (in patients with strabismus, specifically internuclear ophthalmoplegia), dysarthria, pain, and extremity weakness and spasticity. Lhermitte's sign appears in some MS patients and presents as an electrical sensation running down the spine and into the lower extremities with neck flexion. Neurologic symptoms can wax and wane or may be progressive. A history of a separate neurologic attack must often be extracted from the patient, since patients may not initially make a connection between different episodes. Exacerbating factors include infection, heat, trauma, the postpartum period, and vigorous activity. Pregnancy, by contrast, is often associated with a decreased frequency of exacerbations. The risk of UTI may also increase in this population secondary to bladder hypotonia.

Differential. CNS tumors or trauma, multiple CVAs, vasculitis, vitamin B_{12} deficiency, CNS infections (Lyme disease, neurosyphilis), sarcoidosis, and atypical presentations of other autoimmune diseases (e.g., systemic lupus erythematosus [SLE] and Sjögren's syndrome) must be considered.

Workup. In order to make a clinically definitive diagnosis of MS, one must identify the following:

- Two attacks and clinical evidence of two separate lesions, or
- Two attacks with clinical evidence of one lesion and laboratory evidence of another lesion

Laboratory tests include MRI; visual, somatosensory, or brain stem evoked potentials; and spinal fluid analysis. MRI reveals multiple, asymmetric, often periventricular lesions in white matter, called "plaques." Corpus callosum lesions are virtually pathognomonic. Active lesions enhance with gadolinium on MRI. Spinal fluid analysis may show mononuclear pleocytosis (> 5 cells/μL) in 25% of cases, elevated free kappa light chains in 60% of cases, elevated CSF IgG in 80% of cases, and oligoclonal bands in 90% of cases (nonspecific).

Treatment. Although there is no cure for MS, immunomodulatory and immunosuppressive treatments modify the course of relapsing-remitting disease. Immunomodulators include **ABC: A**vonex (β-interferon, interferon-1a), **B**etaseron (β-interferon, interferon-1b), and **C**opaxone (copolymer 1). All these agents can decrease the number of relapses by 30% while also mitigating the severity of the relapses that occur. Steroids should be given during acute exacerbations. Finally, MS patients may benefit greatly from physical therapy and symptomatic treatment of spasticity, pain, fatigue, and depression.

MS treatment is as easy as ABC—

Avonex
Betaseron
Copaxone

Seizures

Seizures are cortical events that are characterized by excessive or hypersynchronous discharge by cortical neurons. The etiology of seizure is multifactorial, depending on a fine balance between (1) seizure threshold, (2) the presence of an epileptogenic focus, and (3) a precipitating factor or provocative event. A change in any of these factors can increase the frequency of seizures. For example, a primary nervous system disorder may induce an epileptogenic focus that has a lower seizure threshold than "healthy tissue." Alternatively, systemic diseases or disturbances can lead to altered seizure threshold. The term *epilepsy* describes the predisposition to recurrent, unprovoked seizures (not everyone with seizures has epilepsy!). Most seizures are self-limited and last less than two minutes; prolonged or repetitive seizures are called "status epilepticus" and constitute a medical emergency.

Not everyone with seizures has epilepsy.

Some definitions related to seizures are essential:

- **Partial (focal) seizures** are seizures arising from a discrete region of one cerebral hemisphere; they can be categorized as simple or complex. Simple seizures do not involve a loss of consciousness; complex seizures cause a loss of consciousness.
- **Generalized seizures** are seizures involving both cerebral hemispheres, with loss of consciousness.

The evaluation and treatment of a patient with a recent history of seizure should seek to answer the following questions:

1. **Did the patient actually have a seizure?** A syncopal event with post-syncopal jerking can easily be confused with a seizure. You should also distinguish pseudoseizures (psychogenic) from true seizures (electrical). Serum prolactin levels are elevated after true tonic-clonic seizures but are unaffected by pseudoseizures. In taking a history from the patient and from observers, ask about possible prodromes, onset, course, and postseizure period (see Table 4.15).

   Tonic-clonic movements do not exclude syncope.

2. **Was the seizure provoked by a systemic process?** It is important to consider the systemic causes of seizure in the workup. If there is a clear, treatable, non-neurologic cause, further neurologic investigation may be unnecessary. Such disorders include hypoglycemia or hyperglycemia, hyponatremia, hypocalcemia, hyperosmolar states, hepatic encephalopathy, uremia, porphyria, drug overdose (especially cocaine, antidepressants, neuroleptics, methylxanthines, and lidocaine), drug withdrawal (especially alcohol and other sedatives), eclampsia, hyperthermia, hypertensive encephalopathy, and cerebral hypoperfusion. Workup should focus on reversible causes and provocative factors first.

3. **Was the seizure caused by an underlying neurologic disorder?** Patients without a known cause for their seizures should undergo neurologic evaluation, particularly for treatable causes (Table 4.16). Seizures with focal onset (or focal postictal deficit) suggest focal CNS pathol-

   Workup should focus on reversible causes of seizure first.

TABLE 4.15. Seizure Versus Syncope.

	Seizure	Syncope
Onset	Sudden onset without prodrome Focal sensory or motor phenomena Sensation of fear, smell, memory	Progressive light-headedness Dimming of vision, faintness
Course	Sudden loss of consciousness (LOC) with tonic-clonic activity May last 1–2 minutes May see tongue laceration, head trauma, and bowel/urinary incontinence	Gradual LOC, limp or with jerking Rarely lasts longer than 15 seconds Less commonly injured
Postspell	Postictal confusion and disorientation; typically immediate return to lucidity	

ogy. Seizures may be the presenting sign of a tumor, stroke, AVM, infection, or hemorrhage, or they may represent the delayed presentation of a developmental abnormality. The history should include past seizures, birth/childhood or recent trauma, and developmental delays. For both treatment and prognosis, it is important to try to determine the etiology. In a patient with a known seizure disorder, you must ask the question, "Why did this seizure occur?" and consider subtherapeutic levels of medications or a new factor, such as infection or trauma.

4. **Is anticonvulsant therapy indicated?** Patients with a first seizure are frequently not treated when the underlying cause is unknown. However, one-third of idiopathic seizures will recur. Recurrence rates are higher in patients with abnormal EEGs or MRIs, with focal exams, and with irreversible predisposing factors (see Figure 4.9).

PARTIAL (OR FOCAL) SEIZURES

Focal seizures arise from a discrete region in one cerebral hemisphere. Such seizures may, however, generalize to involve both hemispheres. Partial seizures are divided into simple and complex seizures.

TABLE 4.16. Common Etiologies of Seizures by Age.

Infant	Child (2–10)	Adolescent	Adult (18–35)	Adult (35+)
Perinatal injury/ ischemia	Idiopathic	Idiopathic	Trauma	Trauma
Infection	Infection	Trauma	Alcoholism	Stroke
Metabolic disturbance	Trauma	Drug withdrawal	Brain tumor	Metabolic disorders
Congenital/genetic disorders	Febrile seizure	AVM	Drug withdrawal	Alcoholism

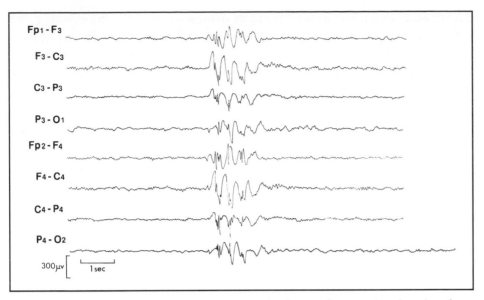

FIGURE 4.9. EEG in idiopathic seizures. Note the burst of generalized epileptiform activity on a relatively normal background. (Reprinted, with permission, from Aminoff MJ et al. *Clinical Neurology*, 3rd ed., Stamford, CT: Appleton & Lange, 1996:241.)

Signs and Symptoms.

- **Simple partial seizures:** The clinical effects of focal seizures depend on the region of the cortex that is affected. Seizure foci in the motor or sensory areas (the frontal or parietal lobes, respectively) cause simple partial seizures and may lead to phenomena such as twitching of the face or tingling of the hand. Involvement of the insular cortex can result in autonomic phenomena such as alterations in blood pressure, heart rate, and peripheral vascular resistance as well as bronchoconstriction.
- **Complex partial seizures:** Involvement of the temporal lobe or medial frontal lobe leads to complex partial seizures, with effects such as memories (déjà vu), feelings of fear, and "complex" actions such as lip smacking or walking.

Postictally, there may be a focal neurologic deficit known as Todd's paralysis that resolves over one to two days and often indicates a focal brain lesion. Todd's paralysis is often confused with acute stroke and can be differentiated by MRI (DWI) imaging.

Differential. When a partial seizure is suspected, consider TIAs, panic attacks, and pseudoseizures as possible diagnoses.

Workup. Perform a detailed neurologic exam. The standard seizure workup includes CBC, electrolytes, calcium, glucose, ABGs, LFTs, a renal panel, RPR, ESR, and a tox screen to rule out systemic causes. Diagnostic tests such as an EEG are often ordered as well to look for epileptiform waveforms and to confirm epileptiform seizures. Rule out a mass by MRI or CT with contrast. MRI is more sensitive and specific in seizure evaluations.

Treatment. Treatment should consist of management of the underlying cause if feasible. Otherwise, phenytoin (Dilantin), carbamazepine (Tegretol), phenobarbital, valproate (Depakote), lamotrigine (Lamictal), or gabapentin (Neurontin) can be administered. In children, phenobarbital is the first-line anticonvulsant. For intractable temporal lobe seizures, surgical options include anterior temporal lobectomy. Prior to surgery, patients undergo Wada testing in which sodium amytal, a brain-numbing agent, is injected into the anterior temporal lobe (via the middle cerebral artery) to determine if there would be a functional deficit associated with the resection.

GENERALIZED SEIZURES

The two most common types of generalized seizures are absence (petit mal) and tonic-clonic (grand mal).

ABSENCE (PETIT MAL) SEIZURES

Absence seizures begin in childhood, are often familial, and typically subside before adulthood.

Signs and Symptoms. Absence seizures are characterized by brief, often unnoticeable episodes of impaired consciousness lasting only seconds and occurring up to hundreds of times per day. There is no loss of muscle tone and no memory of these events. Eye fluttering or lip smacking during absence seizures is common.

Workup. The EEG shows a classic 3-per-second spike-and-wave tracing (see Figure 4.10).

Treatment. Ethosuximide is the first-line agent. Valproic acid or zonisamide may also be used.

TONIC-CLONIC (GRAND MAL) SEIZURES

Signs and Symptoms. Tonic-clonic seizures begin suddenly with loss of consciousness and tonic extension of the back and extremities, continuing with one to two minutes of repetitive, symmetric clonic movements. Seizures are marked by incontinence and tongue biting. Patients may also appear cyanotic during the ictal period owing to poor respiratory function during the seizure. Consciousness is slowly regained in the postictal period. Postictally, the patient may complain of muscle aches and headaches.

Differential. The differential for complex seizures includes syncope, cardiac dysrhythmias, brain stem ischemia, and pseudoseizures.

Treatment. Treatment consists of management of the underlying cause. Otherwise, valproate, phenytoin, and carbamazepine are first-line anticonvulsant therapies. The choice of anticonvulsant depends on EEG, MRI data, and careful history.

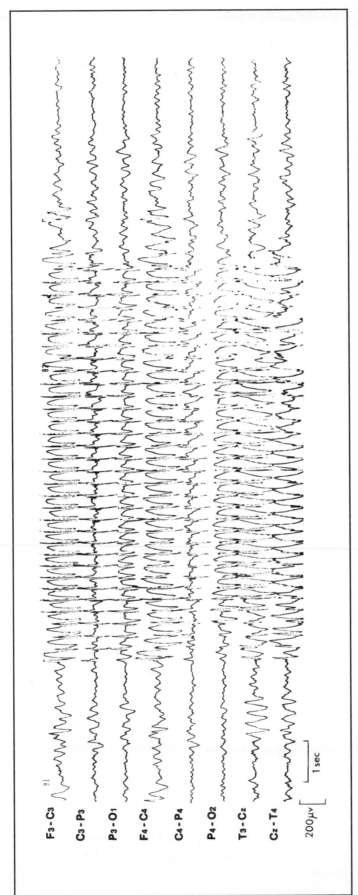

FIGURE 4.10. EEG of absence seizures with the classical 3-spikes-per-second pattern. (Reprinted, with permission, from Aminoff MJ et al., *Clinical Neurology*, 3rd ed., Stamford, CT: Appleton & Lange, 1996:240.)

Neurology

STATUS EPILEPTICUS

Status epilepticus is characterized by prolonged (> 30-minute) or repetitive seizures without a return to baseline consciousness in between. The seizure can be either convulsive or nonconvulsive (a distinction that can be made only by EEG). Common causes include anticonvulsant withdrawal/noncompliance, EtOH/sedative withdrawal or other drug intoxication, metabolic disturbances, trauma, and infection. Although the definition of status epilepticus is a duration greater than 30 minutes, most clinicians start treating status epilepticus after two to three minutes of seizure activity, since brain damage will begin after this short period of time. Status epilepticus is associated with a 20% mortality rate.

Workup. First, protect the airway. Then, check oxygen saturation, CBC, electrolytes, calcium, glucose, ABGs, LFTs, renal panel, ESR, and tox screen.

KEY POINT

EMERGENCY EVALUATION OF STATUS EPILEPTICUS

Treatment with anticonvulsants should be instituted immediately (Table 4.17) while the following measures are taken:

- Check vital signs:
  - **Blood pressure:** Exclude hypertensive encephalopathy and shock.
  - **Temperature:** Exclude hyperthermia.
  - **Pulse:** Exclude life-threatening cardiac arrhythmia with cardiac monitor.
- Draw venous blood for serum glucose, calcium, electrolytes, hepatic and renal function blood studies, CBC, ESR, toxicology, and PT/PTT (in case LP is necessary).

- Insert an IV line.
- Administer glucose (25–50 mL of 50% dextrose) intravenously and thiamine (100 mg).
- Obtain any available history.
- Perform a rapid physical examination, especially for:
  - Signs of trauma
  - Signs of meningeal irritation or systemic infection
  - Papilledema
  - Focal neurologic signs
  - Evidence of metastatic, hepatic, or renal disease
- Obtain ABGs.
- Perform an LP unless the cause of seizures has already been determined or if signs of increased ICP or focal neurologic signs are present (after CT has been done and coagulation studies have been drawn).

- Obtain an ECG.
- Calculate serum osmolality: ≈2 (serum sodium concentration) + serum glucose/20 + serum urea nitrogen/3 (normal range: 270–290).
- Obtain a urine sample for toxicology.

EEG and brain imaging should be deferred until the patient is stabilized. Perform LP in the setting of fever or meningeal signs (only after having done a CT to ensure the safety of the LP).

Treatment. Treatment consists of the following measures:

- On admission, attend to cardiopulmonary status (ABCs).
- Give thiamine (100 mg) and glucose (50 mL of 50% dextrose).
- Give lorazepam (Ativan) at a rate of 2 mg/min up to a total of 6–8 mg.
- Administer a loading dose of phenytoin (50 mg/min) or fos-phenytoin (100–150 mg/min) if available. Begin with a 1-gram loading dose of phenytoin (see Table 4.17).
- If seizures continue, intubate and add IV phenobarbital (at the same dose and rate as phenytoin—first 18 mg/kg, then 7 mg/kg). If the patient fails therapy, admit to the ICU and treat with an IV anesthetic such as midazolam.

TABLE 4.17. Drug Treatment of Status Epilepticus.

Drug	Dosage/Route	Advantages/Disadvantages/Complications
Lorazepam[a] or diazepam	10 mg IV over 2 minutes. 0.1 mg/kg IV rate ≤ 2 mg/min.	Fast-acting. Effective half-life 15 minutes for diazepam and 4 hours for lorazepam. Abrupt respiratory depression or hypotension occurs in 5% of patients, especially when given in combination with other sedatives. Seizure recurrence affects 50% of patients; therefore, one must add maintenance drug (phenytoin or phenobarbital).
Immediately proceed to phenytoin.		
Phenytoin or fos-phenytoin	1000–1500 mg (18 mg/kg), IV rate ≤ 50 mg/min (cannot be given in dextrose solution). Fos-phenytoin at 100–150 mg/min.	Little or no respiratory depression. Drug levels in the brain are therapeutic at the completion of infusion. Effective as maintenance drug. Hypotension and cardiac arrhythmias can occur, probably more often with phenytoin than with fos-phenytoin.
If seizures continue following total dose, proceed immediately to phenobarbital.		
Phenobarbital	1000–1500 mg (18 mg/kg) IV slowly (50 mg/min).	Peak brain levels within 30 minutes. Effective as maintenance drug. Respiratory depression and hypotension common at higher doses. (Intubation and ventilatory support should be immediately available.)
If above is ineffective, proceed immediately to general anesthesia.		
Pentobarbital or midazolam[a]	15 mg/kg IV slowly, followed by 0.5–4 mg/kg/h. 0.2 mg/kg IV slowly, followed by 0.75–10 mg/kg/min.	Intubation and ventilatory support required. Hypotension is limiting factor. Pressors may be required to maintain blood pressure.

[a]Investigational in the United States.

Stroke is a clinical syndrome defined by the acute onset of a focal neurologic deficit as a result of a disturbance in blood flow. The disturbance in blood flow can be either ischemic (85%) or hemorrhagic (15%). A stroke that does not resolve symptomatically is referred to as a cerebrovascular accident. If the deficit reverses within 24 hours, the event is renamed a transient ischemic attack. However, TIA symptoms generally reverse in roughly one hour. TIAs also significantly increase the risk of future stroke.

The workup of stroke is intimately related to the risk factors and common etiologies of stroke. It is therefore essential that you have a good understanding of the epidemiology, risk factors, and causes of "brain attacks."

The risk of stroke increases with age (doubling for every decade over 55), is higher for men than for women, and is higher for African-Americans and Hispanic-Americans than for Caucasians. Intracranial vascular disease is particularly common among Asians. The most important modifiable risk factors for stroke are hypertension and DM. Other modifiable risk factors include smoking, hypercholesterolemia, carotid stenosis, atrial fibrillation, and heavy alcohol intake. Cocaine and IV drug use are also risk factors, particularly in young people.

The most common cause of ischemic stroke is atherothrombosis of the large extracranial vessels (internal and common carotids, basilar and vertebral arteries) and subsequent embolus, which accounts for 35% of all strokes and roughly 40% of ischemic strokes. Lacunar infarcts (the source of 20% of all strokes) occur in regions supplied by small perforating vessels and result from either atherosclerotic or hypertensive occlusion. Other causes include fibromuscular dysplasia, inflammatory diseases, arterial dissection, migraine, and venous thrombosis. Look for lacunar infarcts in the basal ganglia and internal capsules (due to small vessel disease).

Cardiac causes of stroke include atrial fibrillation (the most common cause of cardioembolic stroke) as well as embolism of mural thrombi, thrombi from diseased or prosthetic valves, other arrhythmias, endocarditis (septic, fungal, or marantic emboli), and paradoxic (venous) emboli in patients with right-to-left shunt in the heart (from atrial septal defect or patent foramen ovale). Patients with atrial fibrillation have a five- to sixfold greater risk of stroke than the general population.

Hemorrhagic strokes are far less common than ischemic strokes.

Hematologic disorders implicated in stroke include sickle-cell disease, polycythemia, thrombocytosis, leukocytosis, and other hypercoagulable states (such as those seen in malignancy, hereditary coagulopathies, or collagen vascular diseases).

Intraparenchymal hemorrhage tends to result from hypertensive rupture of small vessels, AVMs, hemorrhage conversion of ischemic strokes, amyloid angiopathy, cocaine use, and bleeding diatheses.

Signs and Symptoms. Remember that the specific signs and symptoms of stroke depend on the location of the stroke; different vascular territories will have different presentations (see Table 4.18). Classically, thrombotic strokes evolve over minutes to hours and may be preceded by TIAs. By contrast, embolic strokes may present with full deficit acutely and do not evolve, while hemorrhagic strokes may be preceded by headache and altered mental status and may have deficits that do not comply with strict vascular territories (although these rules are much too general to be definitive). In all cases, however, one should look for the source of the stroke. A complete physical exam is warranted, with special attention paid to certain key areas. On physical exam, listen carefully to the heart and to the carotid and subclavian arteries, looking specifically for signs of arrhythmias (especially atrial fibrillation) and atherosclerotic disease (bruits). Remember though that the preserve of bruits is not very sensitive for carotid stenosis.

Differential. Todd's paralysis (postictal), subdural or epidural hematoma, brain abscess, brain tumor, MS, metabolic abnormalities, neurosyphilis, and conversion disorder should be considered.

TABLE 4.18. Stroke Sites and Resulting Neurologic Deficits.

Vessel	Region Supplied	Neurologic Deficit
Anterior Circulation		
Middle cerebral (MCA)	Lateral cerebral hemisphere; deep subcortical structures	See deficits of superior/inferior divisions combined; may see coma/symptoms of increased ICP.
Superior division	Motor/sensory cortex of face, arm, hand; Broca's area	Contralateral (CL) hemiparesis of face, arm, and hand; expressive aphasia and hand; expressive aphasia if dominant hemisphere.
Inferior division	Parietal lobe (visual radiations, Wernicke's area), macular visual cortex	Homonymous hemianopsia, receptive aphasia (dominant), impaired cortical sensory functions, gaze preference, apraxias, and neglect.
Anterior cerebral (ACA)	Parasagittal cerebral cortex	CL leg paresis and sensory loss.
Ophthalmic artery	Retina	Monocular blindness.
Posterior circulation		
Posterior cerebral (PCA)	Occipital lobe, thalamus, rostral midbrain, medial temporal lobes	CL homonymous hemianopsia, memory or sensory disturbances.
Basilar	Ventral midbrain, brain stem, postlimb internal capsule, cerebellum, PCA distribution	Coma, cranial nerve palsies, apnea, cardiovascular instability.
Deep circulation		
Lenticulostriate, paramedian, thalamo-perforate, circumferential arteries	Basal ganglia, pons, thalamus, internal capsule, cerebellum	"Lacunes." Pure motor or sensory deficits, ataxic hemiparesis, "dysarthria—clumsy hand" syndrome.

Workup. The workup of a stroke patient seeks to localize the lesion, distinguish between ischemic and hemorrhagic stroke, rule out other lesions, and determine the etiology of the stroke. Remember that the goals of a workup are to determine if ischemic stroke can be reversed within three hours using tissue plasminogen activator (tPA) to salvage ischemic brain, and to prevent further strokes from occurring. Studies include the following:

- CT without contrast to differentiate ischemic from hemorrhagic stroke (see Figure 4.11).
- MRI to identify early ischemic changes (use DWI and the fluid attenuation inversion recovery [FLAIR] sequence to differentiate new from old ischemic regions, respectively), to identify neoplasms, and to adequately image the brain stem and posterior fossa.
- CBC, glucose, coagulation panel, lipid panel, ESR, and hemoglobin A_{1c}.
- ECG; also an echocardiogram if the etiology is suspected to be embolic (transesophageal echo is most sensitive for mural thrombi).
- Vascular studies for extracranial disease by carotid ultrasound; magnetic resonance angiography (MRA) (CT angiography) or traditional angiography looking for intracranial disease.
- Blood cultures; screening for hypercoagulable states (if there is a history of bleeding, this is the first stroke, or the patient is under 50 years of age).

Treatment. Treatment consists of the following measures:

- Reperfusion, neuroprotection, and salvage are the primary goals.
- Antiplatelet agents such as aspirin, clopidogrel (Plavix), and dipyridamole/aspirin are the mainstays of treatment for small-vessel (lacunar) ischemic stroke.
- Heparin and warfarin are used for cardioembolic strokes to prevent further embolization. Hemorrhagic stroke must be ruled out before anticoagulant therapy is initiated. The target INR is 2–3 when Warfarin therapy is initiated.
- Vigilance should be maintained for symptoms or signs of brain swelling, increased ICP, or herniation.
- Avoid hypotension, hypoxemia, and hypoglycemia. Systolic blood pressure (SBP) should generally be maintained approximately 20 mmHg above the patient's normal SBP. The last thing you want to do is starve the brain after it has gone through an ischemic period. It is especially important to maintain blood pressure to ensure adequate cerebral perfusion in light of imminent increases in ICP and possible vasospasm in the first week after hemorrhage.
- Revascularization of thrombotic disease using tPA should be instituted within three hours of ischemia onset. This three-hour period is measured from the last time the patient is confirmed to have been "well." Many people who receive tPA undergo hemorrhagic conversion and may suffer a worse fate. Overall, however, tPA therapy administered in the first three hours improves outcomes. Contraindications to tPA therapy include SBP > 185 or diastolic blood pressure (DBP) > 110 despite aggressive antihypertensive therapy, prior intracranial hemorrhage,

Know the contraindications to thrombolytic therapy.

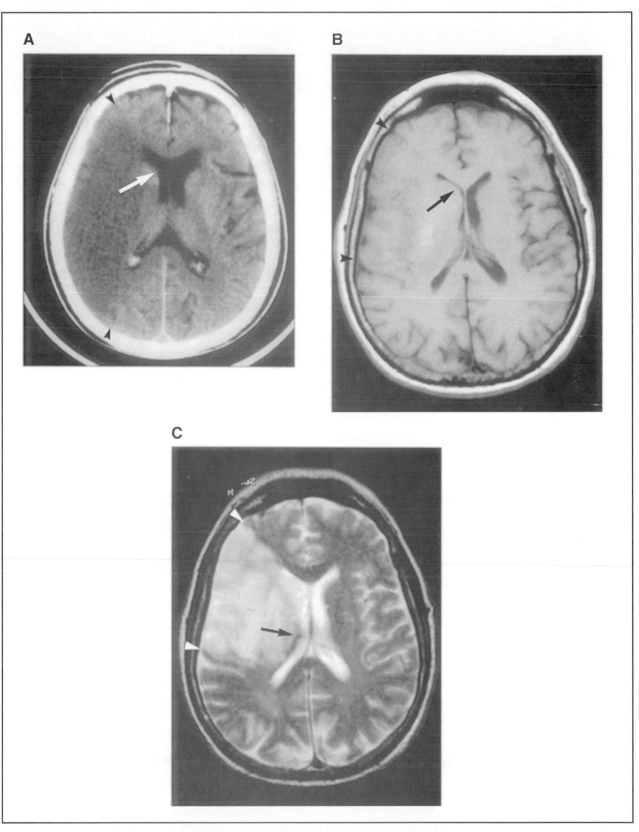

FIGURE 4.11. CT-MRI findings in ischemic stroke in the right MCA territory. (A) CT shows low density and efface-ment of cortical sulci (between arrowheads) and compression of the anterior horn of the lateral ventricle (arrow). (B) T1-weighted MRI shows loss of sulcal markings (between arrowheads) and compression of the anterior horn of the lateral ventricle (arrow). (C) T2-weighted MRI scan shows increased signal intensity (between arrowheads) and ventricular compression (arrow). (Reprinted, with permission, from Aminoff MJ et al. *Clinical Neurology*, 3rd ed., Stamford, CT: Appleton & Lange, 1996:275.)

stroke or head trauma in the last three months, a recent MI, current anticoagulant therapy with INR > 1.7, use of heparin in the last 48 hours with prolonged PTT, a platelet count < 100,000/mm³, major surgery in the past 14 days, GI or urinary bleeding in the past 21 days, seizures present at the onset of stroke, blood glucose < 50 or > 400 mg/dL, and age less than 18.

Preventive and long-term treatments include:

- Aspirin or clopidogrel if stroke is secondary to small-vessel disease or thrombosis or if anticoagulation is contraindicated.
- Anticoagulation (heparin initially, then warfarin) if cardiac emboli, new atrial fibrillation, or a hypercoagulable state is present (possibly for intracranial vascular disease as well).
- Carotid endarterectomy (CEA) for asymptomatic stenosis greater than 60% according to the Asymptomatic Carotid Arteriosclerosis Study (ACAS) criteria. Women may be less likely to benefit from this procedure than men.
- CEA for symptomatic stenosis with greater than 50%–70% stenosis according to the North American Symptomatic Carotid Endarterectomy Trial (NASCET) criteria. CEA is contraindicated in arterial occlusion (100% blockage).
- Management of modifiable risk factors, especially hypertension, DM, and hypercholesterolemia.

Weakness

The key to working up a patient with complaints of weakness is to think anatomically. There are several locations in the chain of executing a movement where pathology can occur, and you should consider them all: the cortex, corticospinal tract (including brain stem pathology), spinal cord, anterior horn cells, nerve roots, plexus, peripheral nerves, neuromuscular junction, and muscle. True weakness involves a loss of motor power or strength and is exclusively a disorder of the motor system, localizing somewhere between the motor cortex and the muscles themselves. It is your job to find a pattern in the patient's weakness and to make an anatomic diagnosis; from there, you can go on to create a differential by etiology.

You should first seek to differentiate upper motor neuron (UMN) from lower motor neuron (LMN) disease (Table 4.19). Then try to pinpoint the location using your exam, thinking about what the affected muscles have in common (e.g., all are proximal, all are innervated by one nerve). As is always the case, the history, the physical, and the remainder of the neurologic examination are crucial in this process. Three common peripheral nervous system disorders with which you should be familiar—carpal tunnel syndrome, GBS, and myasthenia gravis (MG)—are described in further detail below.

TABLE 4.19. Anatomic Localization: Upper Versus Lower Motor Neuron Disease.

Clinical Features	UMN	LMN
Pattern of weakness	Pyramidal (arm extensors, leg flexors)	Variable
Tone	Spastic (increased: initially flaccid)	Flaccid (decreased)
DTRs	Increased (initially decreased)	Normal, decreased, absent
Miscellaneous signs	Babinski's, other CNS signs	Atrophy, fasciculations

Differential. The etiology of weakness is generally classified by anatomic localization. Although in most cases physical exam and history will indicate a certain anatomic level, don't get pigeonholed into a small differential; remember to consider all possible etiologies of weakness each time. Refer to Table 4.20 for the location of lesions, the pattern of weakness expected, and associated etiologies.

Workup. The physical exam and history will largely shape the differential diagnosis and indicate which labs and tests to order. If a central lesion or UMN syndrome is suspected, CT or MRI of the brain (including the brain stem) and MRI of the spinal cord are often ordered. If a peripheral neuropathy or a mus-

TABLE 4.20. Lesions in the Motor Pathways.

Location of Lesion	Disease Term	Weakness Pattern	Etiologies
Intracranial		UMN, as described below	Stroke, neoplasm, MS, hemorrhage, trauma, infection
Spinal cord	Myelopathy	UMN at spinal level	Compression, trauma, MS
Anterior horn cell	Motor neuron disease	UMN/LMN: variable	ALS, spinal muscular atrophy, poliomyelitis
Nerve root	Radiculopathy	LMN at root level	Compression, infection, meningeal mets, trauma
Plexus	Plexopathy	LMN, mixed roots	Trauma, neoplastic infiltration, idiopathic
Peripheral nerve	Neuropathy	LMN, by nerve	Metabolic, toxic, inflammatory, neoplastic
Neuromuscular junction		Diffuse weakness	Myasthenia gravis, Lambert-Eaton syndrome
Muscle	Myopathy	Proximal weakness	Muscular dystrophy, polymyositis, EtOH

cle-related weakness is suspected, tests should include creatine kinase, EMG, nerve conduction velocity (NCV), and laboratory studies for treatable causes of peripheral neuropathy and myopathy. If there is a high index of suspicion for a demyelinating peripheral neuropathy, an LP may also be ordered. In cases of high suspicion of myopathy, a muscle biopsy may be indicated. The pattern of laboratory and test results observed for the different etiologies of weakness are outlined in Table 4.21.

TABLE 4.21. Investigation of Patient with Weakness.

Test	Spinal Cord	Anterior Horn Cell Disorders	Peripheral Nerve or Plexus	Neuromuscular Junction	Myopathy
Serum enzymes	Normal	Normal	Normal	Normal	Normal or increased
Electromyography	Reduced number of motor units under voluntary control. With lesions causing axonal degeneration, may be abnormal spontaneous activity (e.g., fasciculations, fibrillations) if sufficient time has elapsed after onset; with reinnervation, motor units may be large, long, and polyphasic.			Often normal, but individual motor units may show abnormal variability in size.	Small, short, abundant polyphasic motor unit potentials Abnormal spontaneous activity may be conspicuous in myositis.
Nerve conduction velocity	Normal	Normal	Slowed, especially in demyelinative neuropathies. May be normal in axonal neuropathies.	Normal	Normal
Muscle response to repetitive motor nerve stimulation	Normal	Normal, except in active stage of disease	Normal	Abnormal decrement or increment depending on stimulus frequency and disease	Normal
Muscle biopsy	May be normal in acute stage but subsequently suggestive of denervation			Normal	Changes suggestive of myopathy
Myelography or spinal MRI	May be helpful	Helpful in excluding other disorders	Not helpful	Not helpful	Not helpful

Reprinted, with permission, from Aminoff MJ et al. *Clinical Neurology*, 3rd ed., Stamford, CT: Appleton & Lange, 1996:156.

CARPAL TUNNEL SYNDROME

Carpal tunnel syndrome results from compression of the median nerve at the wrist where it passes through the carpal tunnel. It is most commonly seen in women aged 30 to 55. Risk factors include repetitive use injury, pregnancy, diabetes, hypothyroidism, acromegaly, rheumatoid arthritis, and obesity.

Signs and Symptoms. Patients present with wrist pain; numbness and tingling of the thumb, index finger, middle finger, and lateral half of the ring finger; weak grip; and decreased thumb opposition. The pain and symptoms are exacerbated by activities that require wrist flexion, such as holding a cup of coffee or opening a jar. The symptoms may awaken patients at night and are relieved by shaking out the wrists. Patients often complain of nocturnal pain and paresthesias. Thenar atrophy may occur in severe cases.

Workup. Two clinical exams should be performed on suspected carpal tunnel patients: Tinel's sign and Phalen's sign. Tinel's sign (~60% sensitivity and ~65% specificity) involves tapping on the palmaris longus tendon at the wrist over the median nerve to elicit a tingling sensation in the thumb and affected fingers. Phalen's sign (~75% sensitivity and ~35% specificity) requires that the patient appose the dorsal aspects of the hands with the wrists flexed at 90 degrees for at least 30 seconds. The onset of paresthesias confirms the diagnosis. EMG and NCV are used to make a diagnosis, evaluate the degree of neural and motor compromise and assess the severity of compression, especially in patients who exhibit persistent symptoms despite conservative management. Patients should also be evaluated for risk factors, including diabetes and hypothyroidism (myxedema).

Treatment. Patients should be given neutral wrist splints to wear both during the day and at night; should be counseled about modifying repetitive activities and creating a more ergonomic work environment; and should be given NSAIDs to control inflammation of the tendons. Direct injection of corticosteroid into the carpal space may also provide temporary relief. If symptoms persist, surgical division of the transverse carpal ligament is indicated.

GUILLAIN-BARRÉ SYNDROME

Guillain-Barré syndrome is an acute, rapidly progressive, peripheral demyelinating disease. It is believed to be autoimmune in nature and is often associated with a viral upper respiratory infection (URI) prodrome or *Campylobacter jejuni* infection. Approximately 3500 cases occur each year in the United States. Although about 85% of patients make a complete or near-complete recovery, the mortality rate from this disease is roughly 5%.

Signs and Symptoms. GBS is marked by a rapidly progressive course. Classically, weakness and sensory symptoms begin distally (as with all peripheral nerve diseases) and ascend rapidly to involve the trunk, diaphragm, and cranial nerves. Autonomic deficits may also be present. Because this is a peripheral nerve disorder, reflexes are absent. Sensory symptoms such as numbness, tingling, and muscle aching, especially in the low back, are common complaints.

Workup. EMG, NCV, and LP are indicated in suspected GBS. EMG and NCV will be consistent with diffuse demyelination. LP will show CSF protein level > 55 mg/dL with little or no pleocytosis (albuminocytologic dissociation). Depending on the clinical presentation, MRI of the spinal cord may be needed to exclude cord compression.

Treatment. Possible paralysis of the diaphragm and accessory respiratory muscles is the most life-threatening consequence of this rapidly progressive disease. Patients should be admitted to the ICU for close monitoring. Be prepared to intubate patients if they develop impending respiratory failure. Plasmapheresis and IV immunoglobulin are first-line treatments. Most patients will regain premorbid function, but in severe cases this may take up to a year. Aggressive rehabilitation is imperative.

MYASTHENIA GRAVIS

Myasthenia gravis is an autoimmune disease caused by circulating antibodies to postsynaptic acetylcholine receptors. MG occurs at all ages, most often in young adults and in women. The disease can be associated with thymoma, thyrotoxicosis, and autoimmune disorders such as rheumatoid arthritis and SLE.

Signs and Symptoms. Patients most often present with ptosis or double vision due to weakness of the levator palpebrae EOMs. The muscles are notably fatigable, causing weakness to worsen with activity and throughout the day. Difficulty swallowing and proximal muscle weakness can also be present. Respiratory compromise and aspiration are rare but potentially lethal complications and are termed *myasthenic crises*.

Workup. Diagnosis is often made on the basis of clinical findings. On examination, one can test how long patients can keep their eyes open. Carefully monitored edrophonium (Tensilon, a short-acting cholinesterase inhibitor) testing is diagnostic; in a symptomatic patient, IV injection of edrophonium leads to rapid improvement of clinical symptoms. EMG and nerve conduction studies can yield additional confirmation. An assay for circulating acetylcholine antibodies is positive in 85–90% of patients with MG. Antistriational (striated muscle) antibodies are present in 85% of patients with thymoma. CT of the chest is used to evaluate for thymoma.

Treatment. The first line of treatment consists of long-acting anticholinesterase inhibitors, which prolong the action of acetylcholine in the synapse and overcome the antibodies by competition. These medications include neostigmine and pyridostigmine (Mestinon). Persistent weakness after the initiation of therapy may be due to either too much or too little acetylcholinesterase activity. To evaluate, determine if symptoms improve or worsen with the addition of edrophonium. If symptoms improve, the medication dosage should be increased; if symptoms worsen, the medication dosage should be decreased. Prednisone and other immunosuppressive agents are mainstays of treatment. Because symptoms can worsen with prednisone, however, the patient must be closely monitored. In severe cases, plasmapheresis or IV immunoglobulin may provide temporary relief (days to weeks). Thymectomy (regardless of presence of thymoma) is associated with an increased rate of clinical remission and better clinical outcome (especially in younger patients).

IMAGING BASICS

Magnetic Resonance Imaging

The future of magnetic resonance–based techniques in neurology. *Eur J Neurol* 2001;8:17–25. This review highlights the substantial contribution of MRI to clinical neurology and "offers recommendations for maximizing the potential future for magnetic resonance techniques in neurology."

Schaefer PW. Applications of DWI in clinical neurology. *J Neurol Sci* 2001;186:S25–S35. Students will undoubtedly encounter diffusion-weighted imaging (DWI) during the neurology clerkship as part of the evaluation of acute stroke. This article provides a good review of DWI and explains how this particular scan sequence can be useful in evaluating stroke and determining patient prognosis.

LUMBAR PUNCTURE

CSF Profiles

Negrini B, Kelleher KJ, Wald ER. Cerebrospinal fluid findings in aseptic versus bacterial meningitis. *Pediatrics* 2000;105:316–319. A retrospective chart review study that challenges the notion that neutrophil predominance in CSF is indicative of bacterial meningitis. While many may doubt the results, the study provides a good overview of factors to consider when evaluating CSF profiles.

APHASIAS

Code C. Multifactorial processes in recovery from aphasia: developing the foundations for a multileveled framework. *Brain Lang* 200;77:25-44. A discussion of the multifaceted approach (neural, cognitive, and behavioral) currently advocated for recovery from aphasia.

COMA

Teasdale G, Jennett B. Assessment of coma and impaired consciousness: a practical scale. *Lancet* 1974;2:81–84. The classic paper that introduced the now-popular GCS.

Malik K, Hess DC. Evaluating the comatose patient: rapid neurologic assessment is key to appropriate management. *Postgrad Med* 2002;111:38–40, 43–46, 49–50. A well-presented review of the key features involved in the assessment and workup of a comatose patient, with emphasis on obtaining history from eyewitnesses, evaluating key brain stem reflexes, and determining the underlying etiology of the comatose state.

DELIRIUM AND DEMENTIA

Inouye SK. Delirium in hospitalized older patients. *Clin Geriatr Med* 1998;14:745–764. A discussion of the multiple etiologies of delirium in the elderly and both nonpharmacologic and pharmacologic management of delirium in older patients.

McLoughlin DM, Levy R. The differential diagnosis of dementia. *Acta Neurol Scand Suppl* 1996;165:92–100. A review of the differential diagnosis of dementia with particular emphasis on the historical details that should be elicited to differentiate dementia from other neuropsychiatric conditions.

DYSEQUILIBRIUM

Hain TC. Approach to the patient with dizziness and vertigo. In *Practical Neurology* (J Biller, ed). Philadelphia: Lippincott-Raven, 1997:155–169. An excellent step-by-step approach to the assessment and workup of patients with dizziness and vertigo in an easy-to-follow outline format.

HEADACHE

General

Flippen CC. Pearls and pitfalls of headache. *Semin Neurol* 2001;21:371–376. A review of the assessment and management of both typical and atypical headaches using a case study approach. Excellent if you prefer to learn by example.

Migraine Headache

Gallagher RM, Cutrer FM. Migraine: diagnosis, management, and new treatment options. *Am J Manag Care* 2002;8:S58–S73. A review of prophylactic, abortive, and symptomatic treatments of migraines, including a discussion of side effects and evaluating the balance between drug efficacy and tolerability.

INTRACRANIAL HEMORRHAGES

General

Stieg PE, Kase CS. Intracranial hemorrhage: diagnosis and emergency management. *Neurol Clin* 1998;16:373–390. A discussion of the recognition and early treatment of the various types of intracranial hemorrhages.

Dubinsky I, Penello D. Can specific patient variables be used to predict outcome of intracranial hemorrhage? *Am J Emerg Med* 2002;20:26–29. A prospective trial looking at patient outcomes as determined by various patient variables, including GCS scores and the presence or absence of central reflexes. Provides a good review of important physical findings and historical points to note when evaluating and managing a patient with an intracranial hemorrhage. For example, the authors report that the presence of gag in patients with a GCS < 6 is a significant predictor of long-term outcomes.

Subarachnoid Hemorrhage

Ogungbo B, et al. Trends over time in the management of subarachnoid haemorrhage in Newcastle: review of 1609 patients. *Br J Neurosurg* 2001;15:388– 395. A review of the epidemiology, morbidity, mortality, surgical management, and increasing role of endovascular treatment in the management of patients with subarachnoid hemorrhage.

LOW BACK PAIN AND SPINAL CORD INJURIES

Bracken MB, et al. Administration of methylprednisolone for 24 or 48 hours or tirilazad mesylate for 48 hours in the treatment of acute spinal cord injury. *JAMA* 1997;277:1597–1604. Presents the widely debated results of the Third National Acute Spinal Cord Injury study, a randomized controlled trial establishing the use of high-dose steroids (methylprednisolone) in the treatment of acute spinal cord injury.

MOVEMENT DISORDERS

Parkinson's Disease

Hermanoqicz N. Management of Parkinson's disease: strategies, pitfalls, and future directions. *Postgrad Med* 2001;110(6):15–18, 21–23, 28. A review of the symptoms and neurologic findings associated with Parkinson's disease. Also reviews symptomatic therapy, including pharmacotherapy, neurosurgery, and stem cell therapy.

Huntington's Disease

Quinn N, Schrag A. Huntington's disease and other choreas. *J Neurol* 1998;245:709–716. A review of Huntington's disease as the classic choreiform disease as well as a discussion of other diseases manifesting choreas. Although the article stresses theory, it should further students' understanding of the pathophysiology underlying Huntington's disease.

Multiple Sclerosis

Palace J. Making the diagnosis of multiple sclerosis. *J Neurol Neurosurg Psychiatry* 2001;71:ii3–8. Thompson AJ. Symptomatic management and rehabilitation in multiple sclerosis. *J Neurol Neurosurg Psychiatry* 2001;71:ii22–27. Two articles (in series) reviewing the signs, symptoms, and diagnostic criteria for multiple sclerosis and the treatment and management of multiple sclerosis patients.

SEIZURES

Beydoun A, Passaro EA. Appropriate use of medications for seizures: guiding principles on the path of efficacy. *Postgrad Med* 2002;11:69–82. A review of appropriate treatment of seizures and use of antiepileptic drugs in light of seizure type, seizure syndromes, comorbid illnesses, and the psychosocial needs of the patient.

Prego-Lopez M, Devinsky O. Evaluation of a first seizure: is it epilepsy? *Postgrad Med* 2002;111:34–36, 43–48. A review of the assessment and workup of a suspected seizure.

STROKE

Workup, Treatment, and Management

Benavente O, Hart RG. Stroke: Part II. Management of acute ischemic stroke. *Am Fam Physician* 1999;59:2828–2834. A thorough review of the management and treatment of acute ischemic stroke, including a review of both established and investigational protocols.

Executive Committee for the Asymptomatic Carotid Atherosclerosis Study. Endarterectomy for asymptomatic carotid artery stenosis. *JAMA* 1995;273: 1421–1428. The classic and original ACAS trial that established 60% stenosis as the criterion for surgical treatment of an asymptomatic carotid stenosis.

National Institute of Neurological Disorders and Stroke tPA Stroke Study Group. Tissue plasminogen activator for acute ischemic stroke. *N Engl J Med* 1995;333:1581–1587. The original placebo-controlled trial demonstrating the efficacy of tPA for reducing neurologic deficits following ischemic stroke (despite an increase frequency of hemorrhagic conversion) if tPA is administered within four hours of onset of symptoms

North American Symptomatic Carotid Endarterectomy Trial (NASCET) investigators. Clinical alert: benefit of carotid endarterectomy for patients with high-grade stenosis of the internal carotid artery. *Stroke* 1991;22:816–817. The classic and original report of the NASCET trial that established 70% stenosis as the criterion for carotid endarterectomy of symptomatic carotid stenosis. Students who are interested should look into further NASCET trials that were published subsequent to this trial.

WEAKNESS

Guillain-Barré Syndrome

Seneviratne U. Guillain-Barré syndrome. *Postgrad Med J* 2000;76:774–782. A review of the pathophysiology, presentation, treatment, and outcomes associated with Guillain-Barré syndrome.

Myasthenia Gravis

Pascuzzi RM. Pearls and pitfalls in the diagnosis and management of neuromuscular junction disorders. *Semin Neurol* 2001;21:425–440. A review of the clinical features and treatment paradigms for neuromuscular junctions disorders, including both myasthenia gravis and the less common Lambert-Eaton syndrome.

HANDBOOK/POCKETBOOK

Handbook of Symptom-Oriented Neurology
$39.95

Remmel

Mosby, 2002, 3rd edition, 480 pages, ISBN 0323017126

A clinically oriented pocketbook written in outline format. Provides easy, fast access to thorough descriptions of neurologic disease. Appropriate for students who are highly interested in neurology. Contains an extensive number of references.

Neurology (House Officer Series)
$29.95

Weiner

Lippincott Williams & Wilkins, 1999, 6th edition, 300 pages, ISBN 0683304976

A clinically oriented pocketbook organized by signs and symptoms. Concise chapters offer clinically relevant material, although the text is somewhat short on tables and diagrams. Covers most topics thoroughly, but lacks an overwhelming amount of detail. Written for interns and residents, but can be useful for medical students as well during their initial patient encounters.

Manual of Neurologic Therapeutics
$39.95

Samuels

Little, Brown and Company, 1999, 6th edition, 499 pages, ISBN 0781716454

A spiral-bound pocketbook written in expanded outline format and patterned after the *Washington Manual*. Strikes an excellent balance between concise, practical information and reference-level detail. Better for clinical management than for review of pathophysiology. An appendix lists agencies that provide support and education for patients with specific neurologic problems.

Neurologic Pearls
$19.95

Devinsky

F. A. Davis, 2000, 1st edition, 309 pages, ISBN 0803604335

A concise pocketbook that presents simple, clear explanations of the approach to neurologic disorders. Chapters are organized by clinical presentation with useful clinical pearls interspersed throughout. More illustrations of neuroanatomy and pathways would increase the quality of the discussion.

Little Black Book of Neurology
$34.95

Lerner

Mosby, 1995, 3rd edition, 447 pages, ISBN 0815154402

An alphabetically organized pocketbook with a format similar to that of a dictionary. Written in essay format without an index or a table of contents, detracting from its utility as a quick reference. Written more for residents than for medical students. Best used for review by advanced neurology students. New edition available April 2002.

Clinical Neurology $39.95

Greenberg

McGraw-Hill, 2002, 5th edition, 390 pages, ISBN 0071375430

A well organized, clinically oriented reference that is detailed enough to serve as a
student textbook. Emphasizes essential information with excellent usage of tables
and diagrams. A great introductory neurology text for the motivated student. Highly
useful appendices offer guides on how to perform an extensive neurologic exam.

Neurological Examination Made Easy $27.00

Fuller

Churchill Livingstone, 2000, 2nd edition, 220 pages, ISBN 0443061661

A review of the neurologic exam for medical students, written from the author's
perspective of what to do, what you find, and what it means. Excellent flow diagrams guide you through the process of examining the patient. Good for the non-
neurologist who wishes to learn the neurologic exam extremely well or for the serious neurology student who wants to start off with an excellent foundation.

Neurology: Diagnosis in Color $39.95

Parsons

Mosby, 2001, 1st edition, 366 pages, ISBN 0723431795

This quick-reference book provides excellent color photographs of clinical signs and
associated pathology and radiology for common and uncommon neurologic disorders. Figures are accompanied by brief, well-written captions of findings and pathophysiology. Not designed for comprehensive review, but provides excellent examples
of most radiographic pathology and manifestations of disease in neurology.

Neurology and Neurosurgery Illustrated $52.00

Lindsay

Churchill Livingstone, 1999, 3rd edition, 573 pages, ISBN 0443050619

Extensive coverage of a wide variety of topics, with great line drawings illustrating
key aspects of pathophysiology, clinical features, and treatment. Not for reading
cover to cover during a short rotation, but can be used as a reference for the essential features of neurologic disease. Sections are organized both by presenting complaint and by specific disorder.

Underground Clinical Vignettes: Neurology $24.95

Bhushan

Blackwell Science, 2002, 2nd edition, 50 pages, ISBN 0632045671

A well organized review of clinical vignettes commonly encountered on NBME shelf
exam and USMLE Step 2 exams. Includes a focused, high-yield discussion of pathogenesis, epidemiology, management, complications, and associated diseases. Black-and-white
images are included where relevant. Also contains several "mini-cases" in which only
key facts related to each disease are presented. An entertaining, easy-to-use supplement
for studying during your clinical rotation, although it is neither as comprehensive nor as
relevant for day-to-day wards activities. The color atlas supplement may be optionally
purchased or obtained when purchasing the full set of *Underground Clinical Vignettes*.

TOP-RATED BOOKS

Review/Mini-Reference

The Four-Minute Neurologic Exam $12.95

Goldberg

MedMaster, 1999, 1st edition, 58 pages, ISBN 0940780054

A brief, practical guide that is best reviewed before the rotation to help students understand the fundamentals of the neurologic screening examination. Can be read in a few hours to provide a good foundation for physical exam skills, but too simplistic to be of long-term value. Discusses only how to do a physical exam and provides little explanation of what your findings could mean.

 High-Yield Neuroanatomy $19.95

Fix

Lippincott Williams & Wilkins, 1999, 2nd edition, 142 pages, ISBN 0683307215

An outline review designed for USMLE Step 1 exam study. Good for prerotation study for those interested in getting a head start. Not comprehensive, but some students feel that it is a good "minimalist" reference for short neurology rotations. Good for pathways and review of general pathophysiology, but lacks a discussion of management issues.

 Lecture Notes on Neurology $39.95

Ginsberg

Blackwell Science, 1999, 7th edition, 199 pages, ISBN 0632048271

A good, concise review of key points with great tables, figures, and illustrations. May be read from cover to cover during a short rotation. Organized mostly by pathology rather than by presenting complaint.

 Neurology $39.95

Collins

W. B. Saunders, 1997, 1st edition, 201 pages, ISBN 0721659926

A concise, thorough review of neurology that examines the most common symptoms and diseases of the nervous system. A number of tables and interesting historical facts are interspersed throughout the text. The focus on theory may not be practical for wards application but would be of interest to students considering a career in neurology.

 Neurology Secrets $39.95

Rolak

Hanley & Belfus, 2001, 3rd edition, 438 pages, ISBN 1560534656

A quick reference text in question-and-answer format consistent with the *Secrets* series. Although not useful as a comprehensive text, it is of value in helping students prepare for pimping on rounds. Covers the most commonly encountered neurologic disorders. Offers good explanations of clinically relevant questions, although some obscure information is also included.

B **Introduction to the Neurologic Examination**   **$23.95**

Nolan

F. A. Davis, 1996, 1st edition, 224 pages, ISBN 0803600178

An extensive discussion of the neurologic exam, written in essay format. Somewhat verbose, making the text difficult to follow and read. Although a fair number of line illustrations show normal anatomy and pathways, the text would benefit from more drawings that directly illustrate how to perform a neuro exam.

B **Neurology Recall**   **$29.95**

Miller

Lippincott Williams & Wilkins, 1997, 1st edition, 340 pages, ISBN 0683182161

Question-and-answer format typical of the *Recall* series. A good reference for students preparing for pimping on wards, and provides fast, easy-to-read reviews of disorders. Not as detailed as *Neurology Secrets,* so future neurologists will need another reference for in-depth discussion of disease.

B **The Resident's Neurology Book**   **$26.95**

Devinsky

F. A. Davis, 1997, 1st edition, 282 pages, ISBN 0803601867

A comprehensive introductory guide for medical students and residents beginning their training. Offers good descriptions of the most common disorders encountered in neurology. Although the text includes a large number of illustrations of normal neuroanatomy, only a limited number of figures illustrate the localization of pathology and where lesions would be located.

B‒ **Manter and Gantz's Essentials of Clinical Neuroanatomy and Neurophysiology**   **$28.95**

Gilman

F. A. Davis, 1996, 9th edition, 309 pages, ISBN 0803601441

An extensive, in-depth review of neuroanatomy and neurophysiology that is too detailed for most medical students and would be difficult to read during such a short rotation. Offers excellent pathway diagrams. Only for the highly motivated student with a deep interest in the basic sciences.

B‒ **Neurology: An Illustrated Colour Text**   **$32.95**

Fuller

Churchill Livingstone, 1999, 1st edition, 129 pages, ISBN 044305374X

An introductory-level text of common neurologic disorders with good, cartoon-style images illustrating how to evaluate different aspects of the neurologic exam. Includes more color line drawings than color photographs or radiographs of disease. May lack the level of detail necessary for use as a reference during the clinical rotation, particularly with respect to management.

TOP-RATED BOOKS

Review/Mini-Reference

A   **Adams and Victor's Principles of Neurology**   **$89.95**

Victor

McGraw-Hill, 2001, 7th edition, 1692 pages, ISBN 0070674973

A comprehensive reference text with detailed discussions of disease from a clinical perspective. Uniquely organized with chapters transitioning from general patient approach to cardinal manifestations of neurologic disease to specific disease. Tables and figures are somewhat sparse. Most appropriate for students considering neurology as a specialty.

A⁻   **Merritt's Textbook of Neurology**   **$110.00**

Rowland

Lippincott Williams & Wilkins, 2000, 10th edition, 1002 pages, ISBN 0683304747

A reference textbook that covers the entire spectrum of neurologic disease in depth, although not as detailed as *Principles of Neurology*. Concise chapters are accompanied by a number of clinical radiographs.

Obstetrics and Gynecology

Welcome to obstetrics and gynecology! This rotation is dedicated to acquainting future MDs with the basic principles of labor and delivery (L&D) and of managing gynecologic issues, including medical, surgical, and social issues. You will be involved in prenatal care, annual well-woman examinations, contraceptive counseling, and numerous surgical procedures, from cesarean sections to a variety of gynecologic operations. Obstetrician/gynecologists are surgeons by nature who keep extremely demanding schedules and spend minimal time rounding and discussing differentials on a regular basis. For the next few weeks, you will thus be exposed to a whirlwind of activities covering a wide range of issues. Regardless of the field you enter, more than half of your patients will be women with potential gynecologic problems, so take advantage of this learning opportunity and have a good time!

WHAT IS THE ROTATION LIKE?

OB/GYN rotations last approximately six to eight weeks and differ vastly from school to school as well as from site to site. The basic setup consists of inpatient obstetrics, inpatient gynecology, and the outpatient clinic, where both obstetric and gynecologic patients are seen. Obstetrics can be one of the most rewarding and pleasant experiences in medical school, but it is not an easygoing discipline. It will, however, provide you with the opportunity to handle an acute situation primarily on your own (with resident backup), thereby representing perhaps the most responsibility you have had thus far in your medical training.

When you are in the obstetrics portion of your rotation, you will spend much of your time in the L&D suite. Responsibilities in this context include prerounding on postpartum patients and presenting those patients on ward rounds. Other responsibilities include evaluating patients in the triage area, writing the admission history and physical (H&P), working closely with residents and nurses in monitoring the progress of laboring patients, delivering babies, writing delivery notes, and checking labs.

You should get to know the nursing staff very well, as much of the L&D is in many instances handled by nurses or midwives. You should also try to follow the patient from the beginning of her L&D admission to the delivery of her baby and postpartum care. Such longitudinal care will allow you to cultivate a better relationship with your patient while simultaneously enabling you to see the complete picture of labor management. You should also read about the basics of L&D (steps of labor, signs and symptoms of true labor, steps of delivery, fetal heart tracing) and learn about common complications that can arise and their management (failure to progress, hypertension, fetal distress). Always keep in mind that competence is only half the story; knowing your patient well by periodically checking in on her to see if she needs anything—or just to comfort her—will impress not only your patient but your residents and attendings as well.

Obstetrics can be one of the most rewarding and pleasant experiences in medical school.

Try to follow a patient from admission to delivery.

As a surgically oriented specialty, inpatient gynecology is similar to general surgery with the exception of the obvious fact that all of your patients are women. Your responsibilities consist of prerounding on postoperative patients, presenting patients on ward rounds, and writing notes (preoperative, operative, postoperative) on the patients whose surgeries you are involved with. Rounding is early and fast; all the notes, rounding, and daily management planning for the patients must be done prior to the surgeries that are planned for the day, which can start as early as 7:30 AM. When leaving each day, you should thus try to plan out which surgery you want to participate in the next day, read up on the surgery and on relevant anatomy, and learn something about the patient's history. Surgeries will differ depending on the type of hospital with which you are working and can range from a half-hour laparoscopy for tubal ligation to a two-hour hysterectomy to a six-hour gynecologic oncology case.

You should always introduce yourself to the attending surgeon, especially if that surgeon is from a private practice. You should also practice some basic suturing and knot-tying skills in the event that you are presented with a rare opportunity to help close an incision. In addition, you should learn some of the medical jargon common to surgeries and be willing to ask questions pertaining to technique or to the prognosis of the surgery being performed. You should also be ready to answer questions about the basic anatomy, surgical procedure, and prognosis of the surgery being performed.

Outpatient clinics are a great place to see both common and uncommon gynecologic and obstetric cases. Be prepared to perform a very focused H&P. Common gynecologic clinic issues are requests for birth control, routine health maintenance (breast exams, pelvic exams, and Pap smears), abnormal vaginal bleeding, vaginal discharge, and lower abdominal pain. Obstetric patients are seen in the clinic to assess the adequacy of pregnancy progression, to screen for potential maternal-fetal complications, to help mothers adjust to their pregnancies, and to prepare mothers for childbirth. In addition, postpartum patients are seen for their regular six-week checkup or for any postpartum complications that may arise. The clinic experience is extremely helpful in that the skills and knowledge you will acquire there are likely to be applicable to most fields you may ultimately pursue, such as internal medicine, family practice, or surgery.

WHO ARE THE PLAYERS?

Team OB/GYN consists of a senior resident (R3 or R4), at least one junior resident (R2), and an intern (from OB/GYN, family practice, psychiatry, or medicine). There may also be a fourth-year medical student doing his or her senior elective as well as one or two third-year medical students. Usually, there is one ward attending, although there may be several private attendings, subspecialty attendings (maternal-fetal, gynecologic oncology), and fellows as well. Other important players include the nursing staff and midwives (especially in L&D), who can teach you invaluable obstetric skills, and the anesthesiologists, who are needed for pain control both during labor and postoperatively.

Don't wait for residents to call you for deliveries: BE AROUND.

HOW IS THE DAY SET UP?

A typical day on an OB/GYN service may look like this:

	OB Service	GYN	Clinic
5:30–6:30 AM	Prerounds	Prerounds	
6:30–7:30 AM	Work rounds	Work rounds	
7:30 AM–4:00 PM	L&D	OR	Outpatient clinic (8 AM–5 PM)
4:00–6:00 PM	Wrap up work, do PM rounds if on GYN		

Call days are usually busy and are always in-house. After you are done with your regular workday, you start call in the L&D (usually at 5 PM) and see patients in triage while also following any laboring patient you might have. You and your resident will also see and potentially admit patients from the ER for acute obstetric or gynecologic care. You will usually be up all night or, if you are lucky, get one to two hours of sleep. This is because there will often be someone delivering in the early hours of the morning or an emergency to keep you busy.

WHAT DO I DO DURING PREROUNDS?

Depending on the size of your inpatient gynecologic service, prerounds should begin 30 minutes to one hour before work rounds. You should anticipate spending roughly 20 to 30 minutes on each patient you are following, depending on your stage in the year. As in surgery, most of your patients will be postoperative. You will be expected to check vital signs overnight, assess overnight fluid balance ("ins and outs"), check labs, do a quick physical exam, check the surgical wound, review the chart for new notes, and write a concise progress note—all before work rounds. On the obstetrics service, you will preround on your postpartum patients. In addition to your usual preround chores, you will also want to examine your patients' breasts and check fundus size and firmness, the extent of vaginal bleeding, and any wounds, such as sewn lacerations or cesarean incisions. Make sure that your notes are always co-signed by your residents—not only is it good medical practice, but you'll also get helpful feedback on your notes.

HOW DO I DO WELL IN THIS ROTATION?

Don't get shut out of learning the pelvic exam.

Be assertive. Assertiveness is key to furthering your education and to scoring points with the people who evaluate you. So ask good questions (you should know something about the subject matter before asking the questions), know other patients on the service (for your own learning and in case you are asked to fill in), take the initiative to ask for demonstrations of procedures, volunteer for drawing blood (you need to practice anyway), do pelvic exams, and try to dig up interesting/informative articles for the team.

Be the intern for your patients. You will have patients assigned to you by your residents. Among other things, you will be responsible for each patient's H&P, writing progress notes, following up on diagnostic studies and pathology results, and presenting your patients to the team. In order to fulfill your responsibilities diligently, you will need to know and do everything you can for your patient. This means reading up on each case, carefully reviewing your patient's history, and talking to your patient. This will allow you to actively participate in patient care and hence to act as your patient's strongest advocate.

Be knowledgeable in a general sense. It is important to recognize that once residents become involved in a specialty, they spend less time keeping up to date on everything else they learned in medical school. You can thus be a great asset to your team by providing new information about your patients' medical problem (diabetes, hepatitis, hypertension) and recognizing psychiatric or social issues (postpartum depression, drug dependence, domestic violence).

Work quickly, independently, and efficiently. Residents appreciate any student who can effectively contribute to the team. So order lab tests, make necessary phone calls, and write notes for patients. In addition, be focused, organized, and brief when presenting the patient. In many ways, this rotation is similar to surgery. Gynecologic oncology, for example, is really just a surgical subspecialty.

Know the expectations. At the beginning of the rotation, be straightforward and ask the residents on your team exactly what is expected of you. You should also find out your attending's preferred format of patient presentation. Midway through the rotation, it is equally important to get feedback both from residents and from attendings with whom you have worked. Try to be assertive and ask for constructive feedback on what you should continue to do and what you can improve on. Be tactful, and communicate with the goal of maximizing your performance, education, and contribution to the team while on the clerkship.

You may fall in love with OB/GYN and want to pursue it as a career. If this is the case, you should take additional steps. Let your team know of your sincere interest in the field; they will be more than happy to lead you down the right track. Ask the interns and residents for advice on the politics of residency (e.g., which programs are good, who are the key people to get to know better, whom to ask for letters of recommendation, which senior electives to take). If possible, try to work with one of the key faculty members, who can write an influential letter of recommendation or be your adviser in your quest to match into the residency of your choice.

SURVIVAL TIPS

Do not be discouraged if a patient does not want a medical student to deliver her baby or even to be involved in her care. Many mothers want as little intrusion as possible into this sacred, personal moment of their lives, while oth-

Don't be discouraged if the patient initially does not want you in the exam room or delivering her baby.

ers may be concerned about inexperienced students touching their newborn infant. Occasionally, male students may encounter some gynecologic patients who are uncomfortable with the notion of having a male in the examining room, much less a male student. On a rotation such as OB/GYN, in which you will be working very hard with long hours, it can be easy to become frustrated when issues like these arise. It is important, however, to respect a patient's wishes as well as to bear in mind that there may be specific reasons such requests may be made. So do not take it personally if a patient does not want you in the examination room. If this continues to happen frequently, you should discuss it with your resident. Being with an affable yet assertive female resident who cares about your educational experience is of great help in getting your foot in the door as a male medical student.

Here are a few more tips:

- Talk to OB patients early in labor and throughout the delivery. Establishing a rapport early on will increase the likelihood that you will be able to help with the delivery.
- Learn how to "count" and coach a patient through labor. A calm yet clear and assertive voice is usually appreciated.

KEY NOTES

Obstetrics Admission note. The obstetric H&P is similar to a standard H&P but should include the following additional information:

- **Gravida:** The total number of times a patient has been pregnant.
- **Para:** Four numbers that represent term deliveries, preterm deliveries, abortions (including elective, therapeutic, and spontaneous), and number of living children. This is often referred to as TPAL (term, preterm, abortion, living). For example, a pregnant patient with one prior miscarriage and one prior term delivery would be a G3P1011.
- **Gestational age:** Information on gestational age should be included along with information on the last menstrual period (LMP) and estimated date of delivery (EDD, which is the same as the due date and is often referred to as EDC, or estimated date of confinement).
- **Uterine contractions (UCs):** Information on the time of onset, frequency, and intensity of contractions.
- **Rupture of membranes (ROM):** The time of rupture and the color of the fluid.
- **Vaginal bleeding (VB):** This should include the duration of bleeding, its consistency, and the number of pads.
- **Fetal movement (FM):** Notation should be made as to whether fetal movement is normal, decreased, or absent.
- **Ultrasound history:** This should include gestational age at the time of the first ultrasound, whether anatomy was evaluated, and whether the size on ultrasound is equivalent to that expected based on the last menstrual period, or "size equal to dates" (S = D).
- **Prenatal labs (PNL).**

- **Physical exam:** This should include a thorough physical, including a pelvic exam, which is commonly referred to as a sterile vaginal exam (SVE).
- **Fetal heart tracing (FHT):** Record baseline heart rate, variability, accelerations, and decelerations.
- **Tocomonitor (Toco):** Note the frequency of uterine contractions and whether a regular or an irregular pattern is seen.
- **Ultrasound (UTZ or U/S):** Describe findings such as vertex, breech, amniotic fluid index (AFI), and the location of the placenta.
- **Estimated fetal weight (EFW):** Specify whether the EFW was determined by Leopold's (feeling with hands) or measured by ultrasound.

Sample Admission H&P

26 yo G3P1011 at 39½ weeks by LMP 5/11/01 EDD 2/15/02 with ultrasound done at 10½ weeks S = D who presents c/o UCs q3–4min, +FM, –ROM, –VB.

Prenatal care with Dr. Smith since 7 weeks for 11 visits

Pregnancy complicated by:

UTI—treated with Keflex. TOC negative.

Pap smear c/w ASCUS—needs follow-up Pap smear 6 weeks postpartum.

PPD +, CXR–.

PNL: A+/–, RPR neg, rubella immune, HBsAg neg, HIV neg, Pap smear ASCUS, GC neg, chlamydia neg, 1 hour PG 121 (at 26 wks), PPD +, CXR –, MS-AFP neg.

PMH: None.

PSH: Appendectomy age 9.

Meds: PNV, FeSO$_4$.

All: NKDA.

OB/GYN Hx:

Menarche age 13/menses q28 days/lasts 3–5 days.

2000 NSVD, full term, uncomplicated.

1998 SAB in first trimester.

H/O abnormal Pap smears—never had biopsy.

No history of STDs.

SocHx:

Single, father of baby involved & supportive.

Denies T/E/D.

FamHx: Maternal grandmother with hypertension.

AFI = Amniotic fluid index

A/P = Assessment and plan

ASCUS = Atypical squamous cells of undetermined significance

b = Bilateral

c/o = Complaining of

c/w = Consistent with

CTAB = Clear to auscultation bilaterally

CV = Cardiovascular

DTRs = Deep tendon reflexes

FamHx = Family history

FeSO$_4$ = Ferrous sulfate

GC = Gonococcus (gonorrhea) infection

H/O = History of

Hx = History

IUP = Intrauterine pregnancy

LMP = last menstrual period

MS-AFP = Maternal serum α-fetoprotein

NKDA = No known drug allergies

NSVD = Normal spontaneous vaginal delivery

PG = Plasma glucose

PMH = Past medical history

PNV = Prenatal vitamins

PPD = Purified protein derivative

PSH = Past surgical history

RPR = Rapid plasma reagin

RRR = Regular rate and rhythm

S=D = Size equals dates

SAB = Spontaneous abortion

SEM = Systolic ejection murmur

SocHx = Social history

T/E/D = Tobacco/alcohol (EtOH)/drugs

TOC = Test of cure

UTI = Urinary tract infection

Physical exam:

VS: T 37.2 BP 120/70 P 82 RR 18.

Gen: Uncomfortable with UCs.

Lungs: CTAB.

CV: RRR, + II/VI SEM.

Abd: Soft, gravid, nontender.

Ext: 1+ edema, DTRs 2+ b.

SVE: 80% effaced/5cm dilated/0 station.

FHT: 130s, +accels, reactive.

Toco: q4–5 min UCs.

U/S: Vertex, AFI 11.4, placenta fundal.

EFW: 3650 grams.

A/P 26 yo G3P1011 at 39½ weeks with uncomplicated IUP in active labor.

1. Admit to labor and delivery.

2. Obtain routine labs (type and screen, RPR, CBC).

3. Expectant management. Will start pitocin augmentation if UCs decrease in frequency.

4. Fetal heart tracing reassuring. No signs of fetal distress.

5. Anticipate normal spontaneous vaginal delivery.

Prenatal care. Key notes associated with prenatal care should include the following elements on the first visit (see also Table 5.2):

- **Obstetric history:** Dates of pregnancies with gestational age at time of delivery, route (vaginal, C-section), and complications (including preeclampsia, abruption, previa, preterm labor, and unusually long labor).
- **Gynecologic history:** Menstrual history, STDs, oral contraceptive (OCP) use.
- **Family history:** Congenital abnormalities, twins, bleeding disorders, hypertension, diabetes.
- **Social history:** Any tobacco, alcohol, or drug use during pregnancy, occupational exposures (e.g., nurse preparing chemotherapy agents), involvement and/or relationship with the father of the baby. Living situation.
- **Medical history:** Diabetes, hypertension, asthma, lupus, etc.
- **Allergies**
- **Medications:** List and dose of current medications as well as those used during pregnancy.

- **Prenatal labs:** Blood type, Rh type, antibody screen, VDRL/RPR, rubella, glucose testing, hepatitis B surface antigen, urine culture, Pap smear, gonorrhea culture, chlamydia culture, PPD placement, MS-AFP, one hour PG.
- **Diagnostic tests:** Ultrasound, amniocentesis, chorionic villi sampling (CVS).
- **Physical exam:** A thorough exam is critical, particularly evaluation of the thyroid, heart, and lungs and the pelvic exam. It is important to evaluate the size of the uterus on the pelvic exam (to note if it is consistent with gestational weeks). It is also important to document the initial cervical exam (to have a reference point if there are future issues with preterm contractions or preterm labor).

Key notes for all subsequent visits should record the following:

- Fetal heart tones
- Blood pressure
- Urine dip
- Fundal height
- Weight gain
- Fetal movement
- Vaginal bleeding
- Contractions or cramping
- Rupture of membranes

Delivery note. Some hospitals have preprinted delivery forms that allow you to simply fill in the blanks and check off appropriate boxes. If this is not the case, here is a summary of the information that should be included in a delivery note:

- Age, gravida, para, therapeutic abortion (TAB), SAB, gestational age
- Onset of labor, ROM (with or without meconium)
- Indications for induction (if applicable)
- Obstetric, maternal, or fetal complications
- Anesthesia/pain control (IV, epidural, general)
- Time of birth
- Type of birth (NSVD, forceps assist, vacuum suction, C-section)
- Bulb suction, sex, weight, Apgar scores, presence of nuchal cord (tight or loose), number of cord vessels
- Time of placenta delivery, placenta expressed or delivered spontaneously, whether placenta is intact or not
- Episiotomy (how done, degree, how repaired) and/or lacerations (locations, degree, how repaired)
- Estimated blood loss (EBL)
- Disposition—e.g., mother to recovery room in stable condition; infant to newborn nursery in stable condition

Postpartum note. The postpartum note is similar to the routine progress note that is written on most inpatients (subjective, objective—vitals, routine physical exam). Additional items that should be included in the postpartum note are as follows:

- Breast exam (soft, tender, engorged, signs of mastitis [erythema, warmth])
- Fundus check (firmness, location described relative to the umbilicus)
- Lochia (scant, minimal, heavy)
- Perineum (intact or separating)
- Breastfeeding status (problems with feeding, breastfeeding exclusively or supplementing with formula)
- Contraception desired (Depo-Provera injection, OCPs, condoms)

BS = Breath sounds

d/c = Discharge

I/O = Intake/output

NAD = No acute distress

O = Objective

S = Subjective

s/p = Status post

Sample Postpartum Progress Note

S—Eating solid foods. Breastfeeding without difficulty. No urinary complaints. Desires OCPs for contraception.

O—T_{max} 37.2 $T_{current}$ 37.6 BP 120/70   P 82   R 18   I/O 1200/1370.

Gen: NAD, awake and alert.

Lungs: CTAB.

CV: RRR, no murmurs.

Abd: soft, nontender, minimally distended, +BS.

Fundus: firm, at umbilicus.

Perineum: 2nd-degree laceration repair intact.

Lochia: minimal.

Extremities: no edema, no tenderness or evidence of DVT.

A/P—26 yo G3P2012 PPD# 1 s/p NSVD at 39½ weeks with uncomplicated labor course and delivery.

1. Ice packs to perineum.

2. Continue to encourage breastfeeding.

3. OCPs for contraception.

4. Anticipate d/c home tomorrow.

GYN operative note. The gynecology operative note contains the same information as the operative note for any other surgical service. This includes the following:

- Preoperative diagnosis (e.g., fibroids, cervical cancer, ovarian cyst)
- Postoperative diagnosis (usually "same")

- Procedure (e.g., total abdominal hysterectomy, ovarian cystectomy)
- Surgeons
- Anesthesia (e.g., general endotracheal tube)
- EBL
- IV fluids
- Urinary output
- Findings
- Complications (e.g., enterotomy)
- Pathology specimens (e.g., uterus, cervix, ovary)

KEY PROCEDURES

Delivering babies, cervical checks, Pap smears, cervical/vaginal cultures, external fetal monitoring, IV lines, basic suturing and knot tying, and retracting for visualization during procedures are the principal procedures on this rotation. Descriptions of most of these procedures can be found in major textbooks. However, the best way to learn is by observing and practicing. So let your residents know you are interested in these procedures.

WHAT DO I CARRY IN MY POCKETS?

Checklist

- ❏ Pregnancy wheel
- ❏ OB/GYN handbook of your choice
- ❏ Penlight
- ❏ Stethoscope
- ❏ Index cards to keep track of your patients. Create cards with high-yield information, including:
    - ❏ Steps of a vaginal delivery
    - ❏ Normal and abnormal labor patterns (duration, cervical dilation, etc.)
    - ❏ Indications for cesarean section
    - ❏ Outlines of frequently written notes (preop, op, postop, delivery notes)
    - ❏ The diagnosis and management of preeclampsia/eclampsia and other common maternal or obstetrical complications (e.g. abruptio placentae, placenta previa, preterm labor)

Most of the equipment needed for obstetric or gynecologic exams is provided in the examination room.

ROTATION OBJECTIVES

In OB/GYN, you should be able to generate a differential diagnosis for common problems, perfect a systematic way of working up a patient, gain experience in performing a thorough pelvic examination with a Pap smear, and, it is hoped, find an appreciation of the process of birth. You can also learn about commonly used modalities such as ultrasonography, cervical biopsies, and fetal monitoring. The following list outlines common disease entities, conditions, and topics that you are likely to encounter during your OB/GYN rotation. Topics that are further discussed in this chapter are listed in italics.

Obstetrics

- *Normal physiology of pregnancy*
- *Prenatal care*
- *First-trimester bleeding*
- *Ectopic pregnancy*
- *Gestational diabetes*
- *Pregnancy-induced hypertension*
- *Preterm labor*
- *Normal labor*
- *Abnormal labor patterns*
- *Fetal heart rate monitoring*
- *Third-trimester bleeding*
- *Postpartum hemorrhage*

Gynecology

- *Abnormal uterine bleeding*
- *Amenorrhea*
- *Common vaginal infections (vaginitis)*
- *Contraception*
- *Endometriosis*
- *Gynecologic oncology*
- Infertility
- *Menopause*
- *Pelvic inflammatory disease*
- Pelvic relaxation
- Premenstrual syndrome
- *Sexually transmitted diseases (genital herpes, chlamydia, gonorrhea, condylomata acuminata, syphilis)*

NORMAL PHYSIOLOGY OF PREGNANCY

In pregnancy, multiple adaptations occur in each of the mother's organ systems to support the maternal-fetal unit (see Table 5.1).

TABLE 5.1. Maternal Changes During Pregnancy.

System	Changes	Effects
Metabolic	Increased proteins, lipids Increased need for iron, folate Increased insulin sensitivity early in pregnancy; decreased glucose tolerance later in pregnancy	Increased maternal fat deposition Maternal anemia Narrow euglycemic range (normal 84 ± 10)
Blood	Hyperplasia of hematopoietic system 50% increase in plasma volume with corresponding increase of 20–40% in RBC mass	Increased WBCs, fibrinogen, coagulation factors 7, 8, 9, 10 Physiologic anemia of pregnancy
Endocrine	Increased estrogen, progesterone, prolactin, aldosterone Mood changes	Water retention Breast engorgement, preparation for milk production
Skin, hair	Increased estrogen, progesterone Increased testosterone	Increased skin pigmentation (areolae, axillae, vulva) Mild hirsutism
Respiratory	Increase in minute tidal volume; no change in respiratory rate Upward displacement of diaphragm late in pregnancy	Dyspnea Mild respiratory alkalosis
Cardiovascular	Cardiac output increases up to 45% (mostly due to increase in stroke volume) Decreased arterial blood pressure and peripheral vascular resistance	Dependent edema Physiologic flow murmur Decreased blood pressure, supine hypotensive syndrome
Renal	Dilation of collecting system, decreased peristalsis Increased renal blood flow, glomerular filtration rate by 30–50% Decreased renal glucose absorption Increased aldosterone, renin, antidiuretic hormone (ADH)	Increased frequency of UTI, hydroureters Urinary frequency, nocturia Glucosuria Salt and water retention
Gastrointestinal	Decreased muscle tone leading to hypomotility Decreased lower esophageal sphincter tone Bile stasis	Constipation, hemorrhoids Gastric reflux, hiatal hernia Gallstones

PRENATAL CARE

Prenatal care is critical to the uneventful delivery of a healthy baby. Patients with little or no prenatal care can have complications arising from undiagnosed gestational diabetes, pregnancy-induced hypertension (PIH), and intrauterine growth retardation (IUGR) as well as an inability to accurately estimate gestational age.

Frequency of Visits. Once the pregnancy is confirmed, the patient's prenatal visits should be scheduled as follows:

- **0 to 28 weeks' gestation:** Once every four weeks
- **28 to 36 weeks' gestation:** Once every two to three weeks
- **36 weeks' gestation until delivery:** Once every week

Estimated Date of Confinement. The EDC, also referred to as the EDD or due date, is based on the LMP when it is known. The EDC can be determined through use of a pregnancy wheel, or it can be calculated with Nägele's rule: LMP + 7 days – 3 months. For example, if the last menstrual period is April 4, the EDC will be January 11 of the following year.

Accurate determination of the estimated due date is key.

Prenatal Visits. At each prenatal visit, the following subjective and objective findings should be addressed and documented:

Subjective findings:
- Fetal movement
- Vaginal discharge and/or bleeding
- Abdominal cramps or uterine contractions
- Leakage of fluid (LOF) or signs of ROM
- Blurred vision, headache, rapid weight gain, edema

Objective findings:
- Weight
- Blood pressure
- Dipstick urine protein and glucose
- Edema
- DTRs
- Fetal heart tones—heard after 10 to 12 weeks
- Fundal height

Fundal Height. Fundal height is measured with a tape measure from the top of the symphysis pubis to the top of the fundus. At 12 weeks' gestation, the fundal height should be palpable at the pubic symphysis. At 16 weeks, it should be midway between the pubis and the umbilicus (see Figure 5.1) and at 20 weeks at the umbilicus. At 20 to 32 weeks, the fundal height in centimeters above the symphysis should equal the gestational age in weeks (i.e., S = D). See Figure 5.1 for a depiction of typical fundal height measurements.

Nutrition. Nutrition is a crucial factor in ensuring the health of the mother and the fetus. Iron and folate supplementation is recommended. Normal weight gain is roughly 25 to 35 pounds for the entire pregnancy, with a goal of

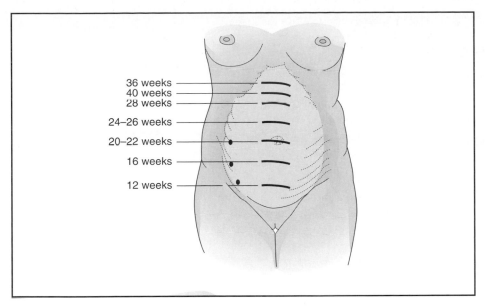

FIGURE 5.1. Height of fundus at various times during pregnancy. (Reprinted, with permission, from DeCherney AH et al. *Current Obstetric and Gynecologic Diagnosis and Treatment*, 8th ed. Stamford, CT: Appleton & Lange, 1994:187.)

a 40-pound weight gain for underweight women and a 15-pound gain for overweight patients. In the first trimester, the patient should gain an average of 2.5 pounds. From 8 to 20 weeks, the patient should gain approximately 0.7 pound a week. From 20 weeks to delivery, she should usually gain roughly one pound a week. Weight gain is excessive when it is greater than four pounds a month and inadequate when it is less than one-half pound a week or less than two pounds a month.

Prenatal Labs. Basic labs should be obtained during the prenatal visits and carefully charted (see Table 5.2).

FIRST-TRIMESTER BLEEDING

First-trimester bleeding, or bleeding that occurs between 0 and 12 weeks' gestational age, complicates some 20–30% of all pregnancies. Approximately 50% of pregnancies with first-trimester bleeding will end in a miscarriage. However, only 5% of cases with the presence of a fetal heart rate on ultrasound end in miscarriage (i.e., abortion). Abortion is the termination of pregnancy at less than 20 weeks' gestational age or with an estimated fetal weight of < 500 g. The different types of abortion are listed in Table 5.3.

Signs and Symptoms. In addition to vaginal bleeding (which can be significant), abortion can be associated with tissue passage, a dilated (opened) cervical os, and hemodynamic instability. Ectopic pregnancy is associated with adnexal mass, cervical motion tenderness (CMT), and bleeding between 6 and 12 weeks' gestational age. A ruptured ectopic pregnancy may present with shock and peritoneal signs.

TABLE 5.2. Standard Prenatal Labs and Studies.

Gestation	Labs to Be Obtained
Initial visit	Type, Rh, and antibody screen CBC Rubella antibody titer (desire immunity) VDRL for syphilis screening Hepatitis B surface antigen test Cervical gonorrhea and chlamydia cultures Pap smear Urinalysis and urine culture PPD Sickle prep in high-risk groups HIV testing (with consent), counseling in high-risk groups Glucose test if patient has risk factors for diabetes Ultrasound for dating purposes if unknown LMP or if discrepancy with exam
15 to 20 weeks	Maternal serum alpha-fetoprotein level should be measured (to screen for any neural tube defect, risk of trisomy 21, or other chromosomal anomaly).
18 to 20 weeks	Ultrasound for anatomy evaluation. If there is only one chance of ultrasound, this is the best time during fetal development to assess both the age and the anatomy of the fetus.
24 to 28 weeks	Glucose test for everyone (risk factors or not).
28 to 30 weeks	RhoGAM administered to patients initially determined to be Rh antibody negative.
34 to 38 weeks	CBC, VDRL (repeated).
36 to 40 weeks	Cervical chlamydia, gonorrhea, and group B streptococcus cultures in high-risk patients.

Differential. The differential diagnosis of first-trimester bleeding includes ectopic pregnancy, complete abortion, incomplete abortion, missed abortion, threatened abortion, septic abortion, intrauterine fetal death, molar pregnancies, and local causes (e.g., cervicitis, genital tract trauma or infection). It is best to place abortion and ectopic pregnancy at the top of your list and rule out one or both of these two most common causes of first-trimester bleeding.

The presence of fetal cardiac activity on ultrasound is reassuring.

Workup. The workup of first-trimester bleeding involves obtaining or performing the following:

- Qualitative/quantitative β-HCG (beta-human chorionic gonadotropin)
- Transvaginal ultrasound
- A pelvic exam to assess cervical dilation and possible ectopic (adnexal mass)
- Consideration of D&C (if the patient does not want the pregnancy)
- Serum progesterone
- Type and screen (for RhoGAM administration if Rh negative)

TABLE 5.3. Types of Spontaneous Abortion.

Abortion	Definition	Treatment
Complete	All products of conception expelled Internal cervical os closed	RhoGAM if appropriate
Incomplete	Some products of conception expelled Internal cervical os open	Dilation and curettage (D&C) RhoGAM if appropriate
Threatened	No products of conception expelled Internal cervical os closed Membranes remain intact Uterine bleeding present Abdominal pain may be present Fetus still viable	Avoid heavy activity Pelvic rest (no intercourse, tampons, etc.) RhoGAM if appropriate
Inevitable	No products of conception expelled Internal cervical os open or Membranes have ruptured Uterine bleeding and cramps	D&C or expectant management RhoGAM if appropriate
Missed	No cardiac activity No products of conception expelled Retained fetal tissue Internal cervical os closed No uterine bleeding	D&C Expectant management RhoGAM if appropriate
Septic	Infection associated with abortion Endometritis leading to septicemia Maternal mortality 10–50%	Complete uterine evacuation D&C IV antibiotics RhoGAM if appropriate

In an abortion, β-HCG is usually not appropriate for gestational age. However, if the abortion is recent or still in the process of expulsion of fetal tissue, β-HCG levels may be within the range of normal values. The progesterone level is usually > 15 ng/mL, and intrauterine pregnancy (i.e., the gestational sac) may be visualized on ultrasound. If a D&C is done, chorionic villi will be evident.

In an ectopic pregnancy, β-HCG is abnormally low for gestational age (80% are < 6500). Ultrasound will not identify an intrauterine pregnancy and may or may not show an adnexal mass. The pelvic and abdominal exam may be significant for an adnexal mass and/or for signs of a "surgical abdomen" (rebound, guarding). No villi are evident on D&C.

If there is a diagnostic dilemma, the β-HCG should be repeated in 48 hours. In a normal intrauterine pregnancy, the β-HCG doubles in 48 hours. An inappropriate rise or plateau of the β-HCG is suspicious for an ectopic pregnancy.

Treatment. As in any case of hemorrhage, the patient needs to be hemodynamically stabilized if there has been significant bleeding. RhoGAM should be given to all antibody-negative patients experiencing abortions or ectopic pregnancy (see Figure 5.2). The treatment for abortions, described above, essentially consists of uterine evacuation and prevention of infection. The treatment for ectopic pregnancy is described below.

ECTOPIC PREGNANCY

An ectopic pregnancy is defined as embryo implantation outside of the uterine cavity, most commonly in the fallopian tubes (98%), and specifically in the ampulla region (90%). The incidence is 17/1000 pregnancies. Etiologies include anything that causes abnormal tubal motility. The primary risk factor for ectopic pregnancy is a history of pelvic inflammatory disease (PID). Other risk factors include prior ectopic pregnancy, tubal/pelvic surgery, diethylstilbestrol (DES) exposure in utero, and intrauterine device (IUD) use.

Signs and Symptoms. The signs and symptoms of an ectopic pregnancy include nausea, vomiting, abdominal and/or pelvic pain (usually on the side of the ectopic pregnancy), abnormal bleeding (including amenorrhea), and a pelvic mass on examination. Ruptured ectopic pregnancies may also present with orthostatic hypotension, tachycardia, local and then generalized abdominal tenderness, shoulder pain, and shock.

Differential. The differential diagnosis of an ectopic pregnancy includes intrauterine pregnancy, threatened abortion, PID, ruptured ovarian cyst, endometriosis, appendicitis, ovarian torsion, renal stones, and diverticulitis.

Workup. A quantitative β-HCG is used to confirm pregnancy and to check for subnormal doubling time and low levels (80% of ectopics have a β-HCG < 6500). Also consider serum progesterone (ectopics usually have < 15 ng/mL).

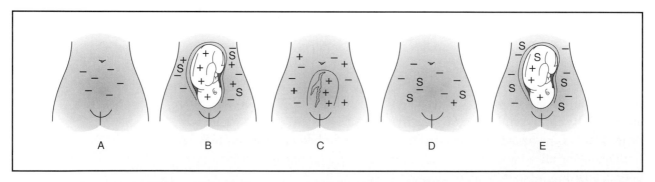

FIGURE 5.2. Why it is important to identify Rh-negative mothers and give RhoGAM. (A) Rh-negative woman before pregnancy. (B) Pregnancy occurs. The fetus is Rh-positive. (C) Separation of the placenta. (D) Following delivery, Rh-isoimmunization occurs in the mother, and she develops antibodies (S = antibodies). (E) The next pregnancy with an Rh-positive fetus. Maternal antibodies cross the placenta, enter the bloodstream, and attach to Rh-positive red cells, causing hemolysis. RhoGAM (Rh IgG) is given to the Rh-negative mother to prevent sensitization. (Reprinted, with permission, from DeCherney AH et al. *Current Obstetric and Gynecologic Diagnosis and Treatment,* 8th ed. Stamford, CT: Appleton & Lange, 1994:339.)

TABLE 5.4. Correlation of Ultrasound Findings, β-HCG Levels, and Time Since Last Menstrual Period.

Transvaginal Ultrasound Findings	β-HCG Level	Time Elapsed Since Last Menstrual Period (days)
Gestational sac[a]	1500	35
Fetal pole	5000	40
Fetal heart motion	11,000	45

[a]For transabdominal ultrasound, the gestational sac should be visualized at a β-HCG level of 6000–6500 and/or 42 days since the last menstrual period.

Transvaginal ultrasound should be performed to identify the possibility of intrauterine gestation. The following possibilities exist:

- The gestational sac is visualized, indicating an intrauterine pregnancy.
- No gestational sac is visualized, in which case the possible scenarios include very early intrauterine pregnancy, ectopic pregnancy, recent abortion, or a false-positive pregnancy test (very rare).

The next step is to correlate the β-HCG level with ultrasound findings and/or with time elapsed since the LMP (see Table 5.4).

On ultrasound, also look for evidence of an ectopic pregnancy (e.g., a noncystic adnexal mass, fluid in the cul-de-sac). Other diagnostic tests include culdocentesis (withdrawal of at least 5 mL of nonclotting blood from the cul-de-sac through the vagina), D&C (only if the patient does not wish to be pregnant) to look for the absence of chorionic villi, and diagnostic laparoscopy.

Maintain a high level of suspicion for ectopic pregnancy.

Treatment. For clinically stable patients in whom the diagnosis of ectopic pregnancy is uncertain and for patients in the "β-HCG discriminatory zone," expectant management of serial β-HCG and ultrasound is warranted.

For patients with confirmed ectopic pregnancy, medical and surgical options are available. For unruptured ectopic pregnancies of < 3 cm with a β-HCG level of < 12,000 in a clinically stable patient, methotrexate can be administered. Surgical options, which depend on the reproductive plans of the patient, the age of the patient, and clinical status, consist of salpingostomy (the tube is incised and only the product of conception is removed), salpingectomy (the entire tube is removed), and salpingo-oophorectomy (both the tube and the ovary are removed).

GESTATIONAL DIABETES

Gestational diabetes occurs in 3–5% of all pregnancies. Physiologically, it is marked by increased insulin release early in pregnancy, although as the pregnancy progresses there is a tendency toward insulin resistance (secondary to the effects of human placental lactogen, progesterone, cortisol, and prolactin).

Risk factors for gestational diabetes include a past history of gestational diabetes, glycosuria or polyuria, obesity, a previous history of a macrosomic baby, habitual abortions or stillbirths, recurrent UTIs, a family history of diabetes, and a fetus that is large for gestational age on ultrasound or by fundal height.

Signs and Symptoms. Gestational diabetes is largely asymptomatic in the mother and is usually noted clinically through the evidence of glycosuria, hyperglycemia, and/or an abnormal glucose tolerance test on routine prenatal screening at 24 to 28 weeks' gestation. Findings may include a fetus that is large for gestational age.

Differential. The differential diagnosis of gestational diabetes includes diabetes mellitus type 1 or 2, volume overload, simple sugar overload, and urinary tract abnormalities.

Workup. All pregnancy patients should be routinely screened for gestational diabetes with a one-hour PG test done between 24 and 28 weeks. For this test, the patient consumes a 50-g glucose load (a special sweet orange liquid) and has her blood glucose level checked one hour later. A value greater than 140 is abnormal and should be followed up with a three-hour glucose test.

In patients with risk factors for gestational diabetes (more than 35 years old, a family/personal history of diabetes, previous delivery of a macrosomic child, obesity, hypertension), a one-hour PG should be checked at the initial intake visit. If the test is normal, the patient should be retested at 24 to 28 weeks' gestation; if it is positive (> 140 mg/dL), she should undergo the three-hour glucose tolerance test.

In the three-hour glucose tolerance test, 100 g of glucose is administered orally, and the blood glucose level is checked at fasting (initial reading) and at one-, two-, and three-hour time intervals:

- **Fasting:** > 95 mg/dL is considered abnormally high serum glucose.
- **One hour:** > 180 mg/dL is considered abnormally high serum glucose.
- **Two hours:** > 155 mg/dL is considered abnormally high serum glucose.
- **Three hours:** > 140 mg/dL is considered abnormally high serum glucose.

The diagnosis of gestational diabetes is established if the patient has abnormally high blood glucose levels at any two of those four time points.

Treatment. For uncomplicated cases, start with the American Diabetic Association (ADA) diet and monitor fasting blood glucose and two-hour postprandial glucose levels. If there is a persistent (one- to two-week) fasting blood glucose level > 95 mg/dL or a two-hour postprandial glucose level > 120 mg/dL despite dietary compliance, then start insulin. Patient education and diabetic clinic/dietitian consults are important in patient management.

Complications. Complications from gestational diabetes can be divided into maternal and fetal (see Table 5.5).

TABLE 5.5. Complications of Gestational Diabetes.

Maternal Complications	Fetal Complications
Preterm labor	Macrosomia
Polyhydramnios	Shoulder dystocia
Cesarean section for macrosomia	Perinatal mortality 2–5%
Preeclampsia/eclampsia, PIH	Congenital defects
Risk of future glucose intolerance or type 1 diabetes mellitus (50% of gestational diabetes patients have impaired glucose tolerance later in life)	

PREGNANCY-INDUCED HYPERTENSION

Hypertension in pregnancy is diagnosed when two blood pressure measurements of 140/90 mmHg are measured two times at least six hours apart. Pregnancy induced hypertension (PIH) is hypertension that is present after 20 weeks' gestation. Hypertension prior to 20 weeks is by definition chronic hypertension.

Preeclampsia is defined as PIH, proteinuria (300 mg/24 hours or > 1+ protein on urine dip), and/or edema. Severe preeclampsia is defined as a blood pressure of > 160/110 (two such values more than six hours apart) or mild preeclampsia with proteinuria > 5 g/day, symptoms (headache, visual changes, epigastric pain), oligohydramnios, and elevated liver enzymes or evidence of IUGR. A variant of preeclampsia with a poor prognosis is known as "HELLP" syndrome (**H**emolysis, **E**levated **L**iver enzymes, **L**ow **P**latelets). Eclampsia manifests as seizures (not due to neurologic disease) in a patient with preeclampsia.

> **HELLP syndrome—**
>
> **H**emolysis
> **E**levated **L**FTs
> **L**ow **P**latelets (thrombocytopenia)

Preeclampsia is thought to result from systemic endothelial damage that causes vascular spasm, capillary hyperpermeability, and an imbalance in which the level of thromboxane (a vasoconstrictor) is much higher than that of prostacyclin (a vasodilator). The pathology is linked to the placenta; the only cure is to remove the placenta (i.e., delivery). Eclampsia results from CNS damage secondary to endothelial damage.

Risk factors for preeclampsia include nulliparity, extremes of age when pregnant (< 15, > 35), multiple gestations, vascular disease (secondary to lupus or diabetes), and chronic hypertension.

Signs and Symptoms. Mild preeclampsia and severe preeclampsia share the same spectrum of signs and symptoms (see Table 5.6). Eclampsia is present if seizures occur in a preeclamptic patient.

Differential. As cited above, the two most common causes of PIH are preeclampsia and eclampsia. A common cause of PIH occurring in the first or second trimester is a molar pregnancy. Other diseases in the differential for preeclampsia include renal disease, renovascular hypertension, primary aldosteronism, Cushing's disease, pheochromocytoma, and systemic lupus erythematosus. Consider primary seizure disorder and thrombotic thrombocytopenic purpura (TTP) in the workup of eclampsia.

Preeclamptic and eclamptic patients are at risk for seizures up to 24 hours postpartum and have been reported up to 7 days out.

Workup. As discussed in Table 5.6, the diagnostic criteria for preeclampsia include two blood pressure readings of 140/90 mmHg or greater measured at least six hours apart, along with proteinuria (300 mg/24 hours or 1 mg/L) and/or edema. The diagnosis of eclampsia is made when seizures that are not due to neurologic disease are present in a patient with preeclampsia.

Labs and diagnostic tests to obtain in the workup of preeclampsia include:

- CBC and platelet count
- BUN/creatinine
- Fibrinogen, fibrinogen split products (where indicated)
- Urinalysis (UA), serial urine protein
- Amniocentesis (to check for fetal lung maturity)
- LFTs
- Prothrombin time/partial thromboplastin time (PT/PTT)
- Urine toxicology screen (if it is possible that blood pressure is secondary to drugs)
- Ultrasound (to rule out oligohydramnios and IUGR)
- Nonstress test
- A biophysical profile as indicated

Treatment. The only cure for preeclampsia is delivery of the fetus and placenta (see Table 5.7).

TABLE 5.6. Signs and Symptoms of Preeclampsia and Eclampsia.

Mild Preeclampsia	Severe Preeclampsia	Eclampsia
BP > 140/90 measured two times six hours apart	Mild preeclampsia plus: BP > 160/110 measured two times six hours apart	The three most common symptoms preceding an eclamptic attack are headache, visual changes, and RUQ/epigastric pain
Proteinuria (>300 mg/day or 1+ on dipstick)	Proteinuria (> 5 g/day or > 3+ on dipstick)	Seizures; severe if not controlled with anticonvulsant therapy
Cerebral changes (headaches, somnolence)	Visual changes (blurred vision, scotomata)	
Rapid weight gain, edema, jugular venous distention	Right upper quadrant (RUQ)/ epigastric pain	
Hyperactive reflexes, clonus, jugular venous distention	Oligohydramnios	
	Elevated liver function tests (LFTs)	
	Thrombocytopenia (< 100)	
	Oliguria	
	Pulmonary edema/cyanosis	
	IUGR	

TABLE 5.7. Management of Preeclampsia and Eclampsia.

Preeclampsia	Eclampsia
If term or fetal lung maturity is demonstrated, deliver.	Insert padded tongue blade.
If severe, expedite delivery regardless of maturity.	Supplemental oxygen.
If mild preeclampsia: Modified bed rest, check blood pressure, reflexes, daily weight, and urine protein output, labs, fetal surveillance, patient education.	Place in lateral decubitus position.
	Prevent maternal trauma.
Control blood pressure with antihypertensives (hydralazine, labetalol, diazoxide) if diastolic blood pressure is higher than 110 mmHg. The goal is to maintain a blood pressure lower than 160/110, preferably with a diastolic blood pressure of 90–100 mmHg.	Control seizure with magnesium sulfate and consider diazepam if seizures are poorly controlled.
	Control blood pressure if severe hypertension (blood pressure > 160/110, or diastolic blood pressure > 110).
If severe, immediately hospitalize, check urine output, check for pulmonary edema, keep diastolic blood pressure 90–105 mmHg with antihypertensive, give magnesium sulfate for seizure prophylaxis, and deliver as soon as possible by labor induction and/or cesarean section.	General measures: Limit fluid intake, Foley catheter, monitor inputs and outputs, monitor magnesium blood level, carefully monitor fetal status, initiate steps to delivery!
	Postpartum: same as preeclampsia.
Postpartum: Continue magnesium sulfate for at least the first 24 hours; check blood pressure, pulmonary status, and fluid retention. Follow heme, renal, and liver labs.	General course of disease: 50% of seizures occur antepartum, 25% occur intrapartum, and 25% occur within 24 hours postpartum.
General course of disease: 30% of preeclampsia cases occur before 30 weeks' gestational age, with the maximum number of cases occurring at 34 weeks' gestational age.	

PRETERM LABOR

Preterm labor complicates 5–10% of all pregnancies. Risk factors for preterm labor can be described by the mnemonic "MAPPS." However, half of all cases of preterm labor occur in patients without any risk factors.

Signs and Symptoms. The signs and symptoms of preterm labor include abdominal or pelvic pain, back pain, vaginal discharge, bloody show, uterine contractions, cervical dilation and/or effacement, and rupture of membranes.

Differential. The differential diagnosis of preterm labor includes false labor (preterm contractions without cervical dilation or change), appendicitis, local causes (cervicitis, trauma, physiologic discharge), and genital tract infections.

Workup. Diagnostic criteria are based on the presence of preterm (< 37 weeks' gestation) and true labor (uterine contractions of sufficient duration and intensity to result in cervical dilation of > 2 cm or effacement of > 80%). A cervical exam is necessary.

Cervical cultures and a wet mount should be obtained to rule out infectious causes of preterm labor. Other possible infectious sources should also be considered, including UTI, pyelonephritis, upper respiratory infection (URI), and chorioamnionitis. Labs to obtain include CBC with differential, urine tox

> **Risk factors for preterm labor—**
>
> **MAPPS**
> **M**ultiple gestations
> **A**bdominal surgery during pregnancy
> **P**revious **P**reterm labor
> **P**revious **P**reterm delivery
> **S**urgery of the cervix

screen, urine culture, vaginal and cervical culture for group B strep/chlamydia/gonorrhea, and a sterile speculum exam if there is suspicion of premature ROM. An ultrasound should be performed to assess estimated fetal weight and presentation.

Treatment. The course of management depends on the gestational age of the fetus. The main goal is to delay delivery until fetal lung maturity has been achieved.

Since dehydration and infectious processes are known to causes preterm contractions and preterm labor, initial therapy should include IV hydration and a workup of possible etiologies. Serial exams—when possible, performed by the same examiner—should be obtained depending on the frequency of uterine contractions. If there is cervical change, tocolytics should be initiated (terbutaline, magnesium sulfate, nifedipine, ritodrine) as long as there are no contraindications (see the mnemonic labeled "CHAMPS"). There is, however, no uncontested evidence that the use of tocolytics prolongs premature delivery; tocolytics are ineffective if the patient is in active labor (cervical dilation ≥ 4 cm). The patient should be observed for possible signs of infection, especially if there is premature ROM. In monitoring the fetus, a daily nonstress test and interval ultrasound should be performed to monitor fetal growth and presentation.

Betamethasone should be considered if the following conditions exist: an estimated gestational age of 24 to 34 weeks (and the possibility of delivery within one week), the absence of chorioamnionitis, the absence of uncontrolled maternal diabetes, and no need for immediate delivery (e.g., placental abruption). Note that betamethasone has been proven most effective with a singleton pregnancy between 28 and 34 weeks' gestational age. Amniocentesis may be considered, especially at 35 to 36 weeks' gestational age, to check for fetal lung maturity (lecithin-sphingomyelin ratio > 2:1). Pediatrics should be notified when the patient is admitted, not only for counseling of the patient as to the expected neonatal outcome but also to ensure that the pediatricians are aware of a potential preterm infant delivery.

NORMAL LABOR

Labor has two components:

- Uterine contractions of sufficient frequency, duration, and intensity
- Cervical changes, including effacement (thinning) and dilation

Cervical dilation that occurs without uterine contractions is not considered true labor. Similarly, uterine contractions without cervical effacement and dilation are referred to as Braxton Hicks contractions, or false labor.

Onset of Labor. Late in pregnancy, patients often report a change in the shape of the abdomen with the sensation that the baby is less heavy. This event, termed *lightening,* results from the descent of the fetal head into the

> **Contraindications for tocolytics—**
>
> **CHAMPS**
> **C**horioamnionitis
> **H**emorrhage
> **A**bruption of placenta
> Fetal **M**aturity
> **P**reeclampsia/ eclampsia
> **S**evere intrauterine growth retardation

pelvis. Another event occurring late in pregnancy is the passage of bloody show, a blood-tinged mucus that is produced when the cervix begins to thin out (effacement). Cervical effacement commonly occurs before the onset of true labor, particularly in nulliparous patients.

Patients are instructed to report to the hospital for evaluation when their contractions occur every five minutes for at least one hour; if they sense that their membranes have ruptured (i.e., there is a large gush of fluid or continuous leakage); if there is significant bleeding; or if there is a significant decrease in fetal movement. At this point, an SVE will be done to assess the amount of effacement (quantified as a percentage of cervix), the amount of cervical dilation (expressed in centimeters), and the station of the fetal head (the relationship of the fetal head to the level of the ischial spines). As the baby descends, he or she moves from station −5 to +5 cm (where 0 is defined to be the fetal head at the level of the ischial spines) or from −3 to +3 station units (still in reference to 0 being the ischial spines, but using "units" rather than centimeters).

Stages of Labor. Labor is divided into three stages, as shown in Table 5.8 and Figure 5.3. The first stage is the onset of labor to the complete (10-cm) dilation of the cervix. The second stage of labor is the time from complete dilation to the delivery of the infant. The third stage of labor is from the delivery of the infant to the delivery of the placenta. The first stage of labor is further divided

TABLE 5.8. The Three Stages of Labor.

Stage	Starts/End	Events	Average Duration (hours)	
			Nulli[a]	Multi[b]
First				
Latent	Regular uterine contractions/ cervix dilated up to 4 cm	Highly variable duration; cervix effaces and slowly dilates	6–20	4–14
Active	4-cm cervical dilation/complete cervical dilation (10 cm)	Regular and intense uterine contractions; cervix effaces and dilates more quickly; fetal head progressively descends into pelvis	4–12	2–5
Second	Complete cervical dilation/ delivery of the baby	Baby undergoes all stages of cardinal movements	1–3	0.5–1.0
Third	Delivery of baby/delivery of placenta	Placenta separates and uterus contracts to establish hemostasis	0–0.5	0–0.5

[a]Nulli = nulliparous (first-time mother).
[b]Multi = multiparous (delivered vaginally before).

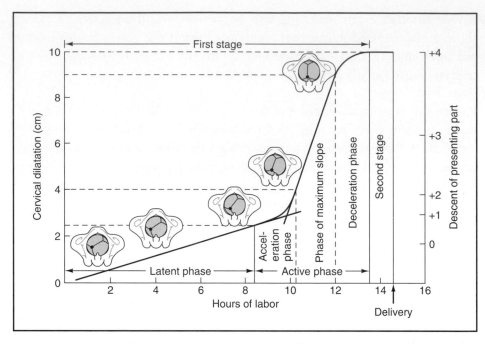

FIGURE 5.3. Cervical dilation, level of descent, and orientation of occipitoanterior presentation during various stages of labor. (Reprinted, with permission, from DeCherney AH et al. *Current Obstetric and Gynecologic Diagnosis and Treatment,* 8th ed. Stamford, CT: Appleton & Lange, 1994:211.)

into the latent phase and the active phase of labor. Latent phase labor involves effacement and the early and slow cervical dilation period. Active labor, which usually begins at approximately 4 cm of dilation, signifies a period of more rapid cervical dilation.

Cardinal Movements. Babies undergo seven stereotypical cardinal movements for successful delivery. These movements, which constitute the second stage of labor, are as follows:

1. Engagement
2. Descent
3. Flexion
4. Internal rotation
5. Extension
6. External rotation
7. Expulsion

Fetal Lie, Presentation, and Position. The orientation of the baby is described in relation to the maternal pelvis in the following manner:

- **Fetal lie:** The long axis of the baby in relation to the long axis of the mother (longitudinal, transverse, oblique).
- **Fetal presentation:** That part of the fetus which enters the pelvis first— e.g., vertex (head first), breech (buttocks or leg first), face, brow.
- **Fetal position:** The reference point of the fetal presenting part (for vertex presentation, the presenting part is the occiput; for breech presentation, the presenting part is the sacrum) to the maternal pelvis (right, left, anterior, posterior).

Note that the most common fetal orientation is longitudinal, vertex, occiput anterior (i.e., the baby's face emerges facing the mom's rectum).

ABNORMAL LABOR PATTERNS

A diagnosis of abnormal labor is considered in any case in which there is a variation in the normal pattern of cervical dilation or descent of the fetal presenting part. It occurs in 8–11% of all cephalic deliveries.

Signs and Symptoms. Labor is abnormal when the duration of an event is too long or too short. Table 5.9 describes patterns of abnormal labor.

Also beware of false labor, which may be confused with arrest of dilation and has the following distinguishing characteristics:

- Irregular intervals and duration of uterine contractions
- Contraction intensity unchanged
- No cervical dilation
- Lower back and abdominal discomfort
- Relief with sedation

TABLE 5.9. Abnormal Labor Patterns.

Abnormal Pattern	Threshold Duration of Labor		Possible Causes
	Nulliparous	**Multiparous**	
Precipitous	Completion of stages 1 and 2 in < 3 hours		Unknown
Prolonged latent phase	> 20 hours	> 14 hours	Ineffective uterine contractions Unripe cervix Abnormal fetal position False labor
Protracted active phase	> 12 hours or rate of cervical dilation: < 1.2 cm/hour or fetal descent: < 1 cm/hour	> 6 hours < 1.5 cm/hour < 2 cm/hour	Abnormal fetal position Fetopelvic disproportion Excess sedation Ineffective uterine contractions
Arrest of dilation in active contractions phase	Cervical dilation stops for > 2 hours		Ineffective uterine contractions Fetopelvic disproportion Abnormal fetal lie, presentation, or position
Arrest of fetal descent (late in active phase and throughout second state)	Fetal descent stops for > 1 hour		Ineffective uterine contractions Fetopelvic disproportion

HIGH-YIELD TOPICS

Obstetrics and Gynecology

Differential. The differential diagnosis of abnormal labor includes normal labor, false labor, ineffective uterine contractions, fetal malposition, and fetopelvic disproportion.

Workup. Workup begins with accurately assessing the specific abnormal pattern the patient is experiencing, which includes:

- Graphic demonstration of cervical dilation and effacement.
- Documenting on each vaginal exam the dilation of the cervix, the station of the fetal presenting part, the presence of the caput or molding of the fetal head, and the position of the fetal presenting part. The results of each examination should be assessed dynamically.

Workup then proceeds with the systematic assessment of the "3 Ps" of labor:

> **Causes of abnormal labor—**
>
> **the "3 Ps"**
> **P**owers (uterine contractions)
> **P**assenger (fetus)
> **P**assage (pelvic)

- **Powers (uterine forces):** Frequency and duration can be evaluated through manual palpation of the gravid abdomen during a contraction; by a tocodynamometer; and by an internal pressure catheter (this is the only way to measure the pressure generated by each uterine contraction).
- **Passenger:** Estimation of fetal weight and clinical evaluation of fetal lie, presentation, and position.
- **Passage:** Measurement of the bony pelvis is often a poor predictor of abnormal labor unless the pelvis is extremely contracted. Also assess for other physical obstacles (distended bladder or colon, uterine myoma, cervical mass).

Treatment. The treatment of abnormal labor is as follows:

- **Precipitous labor:**
  - Tocolytics may be administered to slow down uterine activity.
  - Complications include uterine atony leading to postpartum hemorrhage and genital tract trauma.
- **Prolonged latent phase:**
  - Rest or augmentation of labor with oxytocin if "power" is the problem.
  - Amniotomy (i.e., artificial rupture of membranes [AROM]).
- **Protracted/arrested active phase:**
  - IUPC to measure force of UCs.
  - AROM.
  - Augmentation with oxytocin if "power" is the problem.
  - Cesarean section if there is fetopelvic disproportion or maternal/fetal distress.
- **Arrest in second stage:**
  - Attempt vaginal delivery if the mom and baby are doing well.
  - Give oxytocin augmentation and provide lots of support for mom.
  - Perform operative vaginal delivery (forceps, vacuum) if the vertex is low in the pelvis.
  - Perform a cesarean section if there is maternal/fetal distress, breech, or fetopelvic disproportion.

Prolonged labor predisposes the mother to increased risk of infection, exhaustion, laceration, uterine atony, and operative delivery. The fetus experiences an increased risk of asphyxia, infection, trauma, and possible cerebral damage.

FETAL HEART RATE MONITORING

The fetal heart rate is usually monitored continuously throughout labor to evaluate its effects on fetal intrapartum events. Fetal response to the stress of labor can be assessed by continuously monitoring the fetal heart rate. As described in further detail below, signs of hypoxia and fetal distress may include changes in the baseline fetal heart rate, decreased heart rate variability, and late decelerations.

External monitoring is conducted with an ultrasound transducer affixed to the maternal abdomen. Internal monitoring is done through an electrode attached to the fetal scalp and requires that the membranes have been ruptured.

Baseline Fetal Heart Rate. The normal range of the human fetal heart rate is 110–160 bpm. A baseline heart rate > 160 bpm for more than 10 minutes is referred to as *baseline tachycardia*. Similarly, a baseline heart rate < 110 bpm for more than 10 minutes is classified as a *baseline bradycardia*. Fetal tachycardia and bradycardia are both more likely to be associated with fetal hypoxia than is a normal baseline. Causes of tachycardia other than hypoxia include maternal fever, fetal infection, maternal tachycardia, maternal thyrotoxicosis, fetal anemia, fetal arrhythmias, and the use of β-sympathomimetic drugs such as terbutaline. Fetal bradycardia may signify damage to the conduction system of the fetal heart, maternal autoimmune disease, or treatment with drugs such as beta blockers.

Heart Rate Variability. Heart rate variability represents the interplay between cardioinhibitory and cardioaccelerary centers in the fetal brain stem. Normal beat-to-beat variability is the most reliable indicator of fetal well-being and is one of the best indicators of intact integration between the CNS and heart of the fetus. Short-term variability is the variation on a "beat-to-beat basis" and usually ranges from 3 to 5 bpm. Long-term variability refers to fluctuations with amplitudes of 5–20 bpm occurring at 3–5 cycles per minute.

Periodic Changes. Transient increases in the fetal heart rate are known as accelerations, while transient decreases are referred to as decelerations.

- **Accelerations:** Accelerations are transient increases in the fetal heart rate above the determined baseline. Accelerations are reassuring and usually indicate fetal well-being. For the fetal heart rate to be considered reactive (a sign of fetal well-being), there must be two accelerations of at least 15 beats above the baseline lasting at least 15 seconds during a 20-minute period.
- **Early decelerations:** Early decelerations are decreases in fetal heart rate that begin with a contraction, reach their nadir at the peak of the contraction, and end with the completion of the contraction. As such, they

are essentially mirror images of uterine contractions. The fetal heart rate never falls below 100 bpm. Early decelerations result from pressure on the fetal head through a reflex response mediated by the vagus nerve with release of acetylcholine at the sinoatrial node. Early decelerations are innocuous and can be observed throughout labor without alteration in fetal condition or acid-base status.

- **Variable decelerations:** Variable decelerations are slowings of the heart rate that may start before, during, or after the uterine contraction and are characterized by a rapid fall in fetal heart rate, often below 100 bpm, with a rapid return to baseline. These decelerations are associated with umbilical cord compression and are mediated through the vagus nerve with sudden and often erratic release of acetylcholine at the fetal sinoatrial node. This pattern is often seen with oligohydramnios or after ROM secondary to "decreased cushioning" of the umbilical cord. If the variable decelerations are severe and repetitive, hypoxia and metabolic acidosis may result. Severe variables are those that last longer than 60 seconds or nadir at < 70 bpm. Moderate variable decelerations are those that last between 30 and 60 seconds and nadir between 70 and 80 bpm. Mild variable decelerations are those that last less than 30 seconds and nadir no lower than up to 80 bpm.

- **Late decelerations:** Late decelerations begin after the uterine contraction starts, reach their nadir after the peak of the contraction, and end after the contraction ceases. These may also be mirror images of uterine contractions but occur "late" in timing relative to each contraction. Late decelerations are a sign of uteroplacental insufficiency resulting from decreased uterine perfusion or decreased placental function. Late decelerations are associated with progressive fetal hypoxia and acidemia. This type of deceleration may occur with any process that would predispose to insufficient blood flow and oxygenation of the fetus, such as placental abruption, excessive uterine activity, maternal hypotension, anemia, and IUGR.

THIRD-TRIMESTER BLEEDING

Third-trimester bleeding, which is defined as any bleeding that occurs after 28 weeks' gestation, complicates approximately 5% of all pregnancies.

Signs and Symptoms. Bleeding may range from small amounts of spotting to passage of large clots. It may be preceded or accompanied by cramping or may be painless. See Table 5.10 for a complete description of the characteristics, diagnosis, and management of the two most common causes of third-trimester vaginal bleeding: abruptio placentae and placenta previa (see Figure 5.4).

Differential. The differential diagnosis of third-trimester bleeding includes abruptio placentae (30%), placenta previa (20%), early labor, and genital tract lesions. Other causes of third-trimester bleeding include bloody show (dilation of the cervix and loss of mucous plug associated with cervical dilation during the first stage of labor), ruptured vasa previa (rupture of fetal ves-

TABLE 5.10. Abruptio Placentae Versus Placenta Previa.

	Abruptio Placentae	Placenta Previa
Pathophysiology	Separation of normally implanted placenta from attachment to uterus.	Abnormal implantation of placenta near or at the cervical os, classified as: ■ Total: placenta covers cervical os ■ Partial: placenta partially covers os ■ Marginal: edge of placenta extends to margin of os ■ Low-lying: placenta within reach of the examining finger reached through the cervix
Incidence	1/120 (but accounts for 15% of perinatal mortality).	1/200
Risk factors	Hypertension, abdominal or pelvic trauma, tobacco or cocaine use.	Prior cesarean sections, grand multiparous.
Symptoms	Painful vaginal bleeding (although 10% of the cases are concealed and there will be no bleeding); bleeding usually does not spontaneously cease. Abdominal pain, uterine hypertonicity, tenderness. Fetal distress present.	Painless, bright red bleeding (bleeding source is purely mom's), with the first bleeding episode at roughly 29 to 30 weeks. Bleeding often ceases in one to two hours with or without uterine contractions. Usually no fetal distress present.
Diagnosis	On transabdominal/transvaginal ultrasound, look for retroplacental clot; can only rule in diagnosis but cannot rule out! Not very sensitive. Abdominal exam (tenderness). Signs of fetal distress, frequent uterine contractions, hypertonicity.	On transabdominal ultrasound, look for an abnormally positioned placenta; this test is very sensitive to rule out this diagnosis.
Management	Stable patient with premature fetus: expectant management with continuous monitoring. Moderate to severe abruption: immediate delivery (vaginal delivery if fetal heart rate is stable, cesarean section if mom or fetus is in distress). Close fetal monitoring at all times. Amniocentesis to check fetal lung maturity, if indicated.	No vaginal exam! Premature fetus (stable patient): bed rest, tocolytics, serial ultrasound to check fetal growth, resolution of partial previa. If at or near term, amniocentesis to check fetal lung maturity; betamethasone to augment fetal lung maturity if indicated. Delivery by cesarean section (vaginal route if resolves). Delivery in the presence of persistent labor, unstable bleeding requiring multiple transfusion, coagulation defects, documented fetal lung maturity.
Complications	Hemorrhagic shock. Coagulopathy: Disseminated intravascular coagulation (DIC) complicates 10% of all abruptions. Ischemic necrosis of distal organs. Recurrence risk is 5–16%; this risk increases to 25% after two previous abruptions. Fetal anemia.	Placenta accreta (up to 25% with one previous cesarean section). Vasa previa. Twofold increase in congenital abnormalities. Increased risk of postpartum hemorrhage. Fetal anemia.

HIGH-YIELD TOPICS

Obstetrics and Gynecology

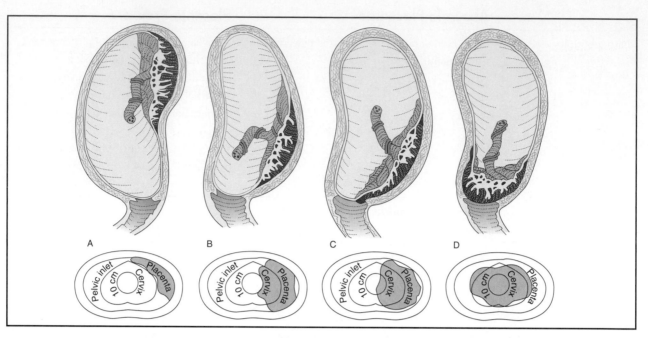

FIGURE 5.4. (A) Normal placenta. (B) Low implantation. (C) Partial placenta previa. (D) Complete placenta previa. (Reprinted, with permission, from DeCherney AH et al. *Current Obstetric and Gynecologic Diagnosis and Treatment,* 8th ed. Stamford, CT: Appleton & Lange, 1994:404.)

sel over the cervical os, which is rare but serious), ruptured uterus, and cervical carcinoma.

Never do a vaginal exam prior to an ultrasound in a patient with third-trimester bleeding.

Workup. The general principles to apply in approaching a patient with third-trimester bleeding are as follows:

- Stat ultrasound to rule out placenta previa before performing a vaginal or speculum exam (Always First!).
- Perform a cautious sterile speculum exam to evaluate the source of bleeding or ruptured membranes if no previa is seen.
- Obtain cervical cultures.
- Perform a vaginal exam (to rule out labor).
- Perform an abdominal exam.
- Check for fetal heart tones and conduct a nonstress test (this should be done while performing the workup).
- Consider amniocentesis for phosphatidylglycerol and a lecithin-sphingomyelin ratio for the assessment of delivery options.

Other tests include type and cross for at least two units of packed RBCs (depending on the amount of bleeding), CBC, type and screen (RhoGAM if Rh negative!), PT/PTT, the Kleihauer-Betke test (a slide test that looks for fetal RBCs among those of the mother), UA, and drug screen.

Treatment. Treatment generally includes bed rest and tocolytics (drugs that arrest uterine contractions) for the stable patient. In a mature fetus or in the presence of severe placental abruption, close fetal monitoring, amniotomy, and cesarean section are indicated, as listed in Table 5.10.

POSTPARTUM HEMORRHAGE

The clinical diagnosis of postpartum hemorrhage is established when there is more than a 500-mL blood loss within the first 24 hours of delivery. Hemorrhage can be sudden and profuse, or blood loss can occur more slowly but persistently. In either case, excessive bleeding is a serious and potentially fatal complication. The following discussion outlines the three most common causes of postpartum hemorrhage together with their diagnosis and management.

Differential. The three most common causes of postpartum hemorrhage are uterine atony (the most common cause), genital tract trauma, and retained placental tissue (see Table 5.11). Other causes of postpartum hemorrhage include uterine inversion, uterine rupture, and cervical carcinoma.

Workup/Treatment. The diagnosis and treatment of the three major causes of postpartum hemorrhage are discussed in Table 5.11.

Don't forget serial hematocrits in postpartum hemorrhage.

Gynecology

ABNORMAL UTERINE BLEEDING

Uterine bleeding is considered abnormal in any postmenopausal woman. In premenopausal women, uterine bleeding is abnormal if any of the following exist: a menstrual cycle lasting more than 8 days, a menstrual interval of less than 21 days, and/or a total blood loss/menstrual cycle > 80 mL (see Table 5.12).

Etiology. Causes of abnormal bleeding during the reproductive years are as follows:

Pregnancy is the most common cause of abnormal uterine bleeding (always check a pregnancy test!).

- Pregnancy is the most common cause. Keep in mind abnormal pregnancies such as ectopic pregnancy, threatened abortion (internal cervical os closed), and incomplete abortion (internal cervical os opened).
- Organic causes such as blood dyscrasias, hypersplenism, hypothyroidism, sepsis, idiopathic thrombocytopenic purpura (ITP), and leukemia.
- Anatomic causes include malignancies, infections, endometriosis, ruptured corpus luteum cyst, fibroids, endometrial polyp, and trauma.
- Dysfunctional uterine bleeding (DUB)—bleeding without any other recognizable cause.

The most common cause of postmenopausal vaginal bleeding is atrophic vaginitis. Other causes of postmenopausal bleeding include endometrial cancer, atrophic endometrium, or hormone replacement therapy (HRT).

Workup. On physical examination, assess rate of bleeding, hemodynamic status, orthostatic vitals, skin and hair changes, thyroid enlargement, galactorrhea, obesity, hirsutism, CMT, uterine size, cervical lesions, and adnexal tenderness. Laboratory tests should include CBC, pregnancy test, coagulation studies if coagulopathy is suspected, endocrine tests (thyroid-stimulating hor-

TABLE 5.11. Common Causes of Postpartum Hemorrhage.

	Uterine Atony	Genital Tract Trauma	Retained Placental Tissue
Risk factors	Overdistention of the uterus (multiple gestations, macrosomia) Abnormal labor (prolonged labor, precipitous labor) Conditions interfering with uterine contractions (uterine myomas, magnesium sulfate, general anesthesia) Uterine infection	Precipitous labor Operative vaginal delivery (forceps, vacuum extraction) Large infant Inadequate laceration repair Unrecognized cervical laceration	Placenta accreta/increta/percreta Preterm delivery Placenta previa Previous cesarean section/curettage Uterine leiomyomas
Diagnosis	Palpation of a softer, flaccid, "boggy" uterus without a firm fundus	Careful visualization of the lower genital tract looking for any laceration > 2 cm in length or bleeding	Careful inspection of the placenta for missing cotyledons Ultrasound may also be used to examine the uterus
Treatment	Most common cause of postpartum hemorrhage (90%) Bimanual uterine massage, is usually successful Oxytocin infusion Empty bladder (overdistended bladder can prevent uterine contractions) Methylergonovine maleate (Methergine) if not hypertensive and/or prostaglandin F2-alpha (Hemabate) if patient is not asthmatic or hypertensive	Surgical repair of the physical defect	Manual removal of the remaining placental tissue Curettage with suctioning may also be used, with care taken to avoid perforating the uterine fundus In cases of true placenta accreta/increta/percreta where the placental villi invade into the uterine tissue, hysterectomy may be required as a life-preserving therapy

mone [TSH], prolactin, luteinizing hormone [LH], follicle-stimulating hormone [FSH]), endometrial biopsy for women more than 35 years old, and transvaginal ultrasound to check for masses/endometrial thickening (normally < 5 mm in postmenopausal women).

To work up abnormal uterine bleeding:

- Obtain a CBC to check hematocrit; do a pregnancy test.
- Determine whether the patient is having ovulatory or anovulatory cycles. The patient is ovulating if she has menstrual cycles at regular intervals.

TABLE 5.12. Abnormal Uterine Bleeding Patterns.

Term	Definition
Menorrhagia	Prolonged cycle (> 8 days) or increased total blood loss (> 80 mL) with regular intervals
Metrorrhagia	Irregular bleeding between menses with frequent intervals
Menometrorrhagia	Irregular, prolonged, and heavy menstrual bleeding with frequent intervals
Polymenorrhea	Regular intervals of < 21 days
Oligomenorrhea	Regular intervals of > 35 days to six months

- If the patient is not ovulating, she has dysfunctional uterine bleeding (irregular, excessive bleeding with no organic cause), most likely secondary to hormonal irregularities.
- If the patient is ovulating, she is having abnormal uterine bleeding, and further workup is required to rule out pathology. Obtain a platelet count, bleeding time, and PT/PTT. Check for cervical masses and polyps, perform a D&C or a hysteroscopy, and obtain a biopsy if necessary.

Treatment. Treatment for abnormal uterine bleeding is as follows:

- **Anovulatory bleeding:** After ruling out pathologies (uterine polyps, endometrial cancer), patients are placed on medroxyprogesterone acetate (Provera) or OCPs. Also consider HRT if the patient is perimenopausal (see Table 5.13).
- **Dysfunctional uterine bleeding:**
  - For mild cases (hemoglobin > 11), treat the patient with iron supplement, docusate (Colace), NSAIDs to reduce menorrhagia, and OCPs. Alternatively, high dose progestins such as norethindrone can be used to normalize menses. In more severe cases (hemoglobin < 7), the patient should be hemodynamically stabilized (blood transfusion, saline) and placed on oral hormone therapy (conjugated estrogen, Provera) or OCPs.

TABLE 5.13. General Management of Abnormal Uterine Bleeding.

Acute Uterine Bleeding	Recurrent Uterine Bleeding
High-dose estrogen OCPs	Gonadotropin-releasing hormone (GnRH) agonists (Lupron) Danazol (multiple side effects) D&C (not recommended) Endometrial ablation Total abdominal hysterectomy

- For recurrent, severe, dysfunctional uterine bleeding, suppression can be achieved by placing the patient on OCPs, Provera, or Depo-Provera with or without an estrogen supplement.
- Surgical options for dysfunctional uterine bleeding include hysteroscopy with D&C, endometrial ablation with laser or electrocautery, and hysterectomy.

AMENORRHEA

Amenorrhea is defined as the complete absence of menstruation and is divided into primary and secondary amenorrhea.

Signs and Symptoms. By definition, primary amenorrhea is the absence of menses by age 16, whereas secondary amenorrhea is the absence of menses for three cycles or for six months with normal prior menses.

Differential. The causes of primary amenorrhea include gonadal failure/agenesis, müllerian abnormality, androgen insensitivity syndrome, pituitary failure, and constitutional delay (physiologic). Common causes of secondary amenorrhea include pregnancy, hypothyroidism, polycystic ovarian syndrome (PCOS), premature menopause (premature ovarian failure), pituitary failure, galactorrhea, hyperprolactinemia, and eating disorders.

Workup/Treatment. The workup of amenorrhea should follow a logical order:

1. Does the patient have primary amenorrhea (see Figure 5.5) or secondary amenorrhea (see Figures 5.6 and 5.7)? Making this distinction will help narrow down the differential workup.
2. The causes of amenorrhea can be systemically broken down into pregnancy, genital tract outflow obstruction, ovarian dysfunction, and hypothalamic-pituitary axis abnormalities.

   - **Pregnancy:** It is essential that pregnancy be ruled out given that it is the most common cause of amenorrhea. A history of breast fullness, weight gain, and morning sickness yields supportive evidence. The diagnosis can be easily and economically confirmed or ruled out with a pregnancy test.
   - **Genital tract outflow obstruction:** Obstruction is a physical cause of amenorrhea and is more common in cases of primary amenorrhea. It commonly results from congenital anomalies in the development and canalization of the müllerian ducts. Physical examination may readily reveal an imperforate hymen or the absence of a uterus and/or a vagina. Occasionally, scarring of the uterus (also known as Asherman's syndrome) may result from uterine D&C or from infection and may subsequently lead to secondary amenorrhea. This information may be elicited from the patient's history. In mild cases of scarring, surgical lysis of the adhesions by D&C or hysteroscopy may be curative; more severe cases may be refractory.
   - **Ovarian-pituitary-hypothalamic axis:** History information should focus on more common problems that can occur in any of these

Pregnancy is a common cause of amenorrhea (always check a pregnancy test).

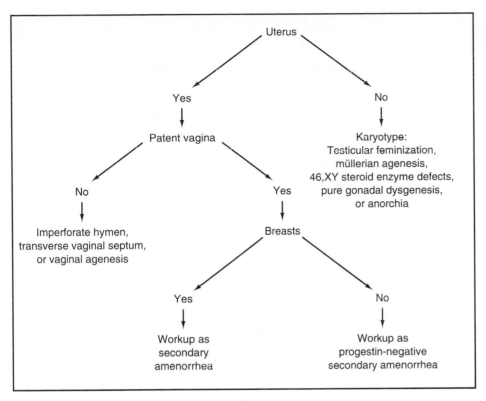

FIGURE 5.5. Workup for primary amenorrhea. (Reprinted, with permission, from DeCherney AH et al. *Current Obstetric and Gynecologic Diagnosis and Treatment,* 8th ed. Stamford, CT: Appleton & Lange, 1994:1010.)

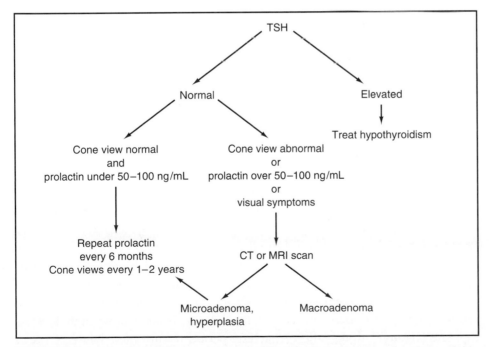

FIGURE 5.6. Workup for patients with secondary amenorrhea and galactorrhea hyperprolactinemia. (Reprinted, with permission, from DeCherney AH et al. *Current Obstetric and Gynecologic Diagnosis and Treatment,* 8th ed. Stamford, CT: Appleton & Lange, 1994:1010.)

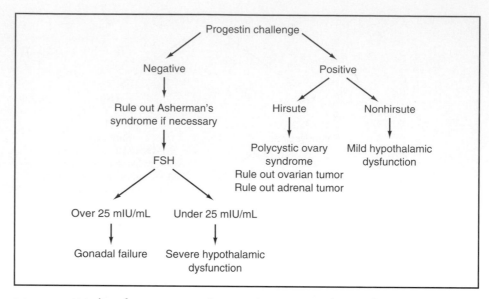

FIGURE 5.7. Workup for patients with secondary amenorrhea without galactorrhea-hyperprolactinemia. (Reprinted, with permission, from DeCherney AH et al. *Current Obstetric and Gynecologic Diagnosis and Treatment,* 8th ed. Stamford, CT: Appleton & Lange, 1994:1010.)

three areas. For primary amenorrhea, look for any incongruence in sexual characteristics and amenorrhea, systemic symptoms suggesting lack of pituitary-regulated hormones, and age. In patients with secondary amenorrhea, check for stress (nutritional, physical, emotional) and for signs and symptoms of hypothyroidism (goiter) or hyperprolactinemia (milky nipple discharge), hirsutism, obesity, and hot flashes/mood changes.

A systematic approach to working up the endocrine axis is much more efficient than a shotgun approach. The following is recommended:

- If the pregnancy test is negative, check blood TSH (if high, evaluate for hypothyroidism) and/or prolactin (if high, evaluate for pituitary tumor and drugs affecting pituitary function).
- If blood TSH/prolactin are normal, do a progesterone challenge (if there is withdrawal bleeding, there is adequate estrogen production and the diagnosis is anovulation).
- If there is no withdrawal bleeding (there is inadequate estrogen production secondary to LH/FSH abnormalities), check LH and FSH levels.

Low to normal levels of LH/FSH indicate that the main problem lies in the hypothalamus-pituitary axis (stress, nutritional imbalance, tumors) or constitutional delay in a patient with primary amenorrhea. High levels of LH/FSH indicate that the problem lies in the ovaries (failure of or resistance to stimulation by gonadotropins). Check the patient's age; if she is more than 40 years old, she is going through the climacteric period toward menopause. If she is less than 40 years old, she is suffering from premature ovarian failure, in which case endocrine disorders must be ruled out.

COMMON VAGINAL INFECTIONS (VAGINITIS)

The normal vaginal flora consist of approximately 25 bacterial species. The vaginal environment is normally acidic (pH 3.3–4.2) secondary to colonizing lactobacilli-producing lactic acid. This acidic environment inhibits the growth of organisms. A less acidic environment can lead to bacterial proliferation and hence to possible clinical infection.

Signs and Symptoms. The signs and symptoms of vaginitis include vulvovaginal itch with or without a burning sensation, abnormal odor, and increased vaginal discharge. Vaginal discharge is occasionally physiologic, although this type of discharge is usually white and odorless, and the patient is asymptomatic. In examining the patient, always check the quantity, odor, and color of vaginal discharge. See Table 5.14 for helpful hints in differentiating the etiologies of vaginitis.

Differential. The differential diagnosis for increased vaginal discharge includes STDs and UTIs.

Workup. Laboratory tests required to establish the diagnosis of vaginitis include slide smears with saline and potassium hydroxide (KOH). In addition, a Gram stain of the vaginal discharge and a gonorrhea and chlamydia antigen test should be performed to rule out STDs. A UA of a clean-catch urine speci-

TABLE 5.14. Causes of Vaginitis.

	Bacterial Vaginosis (usually *Gardnerella*)	*Trichomonas*	Yeast (usually *Candida*)
Relative frequency	50%	25%	25%
Discharge	Homogenous, grayish-white, watery, fishy and stale odor	Profuse malodorous, grayish, frothy, "strawberry spots" on cervix and vaginal wall	Thick, white, cottage-cheese texture
Vaginal pH	> 4.5	> 4.5	Normal vaginal pH
Saline smear[a]	Clue cells (epithelial cells coated with bacteria)	Motile trichomonads	Pseudohyphae Budding yeast
KOH smear	Fishy odor	Nothing	Pseudohyphae Budding yeast
Treatment	Metronidazole[b]	Metronidazole[b] Treat partner; this is considered an STD	Miconazole (Monistat) or Nystatin

[a]Saline smear: if you see lots of WBCs and no organism, suspect chlamydia.
[b]Patients taking metronidazole should not drink alcohol, which would lead to an Antabuse-like effect.

men will rule out UTIs. Table 5.14 describes the three most common causes of vaginitis.

Treatment. Treatments for the specific types of vaginitis are discussed in Table 5.14.

CONTRACEPTION

Table 5.15 summarizes the various forms of contraception available and their failure rates during the first year of use (both "lowest expected" and "typical," meaning the rate you'll actually see in the population!).

TABLE 5.15. Forms of Contraception and Their Failure Rates.

Method	How Used	Percentage of Women with Pregnancy (first year of use)	
		Lowest Expected (%)	Typical (%)
No method	No form of contraception used	85.0	85.0
Combination pill	Once-daily pill	0.1	3.0
Progestin-only pill	Once-daily pill	0.5	3.0
IUD (Copper T)	Inserted every ten years	0.1	0.1
Female sterilization	One-time operation	0.05	0.05
Male sterilization	One-time operation	0.1	0.15
Depo-Provera	IM injection every 12 weeks	0.3	0.3
Spermicides	With each intercourse	6.0	26.0
Periodic abstinence			
Calendar method			9.0
Ovulation method			3.0
Symptothermal			2.0
Postovulation			1.0
Withdrawal	With each intercourse	4.0	19.0
Cervical cap			
Parous	With each intercourse	26.0	40.0
Nulliparous	With each intercourse	9.0	20.0
Diaphragm/spermicide	With each intercourse	6.0	20.0
Condom			
Male	With each intercourse	3.0	14.0
Female	With each intercourse	5.0	21.0

ENDOMETRIOSIS

Endometriosis is characterized by the presence of endometrial glands and stroma outside the uterine cavity. In descending frequency, most endometriosis lesions are found in the ovaries (usually bilateral), broad ligament, and cul-de-sac (see Figure 5.8). Endometriosis afflicts 5–15% of premenopausal women and accounts for 40–50% of all surgeries for infertility. Evidence exists, however, for a genetic disposition in first-degree relatives. Classically, endometriosis lesions have been described as having the appearance of mulberries, raspberries, powder burns, and chocolate cysts found in the ovaries.

Although the exact mechanisms are unknown, the following hypotheses for the pathogenesis of endometriosis have been proposed:

- Direct implantation of endometrial cells by retrograde menstruation
- Vascular and lymphatic dissemination of endometrial cells
- Celomic metaplasia of multipotential cells in the peritoneal cavity

Signs and Symptoms. Classic and often-quoted symptoms of endometriosis are dysmenorrhea (beginning a few days prior to and lasting throughout the entire menstrual cycle), deep dyspareunia, chronic pelvic pain, abnormal bleeding, and infertility. The nature and severity of the symptoms depend on both the extent and the location of the disease. On pelvic examination, findings indicative of more established disease include nodular thickening along the uterosacral ligament; a fixed, retroverted uterus; and tender, fixed adnexal masses (endometriomas). Physical findings in early-stage endometriosis are often subtle and may even be nonexistent despite the patient's complaints.

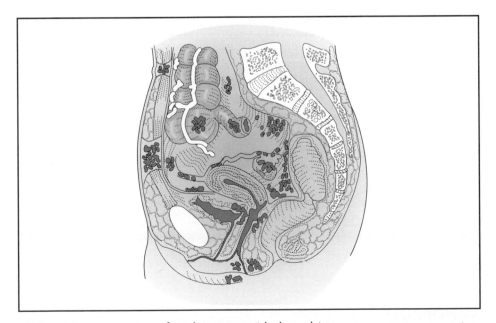

FIGURE 5.8. Common sites of endometriosis (dark ovals). (Reprinted, with permission, from DeCherney AH et al. *Current Obstetric and Gynecologic Diagnosis and Treatment,* 8th ed. Stamford, CT: Appleton & Lange, 1994:802.)

Differential. Patients with endometriosis can present with a wide range of symptoms, and the differential depends on the patient's specific complaints. For chronic abdominal pain, chronic PID and pelvic adhesions should be entertained. In patients presenting with amenorrhea, causes of primary and/or secondary amenorrhea should be on the differential. If sudden-onset lower abdominal pain is the chief complaint, ectopic pregnancy, appendicitis, PID, adnexal torsion, rupture of the corpus luteum, and endometrioma must be considered.

Workup. The definitive diagnosis of endometriosis is established by laparoscopic examination and biopsy of "endometriosis-appearing lesions" that reveal functional endometrial glands and stroma together with hemosiderin-laden macrophages. Laboratory tests to be obtained should include a pregnancy test, UA, CA 125, and ultrasound to rule out differential diagnoses.

Treatment. Treatment should be individualized according to age, reproductive plans, and extent of disease.

- **Medical:** Medical treatment is aimed at inducing inactivity/atrophy of endometrial tissue. These options include hormonal manipulation through use of OCPs, progestin, danazol, and GnRH agonists. All medical treatments are for symptomatic relief, not for cure, as they have no effect on the adhesions and fibrosis caused by endometriosis.
- **Surgical:** Conservative surgical options include laparoscopic removal of implants (excision, electrocauterization, laser ablation) that allows for future pregnancy. Definitive surgeries are appropriate for severe disease that is uncontrolled by medical and conservative surgical treatment or for patients who are willing to forgo future pregnancy. Surgery includes total abdominal hysterectomy, bilateral salpingo-oophorectomy, lysis of adhesions, and removal of all implants. In younger patients, some ovarian tissue may be left intact to prevent early menopause, although there may be a recurrence of endometriosis. In patients without endogenous estrogen production (e.g., patients who have no ovaries), HRT must be instituted.

Note that endometriosis is a chronic disorder that requires long-term therapy. Treatment often improves the chances of successful conception. This disease is hormone dependent and usually improves after menopause. The risk of malignant transformation is very low.

GYNECOLOGIC ONCOLOGY

Table 5.16 summarizes the essentials of the three important gynecologic cancers.

MENOPAUSE

Menopause is the permanent cessation of natural menses and marks the end of a woman's reproductive life. The average age ranges from 45 to 55 years,

TABLE 5.16. Common Gynecologic Cancers.

	Cervical Cancer	**Endometrial Cancer**	**Ovarian Cancer**
Symptoms	Postcoital bleeding Foul discharge May be asymptomatic	Postmenopausal uterine bleeding Palpable abdominal and pelvic masses	Increased abdominal girth (ascites) Often asymptomatic until late stages GI and GU complaints Thrombophlebitis Lower abdominal pain/pressure
Risk factors	Anything that increases the risk of or indication of human papilloma- virus (HPV) infection: ■ Venereal warts ■ Early sexual activity ■ Multiple sexual partners ■ Smoking ■ Family history	Chronic, unopposed estrogen stimulation (e.g., PCOS) Obesity Nulliparity Postmenopausal Diabetes mellitus Hypertension Early menarche Late menopause Anovulation Family history Endometrial hyperplasia	Nulliparity Breast cancer Family history OCPs may have a protective role in decreasing the risk of ovarian cancer
Screening tests	Pap smear (performed at least once a year for sexually active women)	None (Pap smear is only 50% effective in detecting uterine cancer)	None (routine ultrasound, CA 125 are not cost-efficient)
Diagnostic tests	Punch and/or cone biopsy	Endometrial biopsy D&C	Ultrasound, abdominal CT, CA 125 for epithelial cancers; α-fetoprotein and β-HCG for germ cell cancers
Treatment	Early stage: radiotherapy, radical hysterectomy, and lymphadenectomy Advanced stage: irradiation/ chemotherapy only (surgery would harm the bladder and rectum without being effective)	Total abdominal hysterectomy/ bilateral salpingo-oophorectomy (TAH-BSO) and peritoneal washing for cytology ± pelvic and aortic node sampling Radiotherapy Chemotherapy Progesterone	TAH-BSO and peritoneal washing for cytology with or without pelvic and aortic node sampling Tumor debulking Chemotherapy
Prevention	Safe sex (condoms) to decrease risk of HPV infection Smoking cessation Routine Pap smears	Progesterone to oppose estrogen Low-fat diet Weight control	OCPs Oophorectomy in patients with a strong family history of ovarian cancer

HIGH-YIELD TOPICS

Obstetrics and Gynecology

TABLE 5.16 (continued). Common Gynecologic Cancers.

	Cervical Cancer	Endometrial Cancer	Ovarian Cancer
Notes	85% are squamous-cell carcinoma, 15% adenocarcinoma Uremia is the most common cause of of death in patients with end-stage cervical cancer	Most common gynecologic cancer Fourth most common cancer in women (after breast, colorectal, lung) Most are adenocarcinoma Endometrial hyperplasia is the precursor lesion and is treated with progesterone	Most lethal gynecologic cancer Complications of ovarian cancer include ovarian rupture, torsion, hemorrhage, infection, and infarction Most common cause of death in end-stage ovarian cancer is bowel obstruction

with the median age 51 years. The climacteric period is the extended period of decreased ovarian function beginning several years before and lasting years after menopause itself.

Signs and Symptoms. Perimenopausal symptoms include irregular and infrequent menses accompanied by hot flashes, sleep disturbances, vaginal dryness, volatility of affect, sexual dysfunction, and hair and nail brittleness. All of these changes progress over a few months to a few years, and some may continue into the postmenopausal period. Postmenopausal symptoms include genital tract atrophy (e.g., urinary incontinence), osteoporosis, and cardiovascular diseases.

Differential. The differential diagnosis of menopause includes premature ovarian failure (menopause occurring prior to 42 years) due to alkylating chemotherapy, smoking, autoimmune diseases, and hysterectomy.

Workup. Menopause is definitively diagnosed when serum FSH is > 25 mIU/mL at two separate times or when LH/FSH is > 2. Baseline laboratory tests for the workup of menopause include FSH, mammography, Pap smear, LFTs, cholesterol panel, CBC, UA, and a bone density study (to screen for osteoporosis).

Treatment. All of the signs and symptoms of the climacteric period result from declining estrogen production by the ovarian follicles. Exogenous estrogen administration to perimenopausal and postmenopausal women will obviate most of these changes. Because unopposed estrogen can lead to endometrial hyperplasia and adenocarcinoma, it is routine practice to supplement estrogen with progestin in women who still have an intact uterus. Daily administration of estrogen combined with progestin is the most popular regimen to alleviate peri- and postmenopausal changes without subjecting the patient to menstrual cycles. In light of recent reports of increased cardiovascular morbidity and breast cancer with prolonged hormone replacement therapy, hormone replacement should only be used in symptomatic patients for short durations. Patients should also be advised to take calcium supplements, stop smoking, and exercise to prevent/reduce osteoporotic changes. An annual pelvic exam, Pap smear, and mammogram should be performed.

The most common cancers in women:

1. *Breast*

2. *Lung*

3. *Colorectal*

4. *Uterine*

HIGH-YIELD TOPICS

Obstetrics and Gynecology

Common side effects of HRT include irregular bleeding, especially in the first six months. With continuous HRT, the patient may see weight gain, fluid retention, and, endometrial, hyperplasia (rare if the patient is also taking progesterone).

PELVIC INFLAMMATORY DISEASE

Pelvic inflammatory disease is an upper genital tract infection that usually results from an ascending infection from the cervix. Approximately one-third of all cases are caused by *Neisseria gonorrhoeae* alone, another third by *N. gonorrhoeae* and anaerobes/aerobes (including *Chlamydia trachomatis*), and the remaining third by anaerobes/aerobes alone. The lifetime risk is 1–3%. Risk factors for PID include multiple sex partners, a new partner within 30 days before becoming symptomatic, a high frequency of intercourse, young age at first intercourse, and, possibly, IUD use.

Signs and Symptoms. Patients usually present with a one- to three-day history of lower abdominal pain with or without fever, vaginal discharge, recent menses, a history of sexual exposure, and a past history of PID. On physical exam, there is lower abdominal tenderness, cervical motion tenderness (CMT), and possibly an adnexal mass and/or tenderness.

Differential. The differential diagnosis of PID includes ectopic pregnancy, endometriosis, ovarian torsion, hemorrhagic ovarian cyst, appendicitis, UTI, and diverticulitis.

Workup. Specific criteria are required to establish the diagnosis of PID. The following three criteria should be present:

1. A history of abdominal pain and findings of abdominal tenderness with or without rebound (90%)
2. CMT
3. Adnexal tenderness (may be unilateral)

One of the following criteria is also required to establish the diagnosis:

1. A temperature higher than 38°C
2. A WBC greater than 10,000
3. The presence of an inflammatory mass (tubo-ovarian abscess) on exam/sonography
4. Culdocentesis that yields peritoneal fluid with bacteria and WBCs
5. The presence of *N. gonorrhoeae* and/or *C. trachomatis* on the endocervix (mucopurulent cervicitis, evidence of gram-negative diplococci, positive chlamydia antigen test, > 10 WBC/hpf on Gram stain)
6. Erythrocyte sedimentation rate (ESR) > 15 mm/hr

Laboratory tests that should be obtained in the workup of PID include CBC (WBC > 10,000), ESR (> 15 mm/hr), β-HCG (check for pregnancy status), Gram stain of cervical discharge (gram-negative intracellular diplococci),

"Chandelier sign": severe CMT on exam that makes the patient "jump for the chandelier."

RPR/VDRL (to rule out syphilis), HIV, hepatitis screen, and ultrasound (inflammatory mass). Other options for diagnosis determination include culdocentesis (peritoneal fluid with bacteria and WBCs) and laparoscopy (for the definitive diagnosis of edema and erythema of the fallopian tubes and purulent exudate). Note that laparoscopy has been shown to confirm the clinical diagnosis in approximately 60% of cases.

Treatment. PID can usually be treated with a course of outpatient antibiotics (generally cefoxitin or ceftriaxone and doxycycline). If the patient has a temperature > 38.0°C, an uncertain diagnosis, suspected pelvic or tubo-ovarian abscess, nausea and vomiting that would prevent compliance with the administration of oral meds, or upper peritoneal signs—or if the patient is pregnant or shows signs of noncompliance—she should be admitted for IV antibiotics. Surgery is warranted only if there is a complication, such as a tubo-ovarian abscess.

Sequelae of PID include a tenfold increase in the risk of an ectopic pregnancy and a fourfold increase in the risk of chronic pelvic pain, infertility, and recurrent PID. An often-pimped complication of PID is Fitz-Hugh-Curtis syndrome, a perihepatitis that is characterized by inflammation of the liver capsule and the undersurface of the diaphragm. Patients often present with pleuritic right upper quadrant pain limiting chest expansion. Fitz-Hugh-Curtis syndrome complicates 15–30% of PID cases.

Fitz-Hugh-Curtis is a commonly pimped complication of PID.

SEXUALLY TRANSMITTED DISEASES

Taken together, STDs are one of the most common gynecologic problems encountered in the outpatient setting. All sexually active patients must thus be examined with an awareness of a possible STD. Often, patients have had a past history of STDs, which can be elicited through careful and tactful history taking.

On physical examination, the following should be noted:

- **Inguinal area:** Rashes, lesions, adenopathy
- **Vulva:** Lesions, ulcerations, abnormal discharge, abnormal swelling/thickening
- **Vagina/cervix:** Lesions, discharge

Also check out the glands (Bartholin's, Skene's), the urethra, and the perineum and perianal area.

Cultures of the urethra and cervix for chlamydia, gonorrhea, or other infectious agents should be obtained for any suspicious case. It is important to note that 20–50% of patients with an STD have coexisting infections, creating a low threshold for detecting other infectious diseases. All contacts of the patient must be treated.

GENITAL HERPES

Herpes simplex is the most common STD and is highly infectious (75% rate).

Etiology. The etiologic agents are herpes simplex virus type 2 (90%) and type 1 (10%).

Signs and Symptoms. The prodromal phase (mild paresthesia, burning) progresses to painful vesicular lesions three to seven days after exposure; in primary infections, patients may often have malaise, low-grade fever, and adenopathy. Physical findings often reveal clear vesicles that may have lysed, progressing to painful ulcers with red borders that coalesce and become secondarily infected. These lesions can be found on the vulva, vagina, cervix, perineum, and perianal area.

Workup. Workup consists of obtaining a history and physical findings, a Tzanck smear of lesions, and viral cultures.

Treatment. Treatment consists of expectant management (keep lesions dry and clean, use antimicrobial cream to prevent secondary bacterial infections) and administration of acyclovir (ointment for duration of flare-up, oral for decreasing frequency and severity of recurrence, intravenous for hospitalized cases of severe outbreaks).

Pregnant patients with active herpes at the time of labor often require a C-section.

CHLAMYDIA

Chlamydia trachomatis is the second most common STD; is ten times more common than *Neisseria gonorrhoeae*; and has an infection rate five times higher in women with three partners and four times higher in women who use no barrier methods. It can manifest as cervicitis, PID, or lymphogranuloma venereum (rare) and often coexists with gonorrhea.

Etiology. *C. trachomatis* is an obligate intracellular parasite.

Signs and Symptoms. Mild cases can be asymptomatic, or patients may present with dysuria, abnormal vaginal discharge, ectopic pregnancy, or infertility. Physical findings are subtle and nonspecific; mucopurulent cervical discharge is often a clue, but many patients may not have any symptoms or discharge. Findings may be masked by coexisting gonorrheal infection.

Workup. A diagnosis of *C. trachomatis* is usually suspected on clinical grounds; cultures are performed to confirm the diagnosis. Two screening tests are available: a monoclonal antibody test (faster) and an enzyme immunoassay of the cervical secretion (95% specificity). Always check for concomitant gonorrheal infection (cultures, smear).

Treatment. Treatment consists of azithromycin, tetracycline, or doxycycline; erythromycin may be substituted in allergic or pregnant patients. Treatment has a 95% cure rate. The main sequelae from chlamydia infection arise from insidious tubal damage leading to infertility.

GONORRHEA

Gonorrhea is still a very common infection; an increased frequency has also been observed with penicillin-resistant strains in asymptomatic infections.

Etiology. *Neisseria gonorrhoeae*, a gram-negative intracellular diplococcus, is the causative agent.

Signs and Symptoms. *N. gonorrhoeae* lower genital tract infection is characterized by a malodorous, purulent, yellow-green discharge from the cervix, vagina, Skene's ducts, urethra, or anus. In heterosexual women, 10–20% also have gonorrhea infection in the pharynx. Acute upper genital tract infection occurs in approximately 15% of women infected with gonorrhea (see PID section).

Workup. Workup consists of obtaining a Gram stain of discharge for intracellular gram-negative diplococci, cultures from the discharge on Thayer-Martin medium (80–95% sensitivity), and an enzyme immunoassay for gonorrhea antigen.

Treatment. Maintain a low threshold for treating patients for gonorrhea; it is valid to treat on clinical grounds alone. The choice of antibiotics depends on the site of infection: For urethral, cervical, or rectal infection, use ceftriaxone, cefixime, ciprofloxacin, ampicillin, or amoxicillin with probenecid; for pharyngeal infection, use ceftriaxone, ciprofloxacin, aqueous penicillin with probenecid, or tetracycline.

Complications. Infertility occurs in 15% of patients after a single episode and in 75% of patients after three episodes of PID. The risk of ectopic pregnancy is increased seven- to tenfold. Other complications include recurrent infection and chronic pelvic pain.

CONDYLOMATA ACUMINATA (VENEREAL WARTS)

Condylomata acuminata are almost as common as gonorrhea infection. Unlike other STDs, however, the sequelae may take years to manifest.

Etiology. The etiologic agent is HPV. Three subtypes of HPV have a very high association with cervical neoplasia: 16, 18, and 31.

Signs and Symptoms. Patients may present with painless bumps, discharge, and pruritus. Physical findings include soft, fleshy, exophytic, papular, verrucous, flat, or macular growths on the cervix, vagina, vulva, urethral meatus, perineum, or perianal area. Lesions are often symmetrical; coinfection with *Trichomonas* or *Gardnerella* is common.

Workup. Presumptive diagnosis is made with physical findings. The diagnosis can be confirmed with a biopsy of warts following 5% acetic acid staining. Note that Pap smear of the cervix diagnoses only about 5% of patients infected with HPV.

Treatment. External and vaginal lesions are treated with Condylox, cryotherapy, CO_2 laser, or trichloroacetic acid (TCA). Cervical lesions are treated with colposcopy and potential biopsy of the cervix, cryotherapy, laser, or the loop electrosurgical excision procedure (LEEP).

Lesions are often more resistant to therapy during pregnancy, in diabetic patients, or in immunosuppressed patients. Any patient infected with HPV must have at least once-yearly Pap smear evaluation of the cervix.

SYPHILIS

The incidence of syphilis has been rising over the past few years owing to penicillin-resistant gonorrhea strains. In the past, gonorrhea treatment with penicillin would also treat syphilis.

Etiology. *Treponema pallidum*, a motile spirochete, is the etiologic agent.

Signs and Symptoms. The signs and symptoms of syphilis according to the stage of the infection are as follows:

- **Primary (10 to 60 days after infection):** A painless ulcer (chancre) is found in or near the vulva, vagina, cervix, anus, rectum, pharynx, lips, and fingers; it is often missed the first time around. The chancre heals spontaneously in three to nine weeks.
- **Secondary (4 to 8 weeks after the appearance of the chancre):** Symptoms include low-grade fever, headache, malaise, anorexia, and generalized lymphadenopathy, together with a diffuse, symmetric, asymptomatic maculopapular rash on the soles and palms. Highly infective secondary eruptions (mucous patches) can coalesce, forming condylomata lata; lesions heal spontaneously in two to six weeks.
- **Tertiary (1 to 20 years after the initial infection):** Destructive, granulomatous gummas that cause systemic damage to the CNS, heart, or great vessels can be seen.

Workup. Workup consists of VDRL/RPR (rapid, nonspecific screening test); FTA-ABS/MHA-TP (fluorescent treponemal antibody absorption test/microhemagglutination assay—*Treponema pallidum*) specific, diagnostic; and dark-field microscopy (motile spirochetes) of primary or secondary lesions,

Treatment. Penicillin is the treatment of choice for primary, secondary, and tertiary syphilis. Alternatively, tetracycline or penicillin desensitization can be used for allergic patients and erythromycin for pregnant patients. Of note is the fact that transplacental spread can occur at any stage of syphilis, leading to congenital syphilis.

OBSTETRICS

Prenatal Care

Vintzileos AM et al. Prenatal care and black-white death disparity in the United States: heterogeneity by high-risk conditions. *Obstet Gynecol* 2002;99:483–489. A research article that set out (1) to determine the impact of prenatal care in the United States on fetal death rate in the presence and absence of obstetric and medical high-risk conditions; and (2) to explore the role of these high-risk conditions in contributing to the black-white disparity.

First-Trimester Bleeding

McKennett M, Fullerton JT. Vaginal bleeding in pregnancy. *Am Fam Physician* 1995;51:639–646. A review of the process of identifying and evaluating the common causes of vaginal bleeding during pregnancy as the pregnancy progresses to term.

Ectopic Pregnancy

Lipscomb GH et al. Nonsurgical treatment of ectopic pregnancy. *NEJM* 2000; 343:1325–1329. A review article that describes methods of diagnosing ectopic pregnancy as well as surgical and medical management options for treatment once the diagnosis has been made.

Medical Management of Tubal Pregnancy. ACOG Practice Bulletin No. 3, December 1998. This document, published by the American College of Obstetrics and Gynecology, presents evidence (including risks and benefits) on methotrexate as an alternative treatment for selected ectopic pregnancies.

Gestational Diabetes

Kjos SL, Buchanan TA. Gestational diabetes mellitus. *NEJM* 1999;341:1749–1756. A review of gestational diabetes, including its detection, diagnosis, implications, treatment, timing of delivery, and postpartum evaluation.

Pregnancy-Induced Hypertension

Sibai B. Treatment of hypertension in pregnant women. *NEJM* 1996; 335:257–265. A review article defining gestational hypertension, mild preeclampsia, and severe preeclampsia as well as treatment and management guidelines for each.

Lenfant C. Working group report on high blood pressure in pregnancy. *J Clin Hypertens* 2001;3:75–88. A report from the National Education Program Working Group on High Blood Pressure in Pregnancy that focuses on the classification, pathophysiology, and management of hypertensive disorders of pregnancy. Updates contemporary approaches toward hypertension control during pregnancy by expanding on recommendations made in the Sixth Report of the Joint National Committee on Prevention, Detection, Evaluation, and Treatment of High Blood Pressure (JNC VI).

Preterm and Normal Labor

Goldenberg RL et al. Intrauterine infection and preterm delivery. *NEJM* 2000;342:1500–1507. A review article outlining the relationship of intrauterine infections to preterm labor and delivery, specifically the organisms, timing of infection, mechanism, markers of infection, prevention, and treatment.

Norwitz ER et al. The control of labor. *NEJM* 1999;341:660–666. A review article describing the physiologic processes underlying normal term labor and preterm labor.

Abnormal Labor

Gifford DS et al. Lack of progress in labor as a reason for cesarean section. *Obstet Gynecol* 200;95:589–595. An article describing the lack of progress in labor as a reason for cesarean delivery and comparing published diagnostic criteria with the labor characteristics of women with this diagnosis.

Fetal Heart Rate Monitoring

Fetal Heart Rate Patterns: Monitoring, Interpretation, and Management. ACOG Bulletin No. 207, July 1995. A discussion of fetal heart rate monitoring, its physiologic basis, and guidelines for appropriate methods of monitoring and evaluating fetal well-being.

Third-Trimester Bleeding

Sheiner E et al. Placenta previa: obstetric risk factors and pregnancy outcome. *J Matern Fetal Med* 2001;10:414–419. A research article reporting on the incidence, obstetric risk factors, and perinatal outcome of placenta previa.

McKennett M, Fullerton JT. Vaginal bleeding in pregnancy. *Am Fam Physician* 1995;51:639–646. A review of the process of identifying and evaluating the common causes of vaginal bleeding during pregnancy as the pregnancy progresses to term.

Postpartum Hemorrhage

Jackson N, Paterson-Brown S. Postpartum haemorrhage. *Hosp Med* 1999; 60:868–872. A review of factors that may help anticipation of postpartum hemorrhage. Looks at issues involved in the management and treatment of women with this condition.

GYNECOLOGY

Abnormal Uterine Bleeding

Management of Anovulatory Bleeding. ACOG Practice Bulletin No. 14, March 2000. Management guidelines for the treatment of patients with menstrual irregularities associated with anovulation.

Amenorrhea

Pletcher JR, Slap GB. Menstrual disorders: amenorrhea. *Pediatr Clin North Am* 1999;46:505–518. A review of the basic understanding of menstrual and pubertal physiology of amenorrhea, as well as a discussion of an appropriate diagnostic algorithm and management guidelines.

Common Vaginal Infections (Vaginitis)

Sobel J. Vaginitis. *NEJM* 1997;337:1896–1903. A review of *Candida* vulvovaginitis, trichomoniasis, bacterial vaginosis, and atrophic vaginitis.

Contraceptives

Templeman CL et al. Postpartum contraceptive use among adolescent mothers. *Obstet Gynecol* 2000;95:770–776. A comparison of the incidence of repeat pregnancy and method continuation rate at 12 months postpartum in young women who chose either depot medroxyprogesterone acetate (DepoProvera) or OCPs as contraception.

Oral Contraceptives for Adolescents: Benefits and Safety. ACOG Committee Opinion No. 256, December 1999. A discussion of oral contraceptive use in adolescents, specifically focusing on their benefits, potential deterrents, contraindications, and causes of discontinuation.

Vandenbroucke JP et al. Oral contraceptives and the risk of venous thrombosis. *NEJM* 2001;344:1527–1535. A review of the risks associated with oral contraceptives, susceptibility, and mechanism of thrombosis.

Endometriosis

Olive DL, Pritts EA. Treatment of endometriosis. *NEJM* 2001;345:266–275. A review article delineating the evaluation, classification, and treatment of endometriosis.

Gynecologic Oncology

Recommendations on Frequency of Pap Test Screening. ACOG Practice Bulletin No. 152, March 1995. A discussion of recommendations for Pap test screening methods and frequency of screening based on population.

Infertility

Management of Infertility Caused by Ovulatory Dysfunction. ACOG Practice Bulletin No. 34, February 2002. Management guidelines set forth by the American College of Obstetrics and Gynecology for the workup and management of infertility in a patient with anovulation.

Menopause

Dick SE et al. Postmenopausal hormone replacement therapy and major clinical outcomes: a focus on cardiovascular disease, osteoporosis, dementia, and breast and endometrial neoplasia. *Am J Manag Care* 2002;8:95–104; quiz 105–106. A review that evaluates the potential benefits of hormone replacement therapy for cardiovascular disease, osteoporosis, and dementia. Also discusses the potential risks of breast and endometrial neoplasia and an early risk of cardiovascular and thromboembolic disease associated with HRT use.

Pelvic Inflammatory Disease

McCormack W. Pelvic inflammatory disease. *NEJM* 1994;330:115–119. A review article describing PID and its etiology, pathogenesis, clinical characteristics, diagnosis, and management.

Pelvic Relaxation

Koduri S, Sand PK. Recent developments in pelvic organ prolapse. *Curr Opin Obstet Gynecol* 2000;12:399–404. A review of pelvic organ prolapse, particularly its pathophysiology, methods of evaluation, and treatment.

Premenstrual Syndrome

Premenstrual Syndrome. ACOG Practice Bulletin No. 15, April 2000. An examination of the evidence for commonly used approaches in the treatment of PMS; also identifies those that are effective.

Sexually Transmitted Disease

Royce RA et al. Sexual transmission of HIV. *NEJM* 1997;336:1072–1078. A review of HIV transmission, antiretroviral therapy, environmental effects, and prevention.

HANDBOOK/POCKETBOOK

Benson & Pernoll's Handbook of Obstetrics and Gynecology $44.95

Benson

McGraw-Hill, 2001, 10th edition, 908 pages, ISBN 0071356088

A handbook comprehensive enough to serve as a mini-reference. Excellent tables and graphics offer thorough discussions of etiology, pathophysiology, clinical findings, and management. Too bulky to fit in pocket; small print makes for labored reading. Good to have for relatively detailed explanations when you don't feel like carrying a big textbook on the wards. Includes a section on breast disease.

Current Clinical Strategies: Gynecology and Obstetrics $12.95

Chan

Current Clinical Strategies, 2002 edition, 105 pages, ISBN 192962204X

A quick, readable pocketbook containing essential high-yield information. Outline format includes signs and symptoms, differential, treatment, and complications. Inexpensive and remarkably compact. Great for both management and quick review on the wards. Includes an excellent, concise oncology section with classifications.

Manual of Obstetrics $39.95

Evans

Lippincott Williams & Wilkins, 2000, 6th edition, 540 pages, ISBN 078172404X

A good pocketbook in the same format as the *Washington Manual*. Offers a light discussion of pathophysiology, symptoms, and signs but more detailed coverage of diagnostic approach and therapeutics. Covers a broad range of topics on obstetrics; useful for quick review. More appropriate for subinterns than for junior medical students.

Obstetrical Pearls $21.95

Benson

F. A. Davis, 1999, 3rd edition, 225 pages, ISBN 0803604327

A practical, easy-to-read, clinically oriented pocketbook that can be used as prerotation orientation material on the wards. Gives basic wards survival information, but does not cover full spectrum of information necessary for in-depth study or exams. Clinical pearls and current controversies in management are highlighted in text. Contains excellent tidbits that can be read in a few dedicated hours.

Gynecologic Pearls $19.95

Benson

F. A. Davis, 2000, 2nd edition, 243 pages, ISBN 0803605021

Good prerotation introductory material, but not sufficient for exams or the wards. Useful as easy, quick supplementary reading. Requires separate purchase of sister book for obstetrics, which makes the combination expensive. Clinical pearls and current controversies in management are highlighted in text.

B Handbook of Gynecology & Obstetrics $27.95

Brown

McGraw-Hill, 1993, 1st edition, 626 pages, ISBN 0838536085

A concise, easy-to-read pocketbook with a format similar to that of *Benson & Pernoll's Handbook*. Provides good conceptual information with tables, illustrations, and well-written discussions. Its major drawback is that it lacks the most recent advances in the field as it has not been updated for years. Still a good quick reference. Includes a free pregnancy wheel.

B The Johns Hopkins Manual of Gynecology and Obstetrics $39.95

Lambrou

Lippincott Williams & Wilkins, 1999, 1st edition, 453 pages, ISBN 0316467200

A basic pocket guide to providing a practical synopsis of pathophysiology, clinical manifestations, diagnostic approach, and therapeutics. Similar in design to the *Manual of Obstetrics*, this compact book gives a broad overview on many topics pertaining to both obstetrics and gynecology, leaving it a bit short on management details for use on the wards. More algorithms and tables would also be helpful.

B Obstetrics & Gynecology (House Officer Series) $29.95

Carey

Lippincott Williams & Wilkins, 2002, 4th edition, 429 pages, ISBN 078172855X

A good pocketbook for quick reference as you see patients in the hospital. Written in essay form, it is sometimes difficult to sift through for the main points. Offers basic, broad coverage of most conditions encountered on the wards and in outpatient clinics.

B On Call Obstetrics & Gynecology $28.00

Chin

W. B. Saunders, 2001, 2nd edition, 433 pages, ISBN 0721692540

A compact guide with a format similar to that of the rest of the *On Call* series, addressing common problems the on-call physician will encounter on obstetrics and gynecology. Although not comprehensive enough for study, the pocketbook guides your clinical thinking and approach to ward emergent issues. More for residents on call than for medical students.

C+ Obstetrics and Gynecology on Call $24.95

Horowitz

McGraw-Hill, 1993, 1st edition, 640 pages, ISBN 0838571743

Organized by clinical problems with a focus on differential diagnosis; this text assumes a good knowledge base in OB/GYN, making it less useful for students. Minimal discussion in some areas. Includes bonus chapters on diagnostic studies, procedures, and management. Management section is outdated.

Practical Guide to the Care of the Gynecologic/Obstetric Patient

$39.95

Danakas

Mosby, 1997, 1st edition, 800 pages, ISBN 0815123167

Formatted in the same manner as the popular Ferri handbook for medicine, but not as practical. Suffers from some glaring omissions, such as third-trimester bleeding and postpartum care. Placement of sections on lab tests and differential diagnoses of common complaints in the middle of book makes it harder to use. The quality of content varies widely, with some sections seeming incomplete.

Blueprints in Obstetrics and Gynecology $29.95
Callahan

Blackwell Science, 2000, 2nd edition, 207 pages, ISBN 0632044845

A good, concise introductory review for the OB/GYN rotation. Offers an excellent easy-to-read synopsis of major topics as well as good figures and tables. Some students feel this is the best of the *Blueprints* series. Excellent review test for shelf and USMLE Step 2 exams, but students considering a career in OB/GYN will need to find a more detailed textbook as well. Contains a section on breast disease.

 ## First Aid for the Obstetrics & Gynecology Clerkship $29.95
Stead

McGraw-Hill, 2001, 1st edition, 280 pages, ISBN 0071364234

An extremely comprehensive overview of pertinent topics in OB/GYN. Written in a concise outline format that covers essential high-yield information often found on shelf and USMLE Step 2 exams. "Exam tips" and "ward tips" included in the margins of text are too numerous, detracting from their overall utility. Few figures and photographs are provided. A short section at end mentions some general websites, extracurricular activities, and scholarships. Overall, a good review for a busy clerkship. Publication not related to the authors of *First Aid for the Wards*.

 ## Gynaecology Illustrated $54.95
Hart

Churchill Livingstone, 2000, 5th edition, 443 pages, ISBN 044306198X

An excellent mini-reference for gynecology, written at an appropriate level for medical students. Provides high-yield information along with good schematic drawings of anatomy, pathology, and procedures. A bit brief with respect to treatment. The fact that one must find another resource for obstetrics decreases its overall utility. Excellent for reviewing the basics, particularly for those interested in OB/GYN.

Underground Clinical Vignettes: OB/GYN $24.95
Bhushan

Blackwell Science, 2002, 2nd edition, 100 pages, ISBN 0632045698

A well-organized review of clinical vignettes commonly encountered on NBME shelf and USMLE Step 2 exams. Includes a focused, high-yield discussion of pathogenesis, epidemiology, management, complications, and associated diseases. Black-and-white images are included where relevant. Also contains several "mini-cases" in which only key facts related to each disease are presented. An excellent, entertaining, and easy-to-use supplement for studying during your clinical rotation. A color atlas supplement comes with the purchase of the full set of *Underground Clinical Vignettes*.

BRS Obstetrics and Gynecology   **$18.95**

Sakala

Lippincott Williams & Wilkins, 1997, 1st edition, 389 pages, ISBN 1683074989

A general outline review text with questions accompanying each chapter and a comprehensive exam at the end. Appropriate amount of detail for shelf and USMLE Step 2 study. Easy to read with great charts and tables, but few diagrams. An excellent overall review for exams, but you may need to supplement it with a more detailed text for wards work.

 Essentials of Obstetrics & Gynecology   **$49.95**

Hacker

W. B Saunders, 1998, 3rd edition, 737 pages, ISBN 0721674739

A well-organized text written at an appropriate level for medical students. Serves as a good introductory resource for those intending to enter the field, although it may prove difficult to finish on a busy service. Contains excellent discussions on patient workups and good background material. Overall, very readable, but lacks the depth of a true reference book. Compare with Beckmann's *Obstetrics and Gynecology*.

 Obstetrics and Gynecology   **$49.00**

Beckmann

Lippincott Williams & Wilkins, 2002, 4th edition, 896 pages, ISBN 0781724805

A concise textbook intended for medical students on their core OB/GYN rotation, based on the Association of Professors of Gynecology and Obstetrics Instructional Objectives. Features a case-based approach with brief coverage of topics and many questions. Chapters are short enough to finish in one sitting and include some helpful tables, figures, and diagrams. Enough to get by, but lacks the depth of other texts. Some students state it is too simplistic and somewhat disorganized.

 Basic Gynecology & Obstetrics   **$39.95**

Gant

McGraw-Hill, 1993, 1st edition, 472 pages, ISBN 0838596339

An excellent short reference for the core rotation. Thorough and well written, with just enough information for a junior medical student on the wards. Makes good use of graphics to highlight the text. However, contains few references, and the serious OB/GYN student will likely need a more detailed text. Overall, a good introductory text, but very dated in comparison to other books of similar scope.

 Lecture Notes on Obstetrics and Gynaecology   **$39.95**

Chamberlain

Blackwell Science, 1999, 1st edition, 295 pages, ISBN 063204957X

A mini-review text designed for medical students. Offers excellent coverage of basic science, etiology, and clinical presentation, but its discussion of differentials, diagnostic approach, and therapeutic options is only average, limiting its usefulness on the wards. Portable enough to carry around in coat pocket if you desire to use it to study for shelf and USMLE Step 2 exams.

B NMS Obstetrics & Gynecology $32.00
Beck

Lippincott Williams & Wilkins, 1997, 4th edition, 510 pages, ISBN 0683180150

A comprehensive review presented in an outline format that may be too dense for regular use. Well organized, but discussions can be lengthy and boring. An excellent comprehensive exam at the end poses questions similar to those found on the shelf and USMLE Step 2 exams. Few tables and diagrams.

B Obstetrics and Gynecology Secrets $39.00
Fredrickson

Lippincott Williams & Wilkins, 1997, 2nd edition, 380 pages, ISBN 156053205X

A question-and-answer format typical of the *Secrets* series, with good coverage of many high-yield, clinically relevant topics. Detailed, but contains no vignettes or images. Some explanations appear inadequate. Provides a good clinical context for quick self-testing, but does not serve as a formal topic review.

B⁻ Obstetrics and Gynecology Recall $28.00
Bourgeois

Lippincott Williams & Wilkins, 1997, 1st edition, 528 pages, ISBN 0683182145

A *Recall* series–style question-and-answer format set in two columns, making it easy to use for self-quizzing. Reviews many high-yield concepts and facts. Questions emphasize individual facts but do not integrate concepts, and no vignettes or images are included. In addition, some topics are covered only sparingly. Useful as a review of selected material, but not a comprehensive source for wards or end-of-rotation examinations.

B⁻ Oklahoma Notes Obstetrics and Gynecology $17.95
Miles

Springer-Verlag, 1996, 2nd edition, 219 pages, ISBN 0387946322

A rapid review of common topics in OB/GYN presented in outline format. Contains some good charts and illustrations. Variable, spotty coverage of topics.

A⁻ Danforth's Obstetrics & Gynecology $139.00

Danforth

Lippincott Williams & Wilkins, 1999, 8th edition, 715 pages, ISBN 0781712068

An excellent core text for residents and students considering careers in OB/GYN, although too in-depth for most others. A well-organized and comprehensive reference for both obstetrics and gynecology with numerous illustrations. Places increased emphasis on the latest advances, evidence-based medicine, and the most recent clinical guidelines. Also offers good, concise outlines of many diseases, although some key points are not highlighted as well as they should be by virtue of the book's extensive detail.

A⁻ Williams Obstetrics $135.00

Cunningham

McGraw-Hill, 2001, 21st edition, 1668 pages, ISBN 0838596479

The definitive book within its field, meant for the serious OB/GYN student. Organized by organ system and includes good use of graphics to highlight the material. Well referenced with updated guidelines and a strong, evidence-based approach. Its only weakness is that its usefulness is diminished by the need to find another reference for gynecology.

B⁺ Current Obstetric and Gynecologic Diagnosis & Treatment $54.95

DeCherney

McGraw-Hill, 1994, 8th edition, 1230 pages, ISBN 0838514472

A good overall reference book. Makes good use of graphics and tables, but minimal emphasis is placed on differential diagnosis. Good value, but not as "current" any more, especially when compared to other reference textbooks. New edition is expected in October 2002.

Pediatrics

WARD TIPS

Pediatrics

Welcome to pediatrics! The pediatric rotation is a six- to eight-week block at most medical schools. This time is split between the inpatient ward and the outpatient setting. Traditionally, more time has been devoted to the inpatient service, but this may change with the current emphasis on outpatient primary care. The outpatient portion of the rotation may be completed in a community pediatrician's office or in the outpatient service of the hospital. In addition, usually a week or less is devoted to the newborn service. The pediatric rotation emphasizes the care of the ill child as well as that of the healthy child.

WHO ARE THE PLAYERS?

The ward team typically consists of an attending, one to two upper-level residents, two to four interns, and one to four medical students.

Attendings. The attending may be a member of the general pediatric faculty or a member of one of the pediatric subspecialties. The attending is ultimately responsible for patients and generally rounds on a daily basis. This is your opportunity to formally present patients to someone who will be responsible for a large portion of your evaluation. Also note that because some time is usually devoted to didactics, it is important to know your attending's areas of interest, as he or she is likely to focus on those topics during rounds.

Residents. The role of residents is to supervise the interns and medical students. They are responsible for most of the day-to-day teaching you will get on the service. Ask them to give you informal lectures and to show you interesting findings on the ward. Demonstrate your interest in doing procedures. Note that residents are also a good source of articles. Remember that residents play a critical role in your clinical evaluations.

Your daily progress note is a blessing to the intern.

Interns. Interns are responsible for monitoring patients' daily progress and for doing the grunt work. Needless to say, these people are busy—but you can help them by following patients with them and writing a daily progress note. Discuss each patient's assessment and plan with your intern, and make sure you understand the rationale behind all the orders you have written and tests you have ordered; this will make you look more informed when you present to the residents and attending. Interns also play an important role in your evaluations.

Nurses, social workers, child life specialist, etc. As on other services, these specialists are an invaluable source of information about your patients.

HOW IS THE DAY SET UP?

The schedule of a typical day on the ward is as follows:

7:00–8:00 AM	Prerounds: check chart, check labs, check vitals, examine the patient
8:00–9:00 AM	Team rounds
9:00–10:00 AM	Attending rounds
10:00 AM–12:00 NOON	Write progress note, order labs, etc.
NOON–1:00 PM	Lunch or lunch conference
1:00–5:00 PM	Check afternoon labs, sign out to the team members, etc.

WHAT DO I DO DURING PREROUNDS?

Prerounding in pediatrics is similar to prerounding in internal medicine with a few variations. In general, children should be examined during prerounds even if they are still sleeping. However, ask your resident if there are patients who should not be examined prior to rounds in the morning. You may also awaken the parents to ask how their child is doing. Allow yourself some extra time, as there are often calculations that need to be done prior to rounds. Most numbers are reported on a per-kilogram basis. For example, input is reported as cc/kg/day and kcal/kg/day, and urine output is reported as cc/kg/hour. You may need to allow 20 minutes per patient at the beginning until you become more efficient.

HOW DO I DO WELL IN THIS ROTATION?

As you have realized or will soon realize, your grades during the clinical years are more subjective than they were during the preclinical period. Nevertheless, there are some basic rules you can follow to help improve your evaluations.

Know your patient. You've probably heard this at least a thousand times, but this advice is a constant. You have the time to investigate patients thoroughly so that your busy interns, residents, and attendings can turn to you for detailed information they did not obtain during their workups. Important but often not thoroughly investigated aspects of the admission history and physical (H&P) are diet, immunization history, development, and social history.

Communicate with your patient. Although earning the trust of your pediatric patient and parents is no small task, it is a necessity in effectively caring for your patient. You must take every step to ensure that patients know why they are here and what you are doing for them. Take your time when explaining concepts and procedures, and do so at a level that is appropriate to the patient. That may mean using very concrete terms and humor, so try practicing on yourself or on a fellow student, and remember to be very, very patient.

In pediatrics, most numbers are reported on a per-kilogram basis.

Communicate with parents. This rotation is unique in that you will need to interact with concerned (and, unfortunately, sometimes unconcerned) parents who will be in the room with you. You will likely have the most time to speak with a child's family, so you may enjoy the closest relationship with them. It is critical that you maintain an open line of communication regarding a child's condition, prognosis, and any planned procedures. No one knows the patient better than the primary caregiver, so listen carefully. At times, parents may ask you questions that lie beyond your medical knowledge. An incorrect answer could undermine their trust in you, so you should never give an answer if you are unsure of its validity. It is okay to say, "I do not know, but I will find out from the resident for you." In this way, you will help alleviate the family's worries while showing your genuine concern for the child. You will not lose face for not having all of the answers; to the contrary, parents will trust and respect you for being honest and keeping them well informed.

Show genuine interest in patients. Make sure any interest you show is genuine, as nothing is worse than insincerity. Remember how frightened you were of doctors as a child? Try to alleviate some of the patient's fears.

Read about the patients you admitted on a given day as soon as you get the chance. The sooner you read about a patient's problem, the more likely you will be to remember the topic—and the more knowledgeable you will be when you present to your team. During your reading, you will discover questions that you should have asked, new labs to order, and so on. This will allow you to make valuable contributions to the workup and to ask intelligent questions.

Practice your presentation. The only time your attending has the chance to see you at work is during rounds, so use this time to your advantage. Don't stutter and mumble your presentations; instead, make sure they are organized, precise, accurate, and, whenever possible, done from memory. Also make sure that the assessment-and-plan sections are well thought out. Discuss them with the resident beforehand. Handing out a review article about the topic may not hurt either.

Ask for feedback. The attendings and residents will usually schedule a time for feedback halfway through the rotation. If they don't schedule such time, ask for it. Then, when you meet with them, ask them to give you a detailed evaluation of your performance, emphasizing areas in which you can improve. Never accept the answer that you are "doing fine." "Fine" may be average or better—who knows? Ask for feedback on your written work (H&P and progress notes) as well.

Never put down your colleagues. Nothing looks worse than team members criticizing one another, especially in front of a patient. This undermines a patient's trust and can compromise care. So if you need to say something, save it until you leave the patient's room, and then say it tactfully. It is crucial to maintain team morale so that you can work as a cohesive unit. Derogatory remarks are never appropriate on the wards (or anywhere else, for that matter). They're also a surefire way for you to trash your own evaluation.

KEY NOTES

The H&P and daily progress notes for pediatrics are similar to those of medicine, but there are a few variations:

- **Source:** You may obtain the history from the parent, from the patient, or, at times, from a relative or a friend. It is important to include the source of your information as well as your judgment on the reliability of this source (e.g., reliable, vague). This will enable your reader to place the information in context.

- **History of present illness (HPI):** Key pediatric questions include recent eating history (change in appetite, poor feeding), number of wet diapers per day (fewer than three may indicate dehydration), bowel movements, a change in energy or irritability, ill contacts, recent travel, and other environmental changes. Try to present the history chronologically.

- **Past medical history (PMH):** Past medical history should include maternal history (mother's age, gravida, para, abortions, pregnancy course), details on the pregnancy (onset of prenatal care, weight gain, complications such as diabetes or hypertension, blood type, Coombs, rubella immunity status, rapid plasma reagin [RPR]/VDRL), HIV, purified protein derivative [PPD], hepatitis B, blood type, drug/alcohol/tobacco use), details on labor and delivery (spontaneous or induced, duration, complications, presentation, method of delivery, meconium), neonatal history (birth weight, gestational age, complications in the nursery, length of stay), and history of other hospitalizations, surgeries, or injuries. Note that the pregnancy and neonatal history may not be relevant to all admissions (e.g., adolescents admitted for pneumonia).

- **Nutrition:** For infants, include information on breast milk or formula (what type), frequency, and amount; for toddlers, include the introduction of cereal and baby foods as well as milk intake. For older children, discuss appetite and type of food eaten.

- **Immunization:** This is an often-overlooked section that should not be missed in pediatrics. Ask to see the immunization record.

- **Developmental history:** Ask the parents when the child first began to sit, walk, and talk and when he or she completed toilet training. Also ask about school performance.

- **Family history (FH):** Focus on inherited diseases, consanguinity (i.e., inbreeding), miscarriages, early deaths, congenital anomalies, developmental delay, mental retardation, sickle cell disease, asthma, seizure disorders, atopy, and cardiovascular diseases. It is also helpful to include a pedigree chart.

- **Social history (SH):** This is an important section in pediatrics and should include information about the home environment (who lives there, smoking in the home, etc.), the child's interaction with the family, the primary caregiver, and how the parent may be reached. A psychosocial assessment should be tailored to the age of the child; the basic components are outlined in the mnemonic "HEADSS".

Children are not just "little adults."

WARD TIPS

Pediatrics

The psycho-social history—

HEADSS
Home life
Education, employment
Activities (sports, friends)
Drugs (alcohol, tobacco)
Safety (seat belts, guns in the home, abuse)
Suicide, depression

TIPS FOR EXAMINING CHILDREN

Infants from the age of six months on often have anxiety toward strangers. It is thus very common for a child to cry during the exam—but don't take it personally. Here are some tips:

Take time to play with the young patient before attempting a physical exam.

- Anxious children will search your eyes for good intentions. Kind eyes will get you far!
- Take off your white coat before entering the exam room (unless your attending prefers otherwise). Consider wearing a tie with cartoon characters on it—or wear a sticker on your shirt.
- Observe the child's interactions with the parents, primary caregiver, etc.
- For infants and toddlers, do as much of the exam as possible with the child in the parent's lap. If the patient is in respiratory distress, which may worsen with agitation (as would be the case with epiglottitis), the child should be left in the parent's arms.
- Distraction with a toy or even your name badge works well for young children (i.e., those under two years of age). Giving older children a "task" to perform during your exam will also help ensure their cooperation.
- Let the child touch and play with the instruments. Demonstrate what you are about to do on yourself or on a parent to let the child know that the procedure is not painful. Save the invasive and painful parts of the exam for the end.

Check the tympanic membranes last.

- It is best to perform the cardiac and pulmonary portion of the exam first, when the child is still quiet. Once you have accomplished this often-difficult task, move on to the other portions of the physical.
- With newborns, infants, and toddlers, observe, auscultate, and then palpate.
- Use age-appropriate terms.
- Smile and speak in a soft tone. Tell the child how well he or she is doing. Be funny whenever possible.

Variations in the physical exam are as follows:

Report vital signs as ranges with a maximum value.

- **Vital signs:** Information on temperature should include the method by which it was obtained: axillary, rectal, or oral (only in children over age three). Rectal temperatures are the gold standard in pediatrics; axillary temperatures, though often used, are inaccurate and unreliable. Oral temperatures are 1° below rectal. Include weight (in kilograms and percentile range), height (in centimeters and percentile range), and head circumference (in centimeters and percentile range). Head circumference is routinely measured in children up to two years of age. Plot these values on graphs along with old values if available.
- **General appearance:** Be descriptive. Comment on alertness, playfulness, consolability, hydration status (tearing, drooling), respiratory status, development, social interactions, responsiveness (smiling, laughing), and nutritional status.

WARD TIPS

Pediatrics

- **Skin:** Check for jaundice, acrocyanosis, mottling, birthmarks, cradle cap, rashes, and capillary refill.
- **Hair:** Note lanugo and Tanner stage.
- **Head:** Note circumference, sutures, shape, and fontanelles.
- **Eyes:** Note red reflex in the newborn, strabismus (cover test in preschoolers and corneal light reflex in infants), and scleral icterus.
- **Ears:** Use the largest speculum you can. One option to facilitate examining the ear is to have the child held facing you. Ask the parent to cross his or her leg over both of the child's legs. Also ask the parent to wrap one arm around the child's arm and body and to use the other arm to hold the child's head. In an infant, pull the auricle backward and downward. In an older child, pull the external ear backward and upward. Use an insufflator bulb to assess tympanic membrane mobility.
- **Nose:** Look for patent nares and nasal flaring (respiratory distress).
- **Mouth:** Note dentition, palate (cleft), and thrush. Use a gloved finger to evaluate the infant's palate and suck reflex.
- **Heart:** The average heart rate in a newborn is 140–160 bpm; in an older child, it is < 120 bpm. Always check for femoral pulses in infants to exclude coarctation. Innocent murmurs are found in up to 50% of normal children and are characterized by low intensity (I–II/VI), occurrence in systole, variation with position and respiration, and a musical quality.
- **Chest:** The average respiratory rate in a newborn is 40–60; in an older child it is 15–25. Expiration is more prolonged in infants than in adults; in young infants, respiratory movements are produced by abdominal movements. Look for any skin retraction between the rib or above the clavicles (respiratory distress).
- **Abdomen:** Deep palpation should be performed on every infant. Check the umbilicus (or stump), and check for hepatosplenomegaly and masses.
- **Back:** Check for scoliosis, tufts of hair, and deep dimples.
- **Genitalia:** Circumcision, testes (descended bilaterally), hernias, labia (adhesions), hymenal opening, and Tanner stage should be noted.
- **Musculoskeletal:** Check for developmental hip dysplasia. With the infant supine, stabilize the pelvis with one hand, and then flex and adduct the opposite hip and apply gentle posterior pressure on the thigh. Feel for hip dislocation, which will usually relocate spontaneously upon release of pressure (Barlow maneuver). To reduce a dislocated hip, place one finger on the greater trochanter and one on the inner thigh; flex and abduct the hip; and lift the femoral head anteriorly, feeling for a clunk as it relocates into the acetabulum (Ortolani maneuver). Check range of motion, leg length, and symmetry of skin creases.
- **Neurologic:** Check tone, strength, neonatal reflexes (root, suck, grasp, Moro, stepping, etc.), Babinski, deep tendon reflexes (DTRs), and development.

WARD TIPS

Pediatrics

AFOSF = Anterior fontanelle open, soft, and flat

A/P = Assessment and plan

BMP = Basic metabolic panel

BS+ = Bowel sounds present

CC = Chief complaint

c/c/e = Clubbing, cyanosis, and edema

CN = cranial nerve

c/w = consistent with

d/c = Discharge

DOA = Day of admission

EOMI = Extraocular movements intact

F/C = Fever, chills

FM = Fine motor

FROM = Full range of motion

G1P1 = Gravida 1, para 1

GA = Gestational age

GM = Gross motor

HBV = Hepatitis B vaccine

HC = Head circumference

h/o = History of

HSM = Hepatosplenomegaly

ID = Identification

IUTD = Immunizations up to date

IVF = Intravenous fluid

KUB = Kidney, ureter, bladder

LAD = Lymphadenopathy

Sample Pediatric Admit Note

CC: "Throwing up."

ID: 7-week-old previously healthy Caucasian male presents with progressive emesis × 1 week.

Source: Parents, reliable.

Referring physician: Dr. Paul Smith, pediatrician (310) 555-8798.

HPI: This is the first hospital admission for this 7-week-old Caucasian male who was in his USGH until 1 week PTA, when parents describe onset of emesis after feedings. Emesis occurred 1–2 times/day, looked like formula, and was NBNB. In the 3 days PTA, emesis increased in frequency, occurring within 10 minutes of every feeding, and became projectile in nature. On the DOA the mother noted projectile emesis to 2–3 feet of a dark brown color and decided to bring him to the ER. Pt has no prior history of similar symptoms. He feeds avidly and appears hungry after vomiting. Pt had 4 wet diapers in the past 24 hours. Parents deny F/C, diarrhea or constipation, weight loss, irritability, rashes, cough, rhinorrhea, or other URI symptoms. No h/o recent travel or ill contacts. In the ER, pt was given a 20 cc NS bolus × 1 and was admitted to Pediatrics for further evaluation.

PMH:

1. **Past illnesses:** None.

2. **Surgical history:** None.

3. **Medications:** None.

4. **Allergies:** NKDA.

5. **Immunizations:** IUTD. Received HBV at birth. Well-child visit next week for 2-month vaccines.

6. **Birth history:** 3000-g 38-week GA term male born via C-section for failure to progress to a 25 y/o G1P1 Caucasian female at Mercy Hospital. Apgar scores of 7 at 1 min. and 9 at 5 min. Home in 2 days without complications. Pregnancy had been uneventful. Mother denies infections, exposures, tobacco, medication, or drug use.

7. **Diet:** Initial breast-feeding × 4 weeks. Now Enfamil with iron q4h at 2–4 oz per feed.

8. **Developmental history:** Has met developmental milestones. GM: Raises head and chest when prone. FM: Follows objects to midline. Language: Alerts to sound, social smile. Social: Recognizes parents.

FH: Father with pyloric stenosis at age 8 weeks. No other family history of congenital illness, developmental delay, or GI disease.

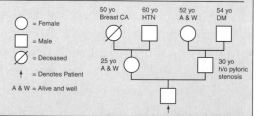

SH: Pt lives with his mother and father in an apartment. There are no siblings (patient is firstborn). Parents are college educated. Father works as an accountant, and mother works part-time as a lawyer. Maternal grandmother baby-sits. No smoking, pets, or firearms in the home.

ROS: Unremarkable except as above.

PE: VS: Temp 98.4°F (rectal), HR 144, RR 48, BP 95/60 (right arm).

Growth: Wt 4.8 kg (50%), length 57 cm (50%), HC 38.7 cm (50–75%).

General: WDWN 7-week-old male resting quietly in NAD.

Skin: Dry, warm, pink, with good turgor. No jaundice, ecchymoses, or rashes.

HEENT:

Head: NC/AT, AFOSF 1 × 1 cm, head shape symmetric.

Eyes: PERRL, EOMI, RR intact bilaterally, anicteric, conjunctiva clear and moist.

Ears: TMs nonerythematous, mobile, normal landmarks bilaterally.

Nose: Patent nares, no nasal flaring or d/c.

Mouth: Palate intact, no thrush, MMM, OP clear without erythema or exudates.

Neck: FROM, no LAD, no thyromegaly.

Chest: No respiratory distress, symmetric excursion, clear in all lung fields, no W/R/R.

Cardiac: RRR, Nl S1S2, no M/R/G, femoral pulses 2+ bilaterally.

Abdomen: ND, occasional peristaltic waves visible, BS+, abdomen soft and NT, no masses or palpable "olive," no HSM.

GU: Nl circumcised male, both testes descended without masses or tenderness.

Back: No dimples or tufts.

Extremities: Brisk cap refill < 2 seconds, no c/c/e. No Barlow's/Ortolani's sign or hip clicks, skin folds symmetric.

Neuro: MS: Alert and active. CNs: pupillary light reflex/face/palate symmetric, tongue midline. Motor: MAE, normal tone and bulk, strong suck; no sensory abnormalities noted. Reflexes: Moro present and symmetric, DTRs 2+ bilaterally, both toes upgoing.

Labs: CBC and BMP pending.

Studies:

KUB: Nonspecific bowel gas pattern. No masses seen.

Abdominal US: Hypoechoic mass > 1.5 cm, c/w pyloric stenosis.

A/P: 7-week-old previously healthy Caucasian male with 1-week h/o progressive, projectile emesis with confirmed pyloric stenosis on US.

1. **Emesis:** The clinical picture of progressive, projectile, nonbilious emesis in a first-born term male is consistent with the diagnosis of pyloric stenosis, which was confirmed on US. Patient does not appear dehydrated. However, prior to surgical intervention must r/o electrolyte abnormalities such as hypokalemic hypochloremic metabolic alkalosis secondary to persistent vomiting.
   - Check BMP results for electrolyte abnormalities
   - Surgery consult to evaluate for pyloromyotomy
   - NPO until surgery
   - IVF at 1 × maintenance for hydration

2. **Routine health maintenance:** Pt is up to date on his vaccinations.
   - Well-child visit for 2-month vaccines is scheduled.

MAE = Moves all extremities

MMM = Mucous membranes moist

M/R/G = Murmurs, rubs, or gallops

MS = Mental status

NAD = No acute distress

NBNB = Nonbilious, nonbloody

NC/AT = Normocephalic, atraumatic

ND = Nondistended

NKDA = No known drug allergies

Nl = Normal

NPO = Nothing by mouth

NS = Normal saline

NT = Nontender

OP = Oropharynx

PERRL = Pupils equal, round, and reactive to light

PTA = Prior to admission

r/o = Rule out

RR = Red reflex

RRR = Regular rate and rhythm

TM = Tympanic membrane

URI = Upper respiratory infection

US = Ultrasound

USGH = Usual state of good health

WDWN = Well developed, well nourished

W/R/R = Wheezes, rhonchi, rales

THE NURSERY ROTATION

Most students will spend a week or less on the nursery service, attending deliveries and working in the newborn nursery. As part of the nursery team, you will be paged to attend deliveries in which newborns may be at risk. The pediatric team is called for factors such as multiple gestations, preterm deliveries, cesarean sections, possible meconium aspiration, and known fetal anomalies. On arrival, the team obtains a brief history, sets up the infant warmer, and prepares resuscitation equipment such as oxygen, suction, and intubation apparatus. The newborn is then shuttled from the obstetrician to the warmer, where the team goes to work. The baby is immediately dried off, the nose and mouth are suctioned, and the baby is rubbed and stimulated. The team provides ventilatory support and/or CPR if necessary. Apgar scores are assessed at one and five minutes, and the baby receives an initial head-to-toe examination. If the baby appears vigorous and healthy, a brief delivery note is written, and the team's role may end there. If there are potential problems, the baby may be taken to the nursery for observation or admitted to the neonatal ICU (NICU).

The laws of neonatal resuscitation: dry, suction, stimulate.

The team will also take care of newborns in the nursery, write daily progress notes, and talk with new mothers. This portion of the pediatric rotation gives you a great opportunity to interact with neonatologists and newborns and to practice physical exams (before the onset of stranger anxiety). Nursery can have a fair amount of down time, so this is a great time to get lectures from your residents.

KEY PROCEDURES

The key procedures in pediatrics are lumbar puncture (LP), urine catheterization, and blood drawing. If the patient needs a painful procedure, parents are sometimes asked to leave the room, depending on the preference of the doctor. Drawing blood in newborns under one month of age is often accomplished with a heel stick. Ask a nurse or a resident to demonstrate the technique for you.

WHAT DO I CARRY IN MY POCKETS?

The white coat is generally not used in pediatrics, so don't rely on those handy oversized pockets to store your peripheral brain and instruments of the trade. Try using a fanny pack or a small over-the-shoulder camera bag.

Checklist

- ❑ Toy for distraction
- ❑ Stethoscope
- ❑ Ophthalmoscope
- ❑ Otoscope with tips of different sizes and an insufflator bulb
- ❑ Penlight
- ❑ Tongue blades

❑ Calculator (to determine dosages for meds)

❑ Optional: stickers for a reward (dinosaurs, Power Rangers, and Barney are very popular), cartoon Band-Aids (Snoopy, Garfield, etc.)

ROTATION OBJECTIVES

The following is a list of core topics that you are likely to encounter in the course of your pediatrics rotation. Conditions and topics discussed in further detail within this chapter are italicized.

Well-Child Care

- Anticipatory guidance and safety
- *Developmental milestones*
- *Growth parameters*
- *Immunizations*
- *Infant nutrition*
- *Tanner staging*

Cardiology

- Arrhythmias (supraventricular tachycardia, long QT syndrome, Wolff-Parkinson-White syndrome) (see Internal Medicine, Chapter 3)
- *Congenital heart disease*
- Congestive heart failure
- Pericardial disease

Dermatology

- Atopic dermatitis
- *Diaper rash*
- Impetigo
- Neonatal rashes (acne neonatorum, erythema toxicum, milia)
- Psoriasis
- Scabies and lice
- Seborrheic dermatitis
- *Viral exanthems*

Endocrinology

- Adrenal dysfunction (congenital adrenal hyperplasia)
- Diabetes
- Thyroid dysfunction

Gastroenterology

- Appendicitis (see Surgery, Chapter 8)
- Constipation

- *Failure to thrive*
- Gastroesophageal reflux
- Hirschsprung's disease
- *Intussusception*
- Malrotation and volvulus
- Meckel's diverticulum
- *Pyloric stenosis*

Genetic Disorders
- *Autosomal trisomies (21, 18, 13)*
- Common associations (CHARGE, VATER)
- Common syndromes (DiGeorge, Marfan, Noonan's, Prader-Willi, Williams)
- Sex chromosome disorders (Turner's, Kleinfelter's, fragile X)

Hematology and Oncology
- Anemia
- *Sickle cell disease*
- Thalassemia
- *Childhood cancers* (acute lymphocytic leukemia, Wilms' tumor, neuroblastoma)

Immunology
- Autoimmune disorders: Henoch-Schönlein purpura, idiopathic thrombocytopenic purpura, *juvenile rheumatoid arthritis, Kawasaki disease*
- *Immunodeficiencies (T-cell, B-cell, combined, complement, phagocytic, HIV)*

Infectious Disease
- Botulism
- Cellulitis
- *Fever management*
- Gastroenteritis
- *Meningitis*
- Orbital and periorbital cellulitis
- *Otitis media*
- *Pneumonia*
- Sexually transmitted diseases (see Obstetrics and Gynecology, Chapter 5)
- Sinusitis
- *Streptococcal pharyngitis*
- *Urinary tract infection*

Neonatology
- *Apgar score*
- *Congenital infections*
- *Neonatal hyperbilirubinemia*

- Prematurity
- *Respiratory distress syndrome*

Nephrology/Urology
- Cryptorchidism
- Fluid and electrolyte management (see Practical Information for All Clerkships, Chapter 2)
- Hematuria and proteinuria
- Hemolytic-uremic syndrome

Neurology
- Cerebral palsy
- *Febrile seizures*
- Hydrocephalus
- Neural tube defects
- Seizure disorders

Psychiatry (see Psychiatry, Chapter 7)
- Attention-deficit hyperactivity disorder
- Learning disorders
- Mental retardation

Orthopedics
- Developmental hip dysplasia
- *Limp*
- Nursemaid's elbow (subluxation of the radial head)
- *Pediatric fractures*

Pulmonology
- Apnea/apparent life-threatening event/sudden infant death syndrome
- *Asthma (reactive airway disease)*
- *Bronchiolitis*
- *Croup*
- *Epiglottitis*
- *Cystic fibrosis*

Toxicology
- Ingestions
- *Lead poisoning*
- Tylenol and salicylate toxicity

Trauma
- *Child abuse*
- Head injury

DEVELOPMENTAL MILESTONES

Language development is the best predictor of future academic achievement.

Pediatricians use a sequence of developmental milestones to monitor children for normal progress and to identify developmental delays. For each milestone, there is an age range for normal acquisition that is based on developmental norms. If a child fails to meet important milestones, it is critical that this be recognized early so that appropriate interventions may be implemented. Assessments are typically divided into gross motor, fine motor, language, and social development. Language is the best predictor of future academic achievement. Table 6.1 summarizes the key developmental milestones. Table 6.2 describes the normal appearance and resolution of neonatal reflexes.

TABLE 6.1. Key Developmental Milestones.

Age	Gross Motor	Fine Motor	Language	Social
1 month	Lifts head when prone	Tracks to midline	Alerts to sound	Regards face
2 months	Lifts chest when prone	Tracks past midline	Coos	Social smile
4 months	Rolls front to back (four months) Rolls back to front (five months)	Grasps objects	Orients to voice (four months) Says "ah-goo," razzes (five months)	Laughs
6 months	Sits upright	Transfers objects	Babbles	Stranger anxiety
9 months	Crawls, pulls to stand	Three-finger pincer grasp	Mama, dada—nonspecific, understands no	Waves bye-bye, plays pat-a-cake
12 months	Cruises (11 months), walks alone	Two-finger pincer grasp	Mama, dada—specific	Imitates actions, comes when called
15 months	Walks backward	Uses a cup	Uses four to six words	Throws temper tantrums
18 months	Runs, kicks a ball	Uses a spoon	Names common objects	May start toilet training
2 years	Goes up and down stairs one step at a time, jumps	Copies a line	Uses two-word sentences, 50-word vocabulary	Follows two-step commands, engages in parallel play
3 years	Goes up and down stairs alternating feet, rides a tricycle	Copies a circle, eats with utensils	Uses three-word sentences	Knows first and last name, shares toys
4 years	Hops, skips, catches a ball	Copies a cross	Counts to 10, knows colors	Engages in cooperative play

TABLE 6.2. Selected Neonatal Reflexes.

Reflex	Description	Age of Appearance/ Disappearance
Moro startle	Head extension causes extension and then flexion of the extremities.	Birth to 4–6 months
Palmar grasp	Infants grasp a finger placed in the palm.	Birth to 4–6 months
Rooting	Infants pursue an object placed around the mouth (e.g., a tongue depressor)	Birth to 4–6 months
Stepping	Infants make a walking movement with the legs when held upright and leaning forward.	Birth to 2 months
Asymmetric tonic neck	Turning the head while supine causes ipsilateral extremity extension and contralateral flexion (fencer position).	2 weeks to 6 months
Parachute	Infants extend the ipsilateral arm to support the body when tilted to one side while sitting.	Appears at 6–8 months

GROWTH PARAMETERS

At each pediatric visit, weight, height, and head circumference are plotted on growth charts specific for gender and age. This enables the clinician to evaluate potential problems such as failure to thrive (FTT) (see later discussion). Some helpful rules of thumb regarding growth are summarized in Table 6.3.

TABLE 6.3. Growth Pearls.

Parameter	Characteristics
Weight	Average birth weight (BW): 3.5 kg (7.7 lb) Formula: weight (lb) = 2.2 × weight (kg) May lose 5–10% BW over first few days; should return to BW by 10–14 days Should double BW by four to five months, triple BW by one year, and quadruple BW by two years Average weights: 10 kg at 1 year; 20 kg at 5 years; 30 kg at 10 years Formula: 2 × (age in years) + 10 = weight (kg) Average weight gain: 30 g/day for 3–4 months; 10–20 g/day for 4–12 months; 5 lbs/year from age 2 to puberty
Height	Average birth length: 50 cm (20 in.) Average height: 30 in. at 1 year; 3 ft at 3 years; 40 in. at 4 years (two times birth length); three times birth length at 13 years Average growth: two to three inches per year from age 4 to puberty
Head circumference	Average birth HC: 35 cm Average HC increase: 1 cm/month for one year; 10 cm over remainder of life span 90% of head growth occurs by two years of age

IMMUNIZATIONS

Keep an immunization schedule handy at all times.

Table 6.4 summarizes the recommended childhood immunization schedule. There are also certain contraindications and precautions to vaccination that are important to understand. Contraindications include the following:

- Pregnancy and immune compromise (oral polio; measles, mumps, rubella [MMR]; varicella)
- Encephalopathy within seven days of prior pertussis vaccination
- Anaphylactic egg allergy for influenza vaccine (must do prior skin testing)
- Current moderate to severe acute illness
- Recent administration of antibody-containing blood products (live injected vaccines)
- Severe allergy to a vaccine component or a prior dose of vaccine
- Precautions include prior reactions to pertussis vaccine, e.g., fever > 105°F, shock-like state, persistent crying for more than three hours within 48 hours of vaccination, or seizure within three days of vaccination

The following are not contraindications:

- The presence of mild illness and/or low-grade fever
- Current antibiotic therapy
- Prematurity

TABLE 6.4. Immunization Schedule.

Vaccine[a, b]	Birth	2 Months	4 Months	6 Months	12–15 Months	15–18 Months	2 Years	4–6 Years
HBV	x	x		x				
DTaP		x	x	x		x		x
Hib		x	x	x	x			
IPV		x	x	x				x
PCV[c]		x	x	x	x			
MMR					x			x
Varicella					x			
HAV[d]							x	

[a]DTaP = diphtheria, tetanus, acellular pertussis; Hib = *Haemophilus influenzae* type b; IPV = inactivated polio; PCV = pneumococcal conjugate vaccine; HAV = hepatitis A vaccine.
[b]Influenza vaccine is indicated in patients over six months with asthma, cystic fibrosis, bronchopulmonary dysplasia, HIV, sickle cell disease, diabetes, and chronic heart disease.
[c]PCV is recommended for all children ages 2 to 23 months; it is also recommended for certain children over 24 months, but fewer doses are needed in older children.
[d]Hepatitis A vaccine is recommended at age two in certain regions and high-risk groups.

INFANT NUTRITION

Human breast milk provides complete nutrition for the first six months of life. Breast-feeding is recommended for almost all children and has some advantages over formula. In addition to encouraging mother-infant bonding, breast-feeding limits exposure to potential antigens, decreases the risk of eczema and cow's-milk protein allergy, and decreases the risk of serious infections. Colostrum, which is produced in the first one to three days postpartum, is high in protein and low in fat and contains immunoglobulins that help limit infection. Mature breast milk is easier to digest and is cheaper (and easier to prepare) than formula. After six months of age, breast-fed infants may require fluoride and iron supplementation.

If a mother chooses to use formula, there are many different types available, but formulas with iron are recommended. Cow's-milk protein formulas include Enfamil, Similac, Carnation Good Start, and Gerber; soy protein formulas include Isomil, ProSobee, Nursoy, and Soyalac. Nutrient formulas for children with special needs include Nutramigen, Alimentum, Pregestamil, and Neocate.

In the first two months of life, babies will eat two to three ounces (or approximately ten to twenty minutes per breast) every two to three hours. After four months of age, the frequency of feedings may be decreased to every four to five hours. As new foods are introduced, milk intake should be decreased proportionately. Keep in mind that new foods should be introduced at a rate of one per week to allow for the identification of allergies. Honey should be avoided in children under one year of age owing to the risk of infant botulism. Also, milk bottles should not be left in the crib overnight, as this may cause "milk bottle caries." Table 6.5 discusses recommended foods for the first year of life.

TABLE 6.5. Infant Nutrition.

Age	Recommended Foods[a]
Birth	Breast milk or formula with iron
4–6 months	Single-grain cereal; supplemental water
6–7 months	Strained fruit
7–8 months	Strained vegetables
8–9 months	Well-chopped meats
9–10 months	Cheese, egg yolk, protein foods
10–12 months	Soft finger foods: cookies, fruits, vegetables, meats
12 months	Soft table foods; may start whole cow's milk

[a]Avoid foods that can lead to choking (e.g., nuts, raisins, hot dogs). Also avoid cow's milk, berries, citrus, corn, shellfish, egg whites, nuts, wheat, orange juice, and honey, until 1 year of age.

TABLE 6.6. Tanner Stages.

Stage	Male Genitalia	Female Breasts	Pubic Hair
I	Childhood-size penis, testes, scrotum	Preadolescent: elevation of papilla only	No pubic hair
II	Enlargement of testes, scrotum	Breast buds: elevation of breast and papilla	Sparse, straight, downy hair on labia/penile base
III	Enlargement of penis	Enlargement of breast and areola, single contour	Darker, coarse, curled hair
IV	Scrotal skin darkens, rugations present	Projection of areola and papilla, separate contour (the secondary mound)	Adult-type hair limited to genital area
V	Adult size and shape	Mature breast	Adult quantity and pattern, spreads to thighs

TANNER STAGING

With each physical exam, it is important to assess the sexual maturity of a child. Puberty follows a predictable sequence in all adolescents, but with variations in timing and rate of change. In males, sexual development begins with testicular enlargement, followed by height growth spurt, penile enlargement, and pubic hair. In females, the sequence begins with thelarche (breast development), followed by growth spurt, pubic hair, and menarche. The Tanner staging system is outlined in Table 6.6.

Cardiology

CONGENITAL HEART DISEASE

Congenital heart disease (CHD) is present in approximately 0.8% of American children and is generally divided into cyanotic and noncyanotic disease. Cardiac defects with right-to-left shunts are categorized as cyanotic and those with left-to-right shunts as noncyanotic. Workup includes an H&P as well as a CXR, an ECG, an echocardiogram, and in some cases angiography. Medical and/or surgical interventions are now available for most of these conditions.

- **Noncyanotic congenital heart conditions:** These include patent ductus arteriosus (PDA), atrial septal defects (ASDs), and ventricular septal defects (VSDs). In these defects, mixing of oxygenated and deoxygenated blood occurs in the pulmonary circulation. Coarctation of the aorta is also noncyanotic, but no mixing occurs. Lesions are often asymptomatic in early childhood, but if severe they can present with symptoms of CHF. Large ASD or VSD lesions may lead to Eisenmenger's syndrome, in which a left-to-right shunt causes pulmonary

Left-to-right shunts—

The 3 Ds
ASD
VSD
PDA

VSD is the most common congenital heart defect.

hypertension and shunt reversal. Many septal lesions close spontaneously, but persistent or large lesions may require surgical intervention.

- **Cyanotic congenital heart conditions:** These include tetralogy of Fallot, transposition of the great vessels, truncus arteriosus, tricuspid atresia, and total anomalous pulmonary venous return. In these defects, nonoxygenated blood is directed into systemic circulation, and infants may present with cyanosis, respiratory distress, or shock either at birth or in the first weeks to months of life. Infants who are unable to establish sufficient circulation will present at or near birth. This is seen in transposition of the great vessels, where systemic and pulmonary circulations occur in parallel rather than in series, necessitating immediate surgical repair to sustain life. In other conditions, symptom onset may be related to the severity of restriction in systemic or pulmonary flow. For example, in tetralogy of Fallot (pulmonic stenosis, overriding aorta, right ventricular hypertrophy, and VSD), severe pulmonic stenosis will dramatically restrict pulmonary flow and lead to an earlier onset of symptoms. In many of these conditions, prostaglandin E_1 (PGE_1) is used to maintain a PDA for collateral flow. The definitive treatment in all cases is surgical repair.

> **Right-to-left shunts—**
>
> **The 5 Ts**
> **T**etralogy
> **T**ransposition
> **T**runcus arteriosus
> **T**ricuspid atresia
> **T**otal anomalous pulmonary venous return

> **Tetralogy of Fallot—**
>
> **PROVe**
> **P**ulmonic stenosis
> **R**ight ventricular hypertrophy
> **O**verriding aorta
> **V**SD

Dermatology

DIAPER RASH

Diaper rash is a common problem seen in outpatient pediatric clinics. It can be caused by fungal infection of the skin with *Candida albicans* or by irritant dermatitis from prolonged skin contact with urine and feces. Note that *Candida* infection and diaper dermatitis often coexist.

Signs and Symptoms. Diaper rash is localized to areas in contact with the diaper, which include the perineum and buttocks. Irritant dermatitis presents with ill-defined erythematous patches or plaques, often with scaling, and usually spares the inguinal folds. *Candida* infection presents with well-demarcated beefy-red erythematous patches surrounded by satellite lesions (erythematous papules or pustules) and can be found within the inguinal folds.

Workup. *Candida* infection can be diagnosed by scraping a satellite lesion, staining with 10% potassium hydroxide (KOH), and observing pseudohyphae under the microscope.

Treatment. The diaper area should be kept clean and dry with frequent diaper changes, air drying, and the use of a barrier cream in moist areas. *Candida* infections may be treated with topical antifungal agents (e.g., clotrimazole bid × 10–14 days). A low-potency topical steroid can be added in severe cases.

VIRAL EXANTHEMS

There are many causes of rash in children. The clinical history is often the key tool needed to make the diagnosis. Common rashes caused by viruses are discussed in Table 6.7. Note that treatment of these conditions involves supportive measures and isolation while contagious.

TABLE 6.7. Viral Exanthems.

Disease	Characteristics
Rubeola (measles)	Agent: paramyxovirus Prodrome: **C**ough, **C**oryza, **C**onjunctivitis (**3 Cs**) for five days Koplik spots: white-gray spots on buccal mucosa; resolve before appearance of the rash Rash: erythematous maculopapular rash that begins on the head and spreads to the body; fades in the same pattern Fever: high fever present Complications: otitis media (common), encephalitis, pneumonia, and subacute sclerosing panencephalitis (rare)
Rubella (German or three-day measles)	Agent: togavirus Prodrome: malaise, then suboccipital lymphadenopathy Rash: maculopapular rash that begins on the face and then generalizes, resolving in three to five days Fever: on the first day of rash only Viral exanthem: petechiae on the palate (Forscheimer's spots)
Roseola infantum (exanthem subitum)	Agent: human herpesvirus 6 and 7 (HHV-6, HHV-7) Fever: abrupt onset of high temperature (> 104°F) for three to five days; child does not feel ill Rash: as fever drops, a maculopapular rash appears on the trunk, spreads peripherally, and resolves in 24 hours Complications: rapid temperature rise associated with febrile seizures
Varicella (chickenpox)	Agent: varicella-zoster virus (VZV) Highly contagious via respiratory droplets and contact with lesions until crusted over Prodrome: fever and malaise for one day Rash: pruritic teardrop vesicles on an erythematous base that start on the face and trunk and spread peripherally. Lesions break and crust over in one week. Classic finding: lesions in different stages of healing Complications: secondary skin infection (most common) and pneumonia Zoster (shingles): reactivation of varicella infection with painful skin lesions in a dermatomal distribution
Erythema infectiosum (fifth disease)	Agent: parvovirus B19 Epidemics occur in the spring Prodrome: mild flulike illness for seven to ten days Rash: "slapped cheek" rash and circumoral pallor; then an erythematous maculopapular rash spreads to the trunk and legs in a lacy, reticular pattern Fever: low-grade or no fever Complications: aplastic crisis (sickle cell disease and other anemias), fetal anemia/hydrops fetalis (in utero infection), and arthritis
Hand, foot, and mouth disease	Agent: coxsackie A virus Contagious by direct contact Rash: vesicles on hands and feet, oral ulcerations; resolves in one week Fever: present

FAILURE TO THRIVE

Failure to thrive, or growth deficiency, refers to an inadequate growth rate in an infant or child. Definitions include weight below the third to fifth percentile for age, weight below 80% of the ideal for age, and falling off the growth curve (crossing two major percentile lines on a growth chart). Cases are identified as organic, in which a medical condition is identified, or nonorganic, in which psychosocial factors are thought to be the cause; nonorganic FTT is more common. Risk factors for FTT include low socioeconomic status, low maternal age, an unstable family environment, chronic illness, genetic disease, inborn errors of metabolism, and HIV infection.

Nonorganic causes are more common in failure to thrive.

Signs and Symptoms. Children are of low weight for their age and height and exhibit minimal weight gain or even weight loss. Other signs and symptoms vary with the underlying cause and may include recurrent infections, GI complaints, and odd eating behavior. In addition to the physical exam, weight, height, and head circumference should be plotted on a growth chart. A comparison of the percentiles may yield valuable information. For example, children receiving inadequate calories may initially show weight loss with preservation of height and head circumference. Children with hypothyroidism, however, may show retarded height growth with normal weight gain. Head circumference is always the last parameter to be affected.

Differential. The differential is extensive, and often no medical cause can be found. Psychosocial factors include poor feeding techniques, inadequate calories, improper mixing of formula, psychological disturbance in the mother or family, and food refusal by the child. Organic factors include mechanical GI dysfunction, structural abnormalities (pyloric stenosis, duodenal atresia), malabsorption, infection, chronic disease, and reduced growth potential (congenital disorders, skeletal dysplasias).

Workup. History, exam, and observation of caregiver-child interaction will help direct further workup. It may also be helpful to observe the child eating or to have the family keep a food diary. Laboratory testing often fails to provide answers, but standard screening tests include CBC, electrolytes, creatinine, albumin, and protein. Other tests may include urinalysis (UA)/urine culture, a sweat chloride test (for CF), and assessment of bone age. If GI symptoms are present, a stool culture, ova and parasites (O&P), tests for malabsorption (stool pH and reducing substances), and tests for stool occult blood may be appropriate.

Treatment. Treatment will vary with the cause and includes the following:

- Give dietary advice, and have caretakers start a food diary and calorie count. Encourage nutritional supplementation if breast-feeding is inadequate.
- Hospitalize for feeding, calorie counts, and observation if there is evidence of neglect or severe malnourishment or if no growth results from dietary modification.

INTUSSUSCEPTION

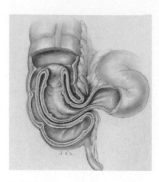

FIGURE 6.1. Intussusception. (Reprinted, with permission, from Way L, Doherty G. *Current Surgical Diagnosis & Treatment*, 11th ed. New York: McGraw-Hill, 2003.)

Intussusception occurs when one portion of the bowel telescopes into an adjacent portion, usually proximal to the ileocecal valve (see Figure 6.1). Intussusception is the most common cause of bowel obstruction in the first two years of life and affects males more often than females. Risk factors include polyps, Meckel's diverticulum, adenovirus or rotavirus infection, Henoch-Schönlein purpura, intestinal lymphoma, celiac disease, and CF.

Signs and Symptoms. Parents may report sudden onset of colicky abdominal pain in an otherwise healthy child. Infants often draw up their legs, cry, and vomit. More ominous signs include red "currant jelly" stools, lethargy, and fever. On abdominal exam, a "sausage-shaped" mass may be palpable. Other signs include abdominal tenderness, positive stool occult blood, and pallor or diaphoresis.

Differential. The differential includes constipation, GI infection, Meckel's diverticulum, lymphoma (in children over six years) and meconium ileus (in neonates).

Workup and Treatment

- Assess and correct any volume or electrolyte abnormalities.
- Abdominal plain films may reveal a mass, an obstruction, or visible intussusception. Ultrasound has recently been used to establish the diagnosis in equivocal cases.
- Air-contrast enema confirms diagnosis and is also curative in 75% of cases.
- If enema reduction is unsuccessful or if the child is unstable, proceed to surgical reduction and resection of gangrenous bowel if present.

PYLORIC STENOSIS

Pyloric stenosis is seen more often in first-born males.

Pyloric stenosis is gastric outlet obstruction caused by hypertrophy of the pyloric sphincter. It is more common in first-born males, exhibiting a male-to-female ratio of 4:1. The incidence is approximately 1/500 births.

Signs and Symptoms. Parents report nonbilious emesis after feedings in the first two to eight weeks of life, which increases in frequency and becomes projectile in nature. Infants appear hungry and feed well but eventually suffer from malnourishment and dehydration. On exam, an olive-shaped mass may be palpable in the epigastric area or gastric peristaltic waves may be visible.

Differential. The differential diagnosis includes pylorospasm, overfeeding, gastroenteritis, hiatal hernia, duodenal atresia ("double bubble" sign on x-ray), esophageal stenosis, malrotation/volvulus, meconium ileus, milk protein allergy, and gastroesophageal reflux disease (GERD).

Workup. The diagnosis can be confirmed by an ultrasound that shows a hypertrophic pylorus. Abdominal plain films may be helpful. Contrast studies, which will show a string sign or a pyloric beak, are occasionally needed as well. Evaluate serum electrolytes for hypochloremic-hypokalemic metabolic alkalosis secondary to persistent emesis.

Treatment. Begin by correcting existing dehydration and electrolyte abnormalities. Definitive treatment then involves surgical intervention with pyloromyotomy. The prognosis is excellent after treatment.

Genetic Disorders

AUTOSOMAL TRISOMIES

There are many important chromosomal defects in pediatrics. Table 6.8 discusses the three major autosomal trisomies that you should know.

TABLE 6.8. Autosomal Trisomies.

Disorder	Clinical Features	Facts and Prognosis
Trisomy 21 (Down syndrome)	Mental retardation, flat facial profile, flat occiput (brachycephaly), upslanted palpebral fissures, prominent epicanthal folds, micrognathia, protruding tongue, downfolding earlobes, excess skin at back of neck, Brushfield spots (speckled irises), transverse palmar crease, short and broad hands (brachydactyly), short stature, small genitalia, sandal gap (between first and second toes), hypotonia at birth, cardiac defects (endocardial cushion defects), duodenal atresia, atlantoaxial instability, increased rates of leukemia (acute lymphocytic leukemia, or ALL), Alzheimer's disease in adults	Most common chromosomal disorder. Incidence of 1/600 (increased with advanced maternal age). 95% of cases are due to meiotic nondisjunction. Life expectancy extends into the 30s and 40s with good medical and social support.
Trisomy 18 (Edwards' syndrome)	Severe mental/growth retardation, rocker-bottom feet, low-set ears, micrognathia, tight palpebral fissures, hypoplastic nasal alae, prominent occiput, cardiac defects, clenched hands with overlapping fingers, hypoplastic nails	Incidence of 1/4000. Male-to-female ratio of 1:3. 30% die before one month and 90% by one year.
Trisomy 13 (Patau's syndrome)	Severe mental/growth retardation, scalp defects (cutis aplasia), microphthalmia, microcephaly, cleft lip/palate, holoprosencephaly, capillary hemangiomas, cardiac defects, polydactyly, hypoplastic nails, renal abnormalities	Incidence of 1/12,000. 60% affected are female. 50% die by one month and 90% by one year.

SICKLE CELL DISEASE

Sickle cell disease is an autosomal-recessive disorder that results in chronic hemolytic anemia with intermittent acute events or "crises." Sickle cell disease is caused by a single amino acid substitution of valine for glutamine in the sixth position on the β-globin chain. As a result, hemoglobin polymers form under deoxygenated conditions, and RBCs assume a sickled shape. The life span of the RBC is shortened, leading to an anemia that is well compensated and usually not transfusion dependent. Deformability of the RBC is also decreased, leading to microvascular obstruction, tissue infarction, pain, and organ dysfunction. Patients are susceptible to life-threatening infections with encapsulated organisms (*Streptococcus pneumoniae, Haemophilus influenzae, Salmonella*) due to splenic dysfunction and autoinfarction by the age of two to four years. Heterozygotes with sickle cell trait generally have no manifestations of disease but may show painless hematuria or inability to concentrate urine. Sickle cell disease is the most common autosomal-recessive disorder in African-Americans.

Any sickle cell patient with fever needs a workup for sepsis.

Signs and Symptoms. A progressive hemolytic anemia develops after four months of age as fetal hemoglobin declines, and patients may exhibit pallor, splenomegaly, jaundice, a systolic ejection murmur, and growth retardation. Given the risk of serious infection, any sickle cell patient with a temperature > 38°C must be evaluated for bacterial sepsis, septic joints, or osteomyelitis. Patients are at increased risk for acute decompensation when exposed to "triggers," which include hypoxia, acidosis, changes in temperature, and dehydration. The main types of sickle cell crises are as follows:

- **Aplastic:** Suppression of RBC precursors in bone marrow, often due to parvovirus B19 infection, results in an acute and reversible reticulocytopenia.
- **Hyperhemolytic:** An acute drop in hemoglobin occurs as a result of exposure to oxidative stress, typically in patients with glucose-6-phosphate dehydrogenase (G6PD) deficiency.
- **Sequestration:** An acute drop in hemoglobin level occurs as a result of splenic pooling of RBCs with splenomegaly and hypovolemic shock. This typically occurs between six months and two years of age.
- **Vaso-occlusive:** Microvascular infarcts occur in any tissue in the body, leading to pain and organ dysfunction. Hand-foot syndrome (dactylitis), priapism, avascular necrosis of the femoral head, and stroke are forms of vaso-occlusive crisis. Acute chest syndrome is a crisis in the lungs that is associated with infection and infarction. Pain crises are the most common vaso-occlusive events and typically occur in bones.

Workup. Newborn screening is generally performed at birth. Diagnosis can be made through use of Sickledex preparations or by hemoglobin electrophoresis to determine the type and amount of hemoglobin present. During an acute crisis, appropriate tests may include blood culture and sensitivity,

CBC, reticulocyte count, UA/urine culture and sensitivity, CXR, serum electrolytes, and type and cross.

Treatment. Treatment for acute disease is as follows:

- Treat pain crises with NSAIDs and/or narcotics, hydration (1.5 to 2.0 times maintenance), and oxygen for hypoxia.
- Treat chest crises with antibiotics, oxygen, fluids, analgesics, incentive spirometry, and exchange transfusion.
- Treat stroke, priapism, and other complications with exchange transfusion to keep HbS below 30%.
- Treat aplastic, sequestration, and hyperhemolytic crises with simple transfusion.

Crisis pain can be severe—don't be stingy with pain medication.

Preventive measures include the following:

- Start prophylactic twice-daily oral penicillin VK at diagnosis and continue until at least age five.
- Vaccinate against *S. pneumoniae, H. influenzae,* hepatitis B, and influenza.
- Hydroxyurea increases the proportion of HbF and decreases the incidence of vaso-occlusive events.
- Bone marrow transplant has been curative in some children.
- Children with a history of stroke are placed on chronic exchange transfusion protocols to prevent future events.
- Deferoxamine (Desferal) is used with transfusion to prevent hemochromatosis.
- Folic acid is given once daily.

CHILDHOOD CANCERS

The most common childhood cancers are acute leukemias, CNS tumors (primarily posterior fossa or cerebellar tumors), and lymphomas. Other common pediatric tumors include Wilms' tumor, neuroblastoma, soft tissue sarcomas, and bone tumors. Although there are many important pediatric cancers, the key features of selected malignancies are discussed here.

Most common cancers in children:

1. Leukemia

2. CNS tumors

3. Lymphoma

4. Neuroblastoma

ACUTE LYMPHOCYTIC LEUKEMIA

Acute lymphocytic leukemia is the most common childhood cancer, exhibiting a peak onset at age four. It results from unregulated proliferation of immature blast cells in the marrow. Pancytopenia may result from marrow invasion.

Signs and Symptoms. Patients often present with fever, bone pain, and limp or refusal to bear weight. Signs include petechiae, purpura and bleeding (from thrombocytopenia), pallor (from anemia), lymphadenopathy, and hepatosplenomegaly.

Differential and Workup. The differential includes aplastic anemia, immune thrombocytopenic purpura, rheumatic diseases, other malignancies, and mononucleosis or other viral infection. Peripheral blood smear reveals large,

HIGH-YIELD TOPICS

Pediatrics

319

immature lymphoblasts, most of which express the common ALL antigen (CALLA). Lactate dehydrogenase (LDH) and uric acid levels are often elevated. A bone marrow biopsy establishes the diagnosis, and flow cytometry identifies the predominant cell type. A workup for metastases includes CXR, LP, and CT scan.

Treatment. Chemotherapy is the treatment of choice, with 85% of children achieving long-term survival. Induction therapy (with three to four drugs), consolidation therapy (with intrathecal chemotherapy with or without cranial irradiation), and maintenance therapy are used for this purpose. Bone marrow transplant can be used for relapses. It is common to see fever in patients who are neutropenic from chemotherapy. Such patients must be assessed for invasive bacterial disease and treated with IV antibiotics.

WILMS' TUMOR (NEPHROBLASTOMA)

Wilms' tumor is a renal tumor of embryonal origin and is the most common renal tumor in children. It is usually seen between the ages of one and four years and is associated with a family history, Beckwith-Wiedemann syndrome (hemihypertrophy, macroglossia, visceromegaly, and embryonal tumors), Denys-Drash syndrome (nephropathy and genital abnormalities), **WAGR** syndrome (**W**ilms', **A**niridia, **G**enitourinary abnormalities, and mental **R**etardation), and neurofibromatosis. A small number of tumors are bilateral.

Signs and Symptoms. Patients may present with complaints of nausea, emesis, bone pain, weight loss, dysuria, and polyuria. Common findings include a painless abdominal/ flank mass (80%), fever, hematuria, and hypertension.

Differential and Workup. Neuroblastoma, polycystic kidneys, hydronephrosis, and other abdominal neoplasms must be excluded. Abdominal ultrasound or CT will show a solid intrarenal mass. CBC, liver function tests (LFTs), and BUN/creatinine can help assess the extent of disease. Since metastases may be present at the time of diagnosis, the workup should include a CXR and/or a chest CT.

Treatment. Treatment involves abdominal exploration with tumor excision and nephrectomy. Postsurgical chemotherapy is with vincristine and dactinomycin. Flank irradiation is sometimes used. The prognosis depends on tumor staging and histology but is generally good.

NEUROBLASTOMA

Neuroblastoma is the most common malignant tumor of infancy.

Neuroblastoma is a tumor of the neural crest cells that make up the adrenal medulla and sympathetic nervous system. It is the most common malignant tumor of infants and most often presents in children under age five. There are familial cases in addition to associations with neurofibromatosis, Hirschsprung's disease, Beckwith-Wiedemann syndrome, and fetal hydantoin syndrome.

Signs and Symptoms. Symptoms depend on the location of the tumor and may include abdominal distention, anorexia, weight loss, and malaise. Neuromuscular symptoms may arise if the tumor is located in the retroperitoneal sympathetic ganglia. Examination may reveal a firm, smooth, nontender abdominal mass as well as hypertension, fever, pallor, and periorbital bruising ("raccoon eyes"). Metastases to the liver, bone, and lymph nodes can result in hepatosplenomegaly, leg swelling, bone pain, or lymphadenopathy. Skin rash, watery diarrhea, and opsoclonus/myoclonus ("dancing eyes/dancing feet") may also be present.

Differential and Workup. Other tumors must be ruled out, including Wilms' tumor, Ewing's sarcoma, rhabdomyosarcoma, and lymphoma. Workup includes CT of the abdomen, chest, and pelvis; a bone scan and bone marrow aspirate; LP; and a 24-hour urine collection for catecholamines (vanillylmandelic acid [VMA] and homovanillic acid [HVA]). Other tests include CBC, LFTs, a coagulation panel, and BUN/creatinine. Staging of the tumor requires cytogenetic analysis for N-myc amplification and evaluation of biopsy specimens.

Treatment. Localized tumors are cured with excision, and some children require no other treatment. More severe disease may require preoperative combination chemotherapy and adjunctive radiation. The prognosis is excellent in stage 1 disease and in a subtype of neuroblastoma that occurs in infants under one year of age.

Immunology

JUVENILE RHEUMATOID ARTHRITIS

Juvenile rheumatoid arthritis (JRA) is a collagen vascular disease that is defined by persistent inflammation in more than one joint for longer than six weeks in a patient under 16 years of age. Onset is most common in children between the ages of one and three. JRA is divided into three types on the basis of clinical symptomatology. Although the nomenclature and classification of JRA are currently under revision, traditional categories are used here.

Signs and Symptoms
- **Pauciarticular** is the most common form of JRA and is characterized by the involvement of four or fewer joints.
  - Adolescents may have involvement of large and small joints and are almost uniformly rheumatoid factor (RF) and antinuclear antibody (ANA) negative.
  - Younger children have involvement of large joints, and young females are more likely to be ANA positive.
  - Chronic asymptomatic uveitis can lead to blindness in young children if not diagnosed by slit-lamp examination; acute-onset uveitis is more common in older children.
  - The prognosis is generally good.
- **Polyarticular** is the second most common form of JRA and is characterized by the involvement of five or more joints.
  - The small joints of the hands and feet are commonly involved.

- Girls are affected more often than boys.
- Systemic illness is common and includes fatigue, anorexia, and fever.
- RF seropositivity is associated with older age of onset, positive ANA, and more severe disease.

- **Systemic** is the least common form of JRA and is known as Still's disease.
  - Arthritis may be present after onset of systemic symptoms and is typically unremitting and severe.
  - Boys and girls are equally affected.
  - A key feature is weeks of high, spiking fevers to > 39.4°C accompanied by an evanescent "salmon-colored" rash that comes and goes with fever.
  - Other symptoms include myalgias, pericarditis, pleuritis, lymphadenopathy, and growth retardation.
  - Patients often have anemia of chronic disease, an elevated WBC, and elevated acute-phase reactants.
  - RF and ANA are negative.
  - Systemic disease carries the worst prognosis.

Systemic JRA is the least common and has the worst prognosis.

Differential and Workup. The differential includes Lyme disease and seronegative spondyloarthropathies (for the pauciarticular type), and rheumatic fever, systemic lupus erythematosus (SLE), occult infection, and malignancy (for the systemic type). The utility of serologies for RF and ANA depend on the category of JRA. X-ray changes may be minimal but can show osteopenia, joint space narrowing, or erosions. MRI is more sensitive for early joint changes.

Treatment. Most cases respond to NSAIDs (aspirin should be avoided because of the risk of Reye syndrome). Methotrexate may be given for more severe disease, and etanercept (Enbrel) has recently been used for refractory polyarticular disease. Systemic steroids are used only for severe systemic disease or severe uveitis. Steroid eye drops and dilating agents are administered for most cases of uveitis. Stretching or a morning bath can be used for morning stiffness. Sufficient calcium intake and weight-bearing exercises are important to prevent osteoporosis. Physical therapy may be used to prevent disability.

KAWASAKI DISEASE (MUCOCUTANEOUS LYMPH NODE SYNDROME)

Kawasaki disease is a multisystem vasculitis that was first described in Japan but has now been diagnosed worldwide. It mainly affects infants and children under age five. The etiology is unknown.

Signs and Symptoms. The disease is divided into three phases. The acute phase lasts approximately ten days and is characterized by high fevers, bilateral nonpurulent conjunctivitis, a rash on the trunk and extremities, cervical lymphadenopathy (> 1.5 cm), inflammation of the oral mucosa, and extremity edema (see the mnemonic "CRASH"). Irritability and aseptic meningitis are also common. The subacute phase lasts ten days and is characterized by a decrease in fever, onset of arthritis, and painless skin desquamation on the hands

Kawasaki disease—

CRASH

Conjunctivitis (bilateral, nonpurulent)

Rash (primarily truncal, evanescent)

Adenopathy (cervical, at least one node > 1.5 cm)

Strawberry tongue, lip fissures, oropharyngeal erythema

Hands and feet (early induration, then desquamation)

Diagnostic criteria:

Fever > 104°F for > 5 days, unresponsive to antibiotics
AND
any 4 of the above criteria

322

and feet by day 14. Thrombocytosis and elevated acute-phase reactants are also present. The convalescent phase begins around day 21 and is characterized by coronary aneurysms on echocardiography. Arthritis and thrombocytosis may persist, and MIs or aneurysm ruptures may occur.

Differential. The differential is broad and includes enterovirus infections, scarlet fever, staphylococcal scalded-skin syndrome, Stevens-Johnson syndrome, leptospirosis, Epstein-Barr virus, JRA, measles, polyarteritis nodosa, Rocky Mountain spotted fever, drug reaction, toxic shock syndrome, and adenovirus.

Workup. Diagnosis is clinical. Tests to order include CBC with platelets, erythrocyte sedimentation rate (ESR), LFTs, blood culture and sensitivity (to rule out infection), and antistreptolysin O (ASO) titer and throat culture for group A streptococcal infection. In the subacute phase, platelet count, ESR, and C-reactive protein (CRP) will be elevated. Echocardiography is used to assess for coronary aneurysms.

Treatment. Treatment consists of the following:

- **Acute phase:** High doses of aspirin (100 mg/kg/day) are given for their anti-inflammatory effect and to treat fever. Intravenous immunoglobulin (IVIG, 2 g/kg) is administered to reduce coronary aneurysm formation. Prednisone is currently contraindicated owing to prior studies that showed worsened disease, although this issue is controversial.
- **Subacute phase:** Low doses of aspirin (3–10 mg/kg/day) are instituted for their antiplatelet effect starting around day 14 until echocardiography is normal (at around six to eight weeks).
- **Convalescent phase:** Evaluate patients one week after discharge and repeat echocardiography at six weeks, six months, and 12 months.

Complications. Serious complications include peripheral aneurysms, coronary artery aneurysms, coronary artery thrombosis, CHF, and death. MI causes death in 0.5% of patients in the early stages of disease. Myocarditis is very common. Hydrops of the gallbladder is a rare complication.

IMMUNODEFICIENCIES

Congenital immunodeficiency disorders are rare, occurring with an overall frequency of 1/10,000. Of these disorders, B-cell deficiencies are the most common and tend to present with recurrent sinopulmonary infections and infections with encapsulated organisms (*S. pneumoniae, H. influenzae*) and *Staphylococcus*. Infections occur after the age of six months, when transplacentally acquired maternal antibodies decline. T-cell deficiencies present with fungal, viral, and intracellular bacterial infections, often between the ages of one and three months, and can cause secondary B-cell dysfunction. Phagocyte deficiencies present with infections of the mucous membranes and poor wound healing. Infections with catalase-positive (*S. aureus* and *Serratia marcescens*) and enteric gram-negative organisms are common. Delayed postnatal umbilical cord separation can be an early sign of these deficiencies. Some common immunodeficiency disorders are listed in Table 6.9.

TABLE 6.9. Pediatric Immunodeficiency Disorders.

Disorder	Description	Treatment
B-cell		
X-linked agammaglobulinemia (Bruton's)	A profound B-cell deficiency found only in males. May present earlier than six months. Characterized by recurrent sinusitis, pneumonia, meningitis, and *Pseudomonas* infections.	Overall treatment is with prophylactic antibiotics. IVIG may also be used in X-linked and combined variable disease.
Common variable immunodeficiency	Initially, children are normal. Immunoglobulin levels drop in the second or third decade of life. Patients have recurrent UTIs, chronic diarrhea, and increased risk of autoimmune disease.	
IgA deficiency	This is the most common immunodeficiency and is often asymptomatic. Patients may have sinopulmonary infections.	
T-cell		
DiGeorge syndrome	**CATCH 22 = C**ardiac anomalies, **A**bnormal facies, **T**hymic hypoplasia, **C**left palate, **H**ypocalcemia, and a deletion on chromosome **22.** Agenesis of the third and fourth pharyngeal pouches causes this syndrome along with severe combined immunodeficiency (SCID).	Severe disease is treated with bone marrow transplant. IVIG can be used for antibody deficiency.
Ataxia-telangiectasia	Cutaneous and conjunctival telangiectasias and cerebellar ataxia with decreased T-cell function and antibody levels. This is a DNA repair defect.	
Combined		
SCID	Patients have a severe lack of B and T cells. They present with frequent, severe bacterial infections, chronic candidiasis, and opportunistic organisms. Eczema can occur as a result of graft-versus-host disease.	Bone marrow or stem cell transplant and IVIG for humoral deficiency.
Wiskott-Aldrich syndrome	X-linked disorder with less severe combined B- and T-cell dysfunction. Patients have thrombocytopenia, eczema, elevated IgE and IgA, and decreased IgM.	
Phagocytic		
Chronic granulomatous disease	An X-linked disorder affecting males only. Deficient superoxide production by neutrophils and macrophages results in chronic bronchitis, GI infection, UTIs, osteomyelitis, and hepatitis. Lymphadenopathy, anemia, and hypergammaglobulinemia may also be present. Diagnosis is made with the nitroblue tetrazolium test.	Treat with antibiotics and surgical debridement of wounds.
Chédiak-Higashi syndrome	An autosomal-recessive disorder causing a defect in neutrophil chemotaxis. The syndrome includes oculocutaneous albinism, neuropathy, and neutropenia.	

TABLE 6.9 (continued). Pediatric Immunodeficiency Disorders.

Disorder	Description	Treatment
Complement		
C1 esterase deficiency (hereditary angioneurotic edema)	An autosomal-dominant disorder with recurrent episodes of angioedema lasting 24 to 72 hours and provoked by stress, trauma, or anxiety. Can result in life-threatening airway edema.	Patients can take daily prophylactic danazol. Purified C1 esterase and fresh frozen plasma (FFP) are available for use prior to surgery.
Terminal complement deficiency (C5–9)	Patients are susceptible to recurrent meningococcal or gonococcal infections and, rarely, SLE or glomerulonephritis.	Meningococcal vaccine and appropriate antibiotics.

Infectious Disease

FEVER MANAGEMENT

The management of a young child with fever depends on the age group of the child. Children are divided into three groups for this purpose: under 28 days, 28 to 90 days, and 3 to 36 months. During your weeks on the pediatric ward, you will be admitting many febrile children. Be thankful that new management guidelines have decreased the number of hospitalizations for fever. To further your understanding of these new guidelines, a few definitions must be explained.

- Fever is defined as a rectal temperature > 38°C (> 100.4°F).
- If one is to diagnose fever without a source, the etiology of the fever must not be evident after a careful H&P. Otitis media is usually not considered a sufficient source.
- "Toxic appearing" describes a clinical picture that includes lethargy, signs of poor perfusion, marked hypoventilation or hyperventilation, and cyanosis.
- "Lethargy" describes an altered level of consciousness characterized by poor or absent eye contact or failure of the child to recognize the parents or to interact with the environment.
- Low-risk criteria include a previously healthy term infant who is non–toxic appearing, has no sign of focal bacterial infection (other than otitis media), has a reliable home environment and follow-up care, and has a negative lab evaluation, including a WBC 5–15,000/mm^3, a total band count < 1500/mm^3, a normal UA (negative dipstick or < 10 WBCs/hpf), a cerebrospinal fluid (CSF) WBC < 10/mm^3, and, if diarrhea is present, < 5 WBCs/hpf.

Management of a febrile infant under 28 days of age. All febrile children under 28 days of age need to be hospitalized to rule out invasive bacterial disease. A complete sepsis evaluation includes cultures of CSF, blood, and urine;

All toxic-appearing children must be hospitalized for antibiotics and a full workup for sepsis.

a CBC with differential; electrolytes, glucose, and BUN/creatinine; CSF analysis for Gram stain, cells, glucose, and protein; a CXR; and a UA. An appropriate parenteral antibiotic regimen must be started while awaiting culture results; one popular choice is ampicillin and gentamicin or cefotaxime. Alternatively, if the infant is categorized as low risk, a full sepsis evaluation is performed and the infant is monitored closely in the hospital without antibiotics while awaiting laboratory results. Herpes simplex virus (HSV) infection should also be considered and should be investigated in the history.

Management of a febrile infant 28 to 90 days of age without a source. All infants at this age who appear toxic need to be hospitalized, given a full workup for sepsis, and started on parenteral antibiotics. For non-toxic-appearing low-risk infants, outpatient management is adequate. There are two options that can be used to approach this problem:

Option 1	Option 2
CBC/blood culture	UA/urine culture
UA/urine culture	Careful observation
LP/CSF culture	If evaluation is normal and low risk, no
Ceftriaxone 50–75 mg/kg IM	antibiotics necessary
Reevaluate in 24 hours	Reevaluate in 24 hours

Management of a febrile child 3 to 36 months old without a source. The risk of bacteremia (mainly *S. pneumoniae*) in this age group is small (1–3%). Again, however, all infants who appear toxic need to be hospitalized, given a complete workup for sepsis, and started on parenteral antibiotics. If the child does not appear toxic and the temperature is < 39.0°C, no diagnostic tests or antibiotics are necessary. The parents should be instructed to give the child acetaminophen 15 mg/kg/4 hours and to return to the office if the fever persists for more than 48 hours or if the clinical condition deteriorates.

A non-toxic-appearing child with a temperature > 39.0°C needs the following:

- A CBC with manual differential.
- For an absolute band count > 1500, a neutrophil count > 10,000/μL, or a WBC > 15,000, a blood culture and empiric ceftriaxone 50 mg/kg IM.
- A catheterized urine culture for males under six months or females under two years of age.
- A stool culture if there is evidence of blood or mucus in the stool or > 5 WBCs/hpf.
- A CXR in children with dyspnea, tachypnea, rales, oxygen saturation < 95%, or decreased breath sounds.
- Acetaminophen 15 mg/kg/4 hours.
- Reevaluation in 24 hours.
- Children who have a positive blood culture and who are still febrile on reevaluation need to have an LP.

MENINGITIS

Meningitis is an inflammation of the leptomeninges that is typically caused by viruses, bacteria, or fungi. Viruses causing meningoencephalitis include enteroviruses, mumps, measles, HSV, VZV, arbovirus, Epstein-Barr virus, rabies, and adenovirus. The most common bacterial pathogens vary with age group (see Table 6.10).

A prompt LP is essential in any patient with possible CNS infection.

Signs and Symptoms. See Table 6.11 for meningitis signs and symptoms according to age.

Differential. The differential diagnosis of meningitis (bacterial and aseptic) includes brain abscess, epidural or subdural empyema, mastoiditis, tumors, cysts, trauma, vasculitis, cysticercosis, Lyme disease, leptospirosis, rickettsial diseases, viral meningitis (enterovirus and arboviruses are the most common), and tuberculous or fungal meningitis.

TABLE 6.10. Common Bacterial Causes and Empiric Therapy for Meningitis.

Age	Potential Bacterial Pathogens	Risk Factors	Treatment	Duration
Neonate (less than one month)	*Streptococcus agalactiae* (group B streptococcus [GBS]) *Escherichia coli* *Listeria monocytogenes* HSV	Maternal exposure, prematurity, obstetric complications	Ampicillin (200 mg/kg) and cefotaxime (100–150 mg/kg) Add acyclovir for suspected HSV.	14–21 days for GBS or *Listeria* Over two weeks after CSF sterilization for gram-negative enteric meningitis
Infant (one to three months)	*S. pneumoniae* *Neisseria meningitidis* *S. agalactiae* *E. coli*	Combined risk factors from younger and older age groups	Cefotaxime (200 mg/kg) or ceftriaxone (100 mg/kg) and ampicillin (200 mg/kg) For *S. pneumoniae*, add vancomycin (40–60 mg/kg).	7–10 days for uncomplicated Hib or *N. meningitidis*. 10–14 days for *S. pneumoniae*
Children (three months– 18 years)	*S. pneumoniae* *N. meningitidis*	Complement defect, unimmunized status, asplenia, complication of skull fracture	Cefotaxime (200 mg/kg) or ceftriaxone (100 mg/kg) For *S. pneumoniae*, add vancomycin (40–60 mg/kg).	7–10 days for uncomplicated Hib or *N. meningitidis* 10–14 days for *S. pneumoniae*

TABLE 6.11. Age-Related Signs and Symptoms of Meningitis.

Age	Symptoms	Early Signs	Late Signs
0–3 months	Paradoxical irritation (irritable when held and less irritable when not held), altered sleep pattern, respiratory distress, vomiting, poor feeding, diarrhea, seizures	Lethargy, irritability, temperature instability	Bulging fontanelle, shock
4–24 months	Altered sleep pattern, lethargy, seizures	Fever, irritability	Nuchal rigidity (after 18 months), coma, shock
more than 24 months	Headache, stiff neck, lethargy, photophobia, myalgia, seizures	Fever, nuchal rigidity, irritability, Kernig's sign, Brudzinski's sign[a, b]	Coma, shock

[a]Kernig's sign = flexion of the hip to 90° with subsequent pain on extension of the leg.
[b]Brudzinski's sign = involuntary flexion of the knees and hips following flexion of the neck while supine.

In aseptic meningitis, many patients feel better after the LP.

Workup

- A CT or MRI will help narrow the differential but is not routinely ordered in cases of meningitis. Get a CT before the LP if there are signs of increased intracranial pressure (ICP) such as focal neurologic findings or papilledema.
- CSF should be sent for a cell count with differential, glucose, protein, Gram stain, and culture. The CSF composition in acute meningitis depends on the etiology of the meningitis (see Table 6.12).
- Blood should be drawn for CBC, electrolytes, glucose, and culture. WBC counts are nonspecific and often unremarkable in aseptic meningitis. For bacterial meningitis, the WBC is usually elevated.
- An EEG may be helpful in patients who present with seizures. Often, the changes are nonspecific and are characterized by generalized slowing. Focal slowing in the temporal area is characteristic of HSV infections.

Treatment. The therapy for meningitis consists of antibiotics and supportive care. The initial choice of antimicrobial is based on the most likely organisms involved given the patient's age group (see Table 6.10). Once the organism has been identified, the antibiotics can be adjusted.

The supportive care of meningitis includes the following:

- Strict fluid balance (owing to the risk of SIADH [syndrome of inappropriate antidiuretic hormone]). Rehydrate with isotonic solution until euvolemic; then switch to 2/3 maintenance fluids.
- Frequent urine-specific gravity assessment.
- Daily weights and daily measurement of head circumference in babies.
- Neurologic assessment.
- Seizure precautions.

TABLE 6.12. CSF Findings in Meningitis.

Component	Normal	Bacterial	Herpes	Viral	Tuberculous
Glucose (mg/dL)	40–80	< 30	> 30	> 30	20–40
Protein (mg/dL)	20–50	> 100	> 75	50–100	100–500[c]
Leukocytes/μL	0–6	> 1000[a]	10–1000	100–500[b]	10–500[d]
Neutrophils (%)	0	> 50	< 50	< 20	< 20
Erythrocytes/μL	0–2	0–10	10–500	0–2	0–2

[a]Mainly PMNs.
[b]Mainly monocytes.
[c]May be higher (500–4000) in the presence of hydrocephalus and obstruction.
[d]PMNs early, with subsequent shift to lymphocyte/monocyte predominance.

- Management of acute complications.
- Isolation until the causative organism has been identified.

Complications. The acute complications of bacterial meningitis include shock, seizures, subdural effusions (common with Hib infection), SIADH, subdural empyema, cerebral edema, ventriculitis, and abscess. Long-term sequelae include deafness, seizure disorder, learning disabilities, blindness, paresis, ataxia, and hydrocephalus. Acute treatment with dexamethasone before or at the time of antibiotic administration may improve neurologic outcome in Hib meningitis but is not indicated in other causes of meningitis.

OTITIS MEDIA

Acute otitis media (AOM) is a suppurative infection of the middle ear cavity. Children are more susceptible to infection owing to the angle of entry and short length of the eustachian tube. Up to 75% of children will have at least three episodes by the age of two. Common pathogens include *S. pneumoniae*, *H. influenzae*, *Moraxella catarrhalis*, and viruses such as influenza A, respiratory syncytial virus (RSV), and parainfluenza virus (PIV). Conditions that predispose children to AOM include viral URIs, passive exposure to tobacco smoke, day care, immunodeficiency, trisomy 21, hypothyroidism, and cleft palate. Breast-feeding reduces the incidence of AOM.

Acute otitis media is an extremely common outpatient diagnosis.

Signs and Symptoms. The presenting symptoms are ear pain, fever, crying, irritability, difficulty sleeping, difficulty feeding, vomiting, and diarrhea. Young children may tug on their ears. The classic physical findings are erythema, opacity, decreased mobility (tested with an insufflator bulb), altered landmarks, and bulging or retraction of the affected tympanic membrane. Erythema alone is not sufficient for diagnosis, as it may result from vigorous crying.

Differential. The differential diagnosis includes otitis externa, mastoiditis, foreign body in the ear, ear trauma, hard cerumen, mumps, toothache, pharyngitis, nasal congestion, and temporomandibular joint dysfunction.

Workup. Diagnosis is based on the physical exam and presenting complaints. Cerumen removal and pneumatic otoscopy must be performed to prevent overdiagnosis of AOM. Tympanocentesis should be attempted in children with multiple episodes of AOM.

Treatment. Most cases resolve spontaneously, but because of the risk of complications, most clinicians treat AOM with antibiotics. The drug of choice for the treatment of otitis media is amoxicillin 40–45 mg/kg/day in two or three divided doses for five to ten days. Children at particular risk for resistant bacteria (e.g., those in day care at under two years of age or those with recent antibiotic exposure) should receive higher doses of amoxicillin (80–100 mg/kg/day for 10 days). For children who fail amoxicillin, other acceptable therapies include amoxicillin/clavulanate (Augmentin), cefuroxime acetil, and parenteral ceftriaxone. Children with more than three infections in six months or four in one year should be considered for referral to an ENT specialist. Persistent infection may warrant tympanostomy tube placement or myringotomy. Topical antipyrine/benzocaine (Auralgan) otic solution can be given to reduce pain.

Complications. Complications include hearing loss, tympanic membrane perforation, scarring (tympanosclerosis), cholesteatoma, chronic otitis media, and mastoiditis.

PNEUMONIA

Viruses are the number-one cause of pneumonia in children.

Pneumonia can be defined as inflammation of the lung parenchyma. It may be classified according to etiologic agent, patient age, host reaction, and anatomic distribution (e.g., lobar, interstitial, bronchopneumonia). Risk factors include anatomic malformations, immunodeficiencies, chronic lung disease secondary to prematurity, and exposure to cigarette smoke. The most common cause of pediatric pneumonia is viral infection (RSV, influenza, PIV, adenovirus). *S. pneumoniae* is the most common bacterial agent. In neonates, GBS and *Listeria* are potential agents. Infants between one and three months may present with *Chlamydia trachomatis* pneumonia, while older children and teenagers are susceptible to *Mycoplasma* and *Chlamydia pneumoniae* infections.

Signs and Symptoms. Common signs and symptoms are tachypnea, cough, shortness of breath, malaise, fever, chest pain, and retractions. However, overall patterns of presentation may vary with the etiologic agent.

- **Viral pneumonia:** Viral infections often present with cough, wheezing or stridor, and low-grade fever. On physical exam, diffuse crackles and wheezes are typical. CXR usually shows diffuse and streaky infiltrates, and the WBC count may be normal or increased with a lymphoctye predominance.
- **Bacterial pneumonia:** Bacterial infections are often more fulminant, presenting with high fever, cough, chills, and dyspnea. Physical exam findings may include focal crackles, decreased breath sounds, dullness to

percussion, and egophony. On CXR, lobar consolidation is common, and the WBC count often shows leukocytosis and neutrophilia.

Presenting symptoms will also differ with age group:

- **Newborns:** Patients usually present with signs of respiratory distress, including tachypnea, cyanosis, nasal flaring, grunting, and retractions. They may also show signs of systemic infection, including poor perfusion, hypotension, acidosis, leukopenia or leukocytosis, and nonspecific signs such as poor feeding, irritability, and lethargy.
- **Young children:** Patients may present with nonspecific complaints such as abdominal pain, fever, malaise, GI symptoms, restlessness, apprehension, and chills. Respiratory signs such as tachypnea, cough, grunting, and nasal flaring may be subtle, and even with a productive cough, children rarely expectorate.
- **Older children:** Patients may present with mild upper respiratory tract symptoms such as cough and rhinitis followed by abrupt fever, chills, tachypnea, chest pain, and productive cough. Adolescents with *Mycoplasma* infections may present with prolonged cough in the absence of fever.

Differential. The differential includes the full spectrum of infectious organisms ranging from viruses to parasites, as well as gastric aspiration, foreign body aspiration, atelectasis, congenital malformation, bronchopulmonary dysplasia, CHF, neoplasm, chronic interstitial lung disease, collagen vascular disease, and pulmonary infarct.

Workup. The diagnosis is usually made on the basis of history and clinical findings, as sputum is difficult to obtain from children. It is important to obtain a CXR in ill-appearing infants and children, patients who need hospitalization, and those who worsen clinically on antibiotics. Pulse oximetry is a useful measure of oxygenation. Helpful laboratory tests include the following:

- CBC for WBC, which is often > 15,000/mL in bacterial pneumonia. A WBC count of < 5000/mL in the newborn period may indicate sepsis.
- Blood culture, which will be positive in < 20% of patients with bacterial pneumonia.
- Viral nasal wash or nasal swab.

Treatment. The treatment of pneumonia should be based on age, clinical and radiographic findings, immune status, and Gram stain of sputum, tracheobronchial secretions, or pleural fluid if available. See Table 6.13 for empiric antibiotic therapy by age group. Criteria for hospitalization include all children under two months of age, or children over two months of age with respiratory distress, hypoxia, inability to take oral medications, failure to respond to oral antibiotics, immunosuppression, underlying cardiopulmonary disease, or evidence of empyema on CXR. Hospitalized children should be treated with IV antibiotics until afebrile and then given oral antibiotics to complete a total of seven to ten days of treatment.

TABLE 6.13. Common Etiologies and Empiric Therapy for Pneumonia.

Age	Organisms	Empiric Coverage
Infants under 6 weeks	GBS, C. *trachomatis*, S. *aureus*, RSV, CMV, HSV, enterovirus	Ampicillin and gentamicin OR Ampicillin and cefotaxime. Add PO erythromycin for suspected C. *trachomatis*. Add IV acyclovir for suspected HSV.
6 weeks–6 months	RSV, S. *pneumoniae*, Hib, group A streptococcus, C. *trachomatis* (until three months of age), S. *aureus*	Supportive care for suspected viral pneumonia. Mild to moderate illness: PO amoxicillin or cefuroxime. Severe illness: IV cefuroxime or ceftriaxone.
6 months to school age	RSV (until two years of age), PIV, influenza virus, adenovirus, S. *pneumoniae*	Supportive care for suspected viral pneumonia. Mild to moderate illness: PO amoxicillin or cefuroxime. Severe illness: IV cefuroxime or ceftriaxone.
School age	*Mycoplasma pneumoniae*, S. *pneumoniae*, adenovirus	Mild to moderate illness: PO erythromycin or clarithromycin if *Mycoplasma* is suspected. Severe illness: IV cefuroxime or ceftriaxone with a macrolide. Vancomycin may be added after 24 to 48 hours if the child has not improved and there is suspicion of drug-resistant S. *pneumoniae*.

Complications. The most common complication is pleural effusion, which can be treated with pleurocentesis and a chest tube. Empyema and lung abscess are also potential complications.

STREPTOCOCCAL PHARYNGITIS

Bacterial pharyngitis in a pediatric population is most commonly caused by group A β-hemolytic streptococcal (*Streptococcus pyogenes*) infection. Streptococcal pharyngitis is important to identify and treat because of its potential complications, which are categorized as suppurative (peritonsillar and retropharyngeal abscesses) and nonsuppurative (acute rheumatic fever, post-infectious glomerulonephritis). Treatment can prevent all the complications except post-infectious glomerulonephritis. Acute rheumatic fever can occur two to six weeks after untreated pharyngitis.

Patients with "strep throat" don't have cough, rhinorrhea, or itchy, watery eyes.

Signs and Symptoms. Patients complain of sore throat, fever, headache, and malaise. Symptoms that are conspicuous in their absence are cough, rhinorrhea, and itchy, watery eyes. Tender anterior cervical lymphadenopathy is found on exam. Tonsils are enlarged and hyperemic with exudates, the pharynx is erythematous, and palatal petechiae may be present. Scarlet fever may be diagnosed in the presence of an erythematous "sandpaper" rash.

Differential and Workup. Viral pharyngitis is often difficult to distinguish from bacterial pharyngitis on a clinical basis. A positive throat culture or streptococcal antigen detection test ("rapid strep test") is diagnostic.

Treatment. Patients with a positive test for streptococcal infection should be treated with PO penicillin VK for ten days or azithromycin for five days to prevent rheumatic fever. Empiric therapy is sometimes initiated (after a culture has been sent) if there is a high index of suspicion for streptococcal infection.

Complications

- **Post-infectious glomerulonephritis:** Onset may follow pharyngitis or skin infections within one to two weeks. Antibiotic treatment is not preventive, but the disease is typically self-limited and does not recur. Signs include hematuria, proteinuria, decreased urination, hypertension, pulmonary edema, and peripheral edema.
- **Acute rheumatic fever (ARF):** ARF is an immune reaction that may arise two to six weeks after untreated streptococcal pharyngitis. Diagnosis is made using the Jones criteria, which can be remembered by the mnemonic "J♥NES". Major manifestations include:
  - Migratory polyarthritis involving more than two joints
  - Active carditis evidenced by a new murmur (mitral or aortic insufficiency or Carey Coombs murmur), pericarditis, or symptoms of CHF
  - Nontender subcutaneous nodules over the joints, scalp, or spine
  - Erythema marginatum, a circinate erythematous maculopapular rash on the trunk and extremities
  - Chorea characterized by emotional instability and involuntary movements

Treatment involves penicillin, anti-inflammatory medications, and supportive therapy. Owing to the high rate of recurrence, indefinite daily prophylactic penicillin should be started.

URINARY TRACT INFECTION

Urine should be sterile. The simple definition of UTI is growth of an abnormal number of bacterial colonies from the urine. UTI can be classified as lower (cystitis) or upper (pyelonephritis). Organisms usually infect the urinary tract from below except in neonates, where they can also reach the urinary tract via hematogenous spread. During the newborn period, the incidence of UTI is slightly higher in males; during childhood, it becomes ten times more common in females. The predominant organisms responsible for UTI are *E. coli, Proteus, Klebsiella, Staphylococcus saprophyticus* (especially in adolescent females), and the enteric streptococci. Risk factors include vesicoureteral reflux, obstructive uropathy, renal calculi, bladder dysfunction, and intermittent catheterization. Infection in a small child should make you consider the possibility of abnormal anatomy.

Jones criteria for ARF—

J♥NES (major criteria)
Joints
♥ Pancarditis
Nodules
Erythema marginatum
Sydenham's chorea

Minor criteria:
Fever, arthralgias, prior rheumatic fever, leukocytosis, elevated ESR/CRP, prolonged PR interval.

Diagnosis:
Two major or one major and two minor criteria PLUS evidence of recent streptococcal disease (scarlet fever, positive culture or increased ASO titer).

UTI pathogens—

SEEKS PP
S. saprophyticus
E. coli
Enterobacter
Klebsiella
Serratia
Proteus
Pseudomonas

Signs and Symptoms. The signs and symptoms of a UTI in the pediatric population are often different from those in the adult population (see Table 6.14). Upper UTIs are more likely to produce constitutional symptoms such as fever, chills, flank pain, nausea, vomiting, costovertebral tenderness (flank pain), and dehydration.

Differential and Workup. Although a UA can suggest a UTI, definitive diagnosis requires a positive urine culture. A urine sample may be obtained as a clean-catch midstream specimen or via catheter or suprapubic aspiration. The method employed depends on the age of the child and on the clinical suspicion of infection. Criteria for a positive culture differ according to the method used to obtain the sample. A culture is positive if:

- More than 10^5 colonies/mL are obtained from a midstream clean-catch sample.
- More than 10^4 colonies/mL are obtained from an intermittent ("in and out") catheterization sample.
- Any colonies are obtained from a suprapubic tap sample.

If diphtheroid bacilli, *Staphylococcus*, or multiple organisms are present in the sample, suspect contamination and repeat the urine culture. Finally, any toxic-appearing child should have blood cultures, CBC with differential, electrolytes, and BUN/creatinine to rule out pyelonephritis and sepsis.

Treatment. Empiric antibiotic treatment is begun while awaiting sensitivity results. Uncomplicated cystitis in children can be treated with a single agent such as cephalexin or trimethoprim-sulfamethoxazole (TMP-SMX) for five to ten days. In neonates, toxic-appearing patients, or children with suspected pyelonephritis, IV antibiotics (e.g., ampicillin plus gentamicin or cefuroxime) are indicated. Neonates automatically receive 10 to 14 days of parenteral antibiotics. Once older patients have clinically improved and are afebrile, switch to oral antibiotics to complete a 14-day course. A repeat urine culture is performed 48 hours after therapy begins (or after the patient is afebrile) to ensure adequate treatment.

TABLE 6.14. Signs and Symptoms of UTI.

Newborns	Infants	Preschool	School age
Fever	Fever	Fever	Fever/chills
Hypothermia	Irritability	Enuresis	Enuresis
Poor feeding	Poor feeding	Dysuria	Dysuria
Vomiting	FTT	Urgency	Urgency
Jaundice	Diarrhea	Urinary frequency	Urinary frequency
FTT		Abdominal pain	Costovertebral
Sepsis		Vomiting	tenderness
Apnea			Hematuria
Diarrhea			

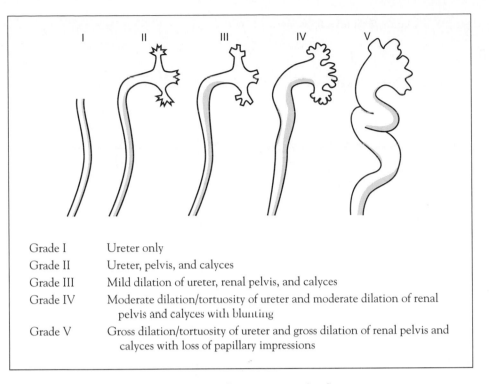

Grade I	Ureter only
Grade II	Ureter, pelvis, and calyces
Grade III	Mild dilation of ureter, renal pelvis, and calyces
Grade IV	Moderate dilation/tortuosity of ureter and moderate dilation of renal pelvis and calyces with blunting
Grade V	Gross dilation/tortuosity of ureter and gross dilation of renal pelvis and calyces with loss of papillary impressions

FIGURE 6.2. International classification of vesicoureteral reflux.

Indications for further workup with renal ultrasound (to evaluate the urinary tract anatomy) and a voiding cystourethrogram (VCUG) (to evaluate reflux) include all boys with a UTI, all girls under age five, and prepubertal girls under age ten. Prophylactic therapy is indicated in the following situations:

- Prior to undergoing a VCUG
- Reflux of any grade (grades I–V) in infancy and early childhood (see Figure 6.2)
- Reflux of grades III–V in children over five years of age
- More than three UTIs per year

Neonatology

APGAR SCORE

The Apgar score is an objective method for evaluating the need to resuscitate a newborn, and it is determined at one and five minutes after birth. However, assessment of the infant should begin immediately at birth, and the Apgar score alone should not be used to determine when to initiate resuscitation. In general, scores of 8–10 indicate no need for resuscitation. Scores of 4–7 indicate a potential need for resuscitation, and infants should be carefully observed, stimulated, and given ventilatory support as needed. Scores of 0–3 indicate severe distress and the need for immediate resuscitation (see Table 6.15).

> **APGAR—**
>
> **A**ppearance (color)
> **P**ulse (heart rate)
> **G**rimace (reflex irritability)
> **A**ctivity (muscle tone)
> **R**espiratory effort

TABLE 6.15. Apgar Score.

	0	1	2
Color	Blue, pale	Body pink, extremities blue	Body and extremities pink
Heart rate	Absent	< 100/min	> 100/min
Reflex irritability	No response	Grimace	Cough or sneeze
Muscle tone	Limp	Some extremity flexion	Full extremity flexion
Respiratory effort	Absent	Weak cry	Strong cry

CONGENITAL INFECTIONS

Infections acquired in utero or in the perinatal period are commonly referred to by the acronym **TORCHeS.** This includes **T**oxoplasmosis, **O**ther (including HIV, hepatitis B and C, parvovirus, *Borrelia burgdorferi*, and VZV), **R**ubella, **C**ytomegalovirus (CMV), **H**SV, and **S**yphilis. Clinical findings common to many of these infections are intrauterine growth restriction, anemia and thrombocytopenia, hepatosplenomegaly, hydrops fetalis, jaundice, and chorioretinitis. Each infection also has distinctive clinical signs and symptoms, which are listed in Table 6.16.

NEONATAL HYPERBILIRUBINEMIA

Conjugated hyperbilirubinemia is always pathologic.

Hyperbilirubinemia is a condition defined by excessive concentration of bilirubin in the blood. Unconjugated (indirect) hyperbilirubinemia can be of physiologic or pathologic origin. Conjugated (direct) hyperbilirubinemia is always of pathologic origin.

Signs and Symptoms. Babies will develop visible jaundice at 5–10 mg/dL (higher levels than in adults). Jaundice typically follows a cephalopedal progression as concentration increases, although the physical exam is notoriously inaccurate for estimating the bilirubin levels.

Differential. The differential includes the following:
- **Unconjugated:** Physiologic jaundice, breast-milk jaundice, hemolysis (blood group incompatibility, infection), internal bleeding, polycythemia, infant of a diabetic mother, defective clearance of bilirubin from the blood, defective bilirubin conjugation in the liver (Crigler-Najjar, Gilbert syndromes), and other rare causes. Features of physiologic versus pathologic jaundice are discussed in Table 6.17.
- **Conjugated:** TORCHeS infections, metabolic disorders, bacterial sepsis, obstructive jaundice, prolonged administration of total parenteral nutrition (TPN), and neonatal hepatitis.

Workup. The workup should be guided by the type of hyperbilirubinemia and other clinical information. The workup of unconjugated hyperbilirubine-

TABLE 6.16. TORCHeS Infections.

Infection	Epidemiology	Clinical Features
Toxoplasma gondii	Maternal exposure to cat feces or poorly cooked meat. Fetal disease with primary infection only. Highest risk of exposure at 10–24 weeks' gestation.	Hydrocephalus, microcephaly, severe mental retardation, epilepsy, diffuse intracranial calcifications. Infants may be asymptomatic at birth. Treatment: pyrimethamine + sulfadiazine.
HIV	Most mothers are asymptomatic with a high-risk history: prostitution, drug abuse, hemophilia.	Recurrent infections, hepatosplenomegaly, neurologic abnormalities, FTT. 10–25% develop AIDS symptoms between three and six months, depending on the use of perinatal anti-retrovirals. Prevention: maternal pre/intra/postpartum AZT; avoid breast-feeding. Treatment: TMP-SMX, AZT, and other agents.
VZV	First-trimester maternal chickenpox infection. Infections that develop within one week before or after delivery are associated with severe disseminated disease.	Microphthalmia, cataracts, cutaneous and bony abnormalities. Risk of zoster as an older child. Prevention: varicella-zoster immune globulin, or VZIG (after exposure to VZV). Treatment: acyclovir.
Rubella virus	Non-rubella-immune mother. Fever and rash in mother. Highest transmission risk in first trimester (80%). Virus may persist in infant's oropharynx for one year.	Microcephaly, cataracts, glaucoma, microphthalmia, "salt-and-pepper" chorioretinitis, "blueberry muffin" rash, B- and T-cell deficiencies, deafness, PDA, ASD, VSD. Infants may be asymptomatic at birth. No treatment; vaccine preventable.
CMV	Most common congenital infection. Sexually transmitted. Primary infection has worst outcome, but reinfection can produce disease. Infant may shed virus in urine for one to six years.	Sepsis, periventricular calcifications, microcephaly, pneumonia, deafness, severe mental retardation. Infants may be asymptomatic at birth with late neurologic sequelae. Prevention: CMV-negative blood products. Treatment: possible ganciclovir.

TABLE 6.16 (continued). TORCHeS Infections.

Infection	Epidemiology	Clinical Features
HSV	Sexually transmitted. Primary infection may be asymptomatic. In utero infection rare; common transmission at time of delivery; C-section for active lesions.	Intrauterine: skin lesions, microcephaly, chorioretinitis. Postnatal: encephalitis, keratoconjunctivitis, seizures, pneumonia, skin vesicles, hepatitis, and disseminated disease. Treatment: acyclovir.
Syphilis (*Treponema pallidum*)	Sexually transmitted. In utero infection usually after first trimester. Penicillin (but not erythromycin) prevents fetal infection.	Early: jaundice, hemolytic anemia, prematurity, hepatitis, pneumonia, rash, saddle nose, keratitis, snuffles, osteochondritis, condylomata lata, CSF pleocytosis. Late: Hutchinson's teeth, mulberry molars, saber shins, frontal bossing. Diagnosis: RPR/VDRL and fluorescent treponemal antibody (FTA) serologies in mother. Treatment: procaine penicillin G for 10 to 14 days.

mia may include indirect and direct bilirubin levels, blood typing, Coombs' test, CBC, blood smear, and reticulocyte count. The workup of conjugated hyperbilirubinemia may include LFTs, bacterial and viral cultures, metabolic screening tests, hepatic ultrasound, and a sweat chloride test.

Treatment. Phototherapy is initiated in term infants at bilirubin levels of approximately 15–20 mg/dL, depending on the infant's age and the cause of hyperbilirubinemia. Premature infants are more susceptible to kernicterus, so phototherapy is initiated at lower levels, which are determined by birth weight. Exchange transfusions may be used for bilirubin levels > 20 mg/dL if phototherapy fails. Skin bronzing may be seen after phototherapy in infants with direct hyperbilirubinemia.

KEY POINT

BREAST-MILK VERSUS BREAST-FEEDING JAUNDICE

Breast-milk jaundice is a syndrome of prolonged unconjugated hyperbilirubinemia that is thought to be due to an inhibitor of bilirubin conjugation in the breast milk of some mothers. It is an extension of physiologic jaundice, peaks at 10 to 15 days of age, and declines slowly by 3 to 12 weeks of age. Breast-feeding jaundice is attributed to poor feeding or inadequate breast-milk supply and increased enterohepatic circulation of bilirubin. It usually occurs during the first week of life and resolves when enteral intake improves. Treatment involves evaluating the breast-feeding pair and encouraging more feeding.

TABLE 6.17. Differentiating Physiologic and Pathologic Jaundice.

Physiologic Jaundice	Pathologic Jaundice
Not present until 72 hours after birth.	Present in the first 24 hours of life.
Bilirubin increases < 5 mg/dL/day.	Bilirubin increases > 0.5 mg/dL/hour.
Bilirubin peaks at < 14–15 mg/dL.	Bilirubin rises to > 15 mg/dL in formula-fed term and preterm infants. Bilirubin can rise to > 17 mg/dL in breast-fed or full-term infants.
Direct bilirubin < 10% of total.	Direct bilirubin > 10% of total.
Jaundice resolves by one week in term infants and two weeks in preterm infants.	Jaundice persists beyond one week in term infants and two weeks in preterm infants.

Complications. The primary concern with unconjugated hyperbilirubinemia is the development of kernicterus (bilirubin encephalopathy). Unconjugated bilirubin is fat soluble and, when it exceeds the binding capacity of albumin, can deposit in brain cells to cause permanent neurologic damage. The basal ganglia are particularly affected. Kernicterus typically occurs at levels > 20–25 mg/dL but can occur at lower levels in the presence of factors such as prematurity, asphyxia, hemolysis, and sepsis. Infants who survive the initial insult often develop a neurologic syndrome characterized by seizures, mental retardation, chorioathetoid movements, deafness, and decreased upward movement of the eyes.

Premature infants are more susceptible to kernicterus.

RESPIRATORY DISTRESS SYNDROME

Respiratory distress syndrome (RDS) is the most common form of respiratory failure in preterm infants. It results from a deficiency of surfactant, which causes poor lung compliance, atelectasis, and hyaline membrane formation in the alveoli. Risk factors include maternal diabetes, hypothermia, asphyxia, and prematurity. RDS is seen in 65% of infants born at 29 to 30 weeks' gestation.

Signs and Symptoms. Patients present with tachypnea (respiratory rate > 60), progressive hypoxemia, cyanosis, nasal flaring, intercostal retractions, and grunting in the first 24 to 72 hours of life.

Differential and Workup. The differential includes transient tachypnea of the newborn (TTN), meconium aspiration syndrome, congenital pneumonia, spontaneous pneumothorax, diaphragmatic hernia, and cyanotic heart disease. Typical patterns seen on CXR include the following:

- **RDS:** Bilateral atelectasis leads to a "ground glass" appearance and air bronchograms. Severe RDS may present as "white out" or an airless lung.
- **TTN:** Retained amniotic fluid leads to perihilar streaking in the interlobular fissures.
- **Meconium aspiration:** Coarse, irregular infiltrates, hyperexpansion, and pneumothoraces are seen.

■ **Congenital pneumonia:** CXR findings are not specific. Gram stain, WBC, and tracheal aspirate suggest the diagnosis.

Treatment

■ Intubation and ventilation (conventional, high-frequency, or oscillator) may be required to maintain oxygenation.
■ Surfactant replacement therapy decreases mortality.
■ Supportive care in a NICU is required.
■ RDS can be avoided by preventing premature birth or by pretreating at-risk mothers with corticosteroids.
■ Fetal lung maturity can be monitored in utero with the amniotic fluid lecithin-to-sphingomyelin ratio and the presence of phosphatidylglycerol (PG).

Complications. Complications include a persistent PDA, development of bronchopulmonary dysplasia (BPD), pulmonary air leaks (pneumothorax, interstitial emphysema), and retinopathy of prematurity (due to oxygen toxicity).

Neurology

FEBRILE SEIZURES

Febrile seizures are seizures that occur in association with fever. They generally occur in children between the ages of six months and six years with an incidence of 3–4%.

Signs and Symptoms. Febrile seizures are associated with a rapid rise in temperature. They generally occur when the temperature reaches 39°C or higher but may also occur at lower temperatures. Febrile seizures are classified as simple or complex (see Table 6.18).

Workup. When taking the history, it is important to ask the parents to describe the nature of the seizure (focal vs. generalized), its duration (keep in mind that parents often overestimate duration), the number of seizures, the postictal state, events preceding the seizure, history of previous seizure, family history of febrile and afebrile seizure, history of trauma or ingestions, and the child's neurologic development and medication exposure.

During the physical exam, pay special attention to rectal temperature, vital signs, mental status, nuchal rigidity (note that this is valid only for children

TABLE 6.18. Febrile Seizures.

Simple Febrile Seizure	Complex Febrile Seizure
Short duration (< 15 minutes)	Long duration (> 15 minutes)
Generalized seizure	Focal seizure
One seizure in a 24-hour period	More than one seizure in a 24-hour period

over 18 months), fullness of the fontanelle, and abnormalities or focal differences in muscle strength and tone. The following laboratory tests are helpful:

- In younger children (under 12 months), a workup for sepsis should be performed, including CBC/blood culture, CSF culture, and UA/urine culture.
- An LP is necessary if CNS infection is suspected in children over one year.
- A serum glucose determination by Dextrostix is indicated in all seizure patients.
- A head CT is indicated only if CNS disease is suspected.
- An EEG should be considered for complex febrile seizures.

Treatment. The therapy for simple febrile seizures consists of antipyretics and appropriate treatment of any underlying illness. Reassurance and parental education about febrile seizures are essential. Thermometer use and antipyretic dosing should be reviewed.

Diazepam per rectum may be used to stop a prolonged seizure. For children with complex febrile seizures, daily prophylactic therapy may be necessary with phenobarbital or valproic acid. However, these treatments have significant side effects and are infrequently used in the treatment of complex febrile seizures. Anticonvulsants have no role in the prophylaxis of simple febrile seizures.

Complications. Approximately 30% of children will have a recurrent febrile seizure, with a higher recurrence rate found in children under one year of age. The majority of recurrent seizures take place within one year of the initial episode. For simple febrile seizures, there is no increased risk of developmental, intellectual, or growth abnormalities, and the risk of developing epilepsy, at 1%, is no greater than that of the general population. The risk of developing epilepsy is higher if there is a neurologic or developmental abnormality, a complex seizure, an abnormal neurologic exam, or a family history of epilepsy.

Orthopedics

LIMP

Disturbances in gait are common in children and may present with a limp or refusal to bear weight. A painful limp is typically acute in onset and may be accompanied by fever and irritability. A painless limp is usually slow in onset and may be associated with weakness or limb deformity. The causes of limp are listed in Table 6.19 and can be remembered with the mnemonic "STARTS HOTT."

PEDIATRIC FRACTURES

A number of fracture types are specific to pediatrics. Torus fractures involve "buckling" of the cortex with compression of the bone. Greenstick fractures

Simple febrile seizures carry a better prognosis.

Table 6.19. Causes of Pediatric Limp.

Septic arthritis	Most common cause of painful limp in a one- to three-year-old; usually monoarticular (hip, knee, ankle).
	Agents: *S. aureus* (most common), group A streptococcus, *Neisseria gonorrhoeae* (in sexually active teenagers).
	Acute onset of pain, fever, warmth, swelling, reduced joint mobility, leukocytosis, increased ESR.
	X-ray: joint space widening.
	Joint aspiration shows turbid fluid with low glucose, WBC > 10,000 with neutrophilia.
	Treatment: drainage and antibiotics.
Transient synovitis	Most common in three- to eight-year-old males; may follow a viral URI.
	Acute onset of pain, limp, and reduced joint mobility in hip. Afebrile or low-grade fever; no tenderness, warmth, or joint swelling; normal WBC and ESR. Can be difficult to differentiate from septic arthritis.
	X-ray: normal; ultrasound may show effusion.
	Treatment: bed rest and NSAIDs.
Aseptic vascular necrosis	Legg-Calvé-Perthes disease (LCPD)—femoral head; Köhler's disease—navicular bone; Sever's disease—calcaneus.
	LCPD occurs in four- to nine-year-old boys after interrupted blood supply to the femoral head; may be bilateral.
	Painless limp or pain in inner thigh, restricted motion, short stature, muscle spasm. Afebrile, normal WBC and ESR.
	X-ray (anterior-posterior [AP] and frog-leg lateral): sclerosis of femoral head, widened femoral neck.
	Treatment: surgical or cast containment of femoral head to prevent deformity and osteoarthritis.
Rheumatoid arthritis (juvenile)	See discussion of JRA.
Trauma	Obtain from history.
Slipped capital femoral epiphysis	Often seen in obese male adolescents or children in their growth spurts; may be bilateral; mostly gradual onset and progressive.
	Dull pain referred to thigh or knee; worse with activity.
	X-ray (AP and frog-leg lateral): widened physis, posterior and medial displacement of the femoral head relative to the femoral neck (Klein's line).
	Treatment: pinning and cast immobilization.
Henoch-Schönlein purpura	Vasculitis in four- to ten-year-old children.
	Asymmetric migratory periarticular swelling, palpable purpura on buttocks and legs, and abdominal pain. Complications include GI bleeding, intussusception (monitor for stool occult blood), and glomerulonephritis (monitor for hematuria/proteinuria).
	Treatment: self-limiting disease; treat symptoms (NSAIDs for arthralgias) and complications (steroids for intestinal and CNS complications).

Table 6.19 (continued). Causes of Pediatric Limp.

Osteomyelitis	Most common in three to twelve-year-old boys; results from hematogenous (younger children) or direct spread.
	Agents: *S. aureus* (most common); neonates are at risk for GBS, *E. coli*, and anaerobic organisms; children are at risk for *Streptococcus, Pseudomonas* (foot puncture wounds in tennis shoes), *Pasteurella multocida* (dog and cat bites), and *Salmonella* (sickle cell patients).
	Young infants may have fever only; children may have fever, localized pain, decreased mobility, erythema, and edema.
	X-ray: normal for one to two weeks.
	Diagnosis: neutrophilic leukocytosis, elevated ESR, positive blood culture (approximately 50% are positive), bone scan, and MRI (gold standard).
	Treatment: IV and PO antibiotics for a total of four to six weeks.
Tumor	Must rule out malignant pediatric bone tumors.
	Ewing's sarcoma: small, round blue-cell tumor found in femur and pelvis with early metastases.
	X-ray: "onion-skin" appearance.
	Treatment: chemotherapy; highly sensitive to radiation.
	Osteogenic sarcoma: seen in adolescent boys more often than girls; often metastasizes to the lung. Located in the distal femur, proximal tibia, and proximal humerus; presents with pain, palpable mass.
	X-ray: Codman's triangle (periosteal elevation) and "sunburst sign" (calcification in soft tissues).
	Treatment: surgical and adjuvant chemotherapy.
Tuberculosis	Skeletal TB results from hematogenous or direct spread from lymph nodes. Affects vertebrae (Pott's disease), hips, fingers, and toes.
	Diagnosis: biopsy and culture of affected bone.
	X-ray: destruction of cortex.
	Treatment: four-drug regimen for two months; then two-drug regimen for seven to ten months (depends on local sensitivities).

are incomplete fractures involving disruption of the cortex on one side of the bone. Bowing occurs when a bone receives angular stress but the cortex does not break. Epiphyseal fractures involve the growth plate and are classified into five groups by the Salter-Harris system, which predicts the prognosis for a given fracture (see Figure 6.3).

Pulmonology

ASTHMA (REACTIVE AIRWAY DISEASE)

Asthma is a bronchial disorder characterized by inflammation, reversible smooth muscle constriction, and mucus production. This leads to airway obstruction and difficulty breathing. It is the most common chronic condition of childhood.

Signs and Symptoms. Asthma may present suddenly or gradually. Cases that present gradually are often associated with respiratory tract infection,

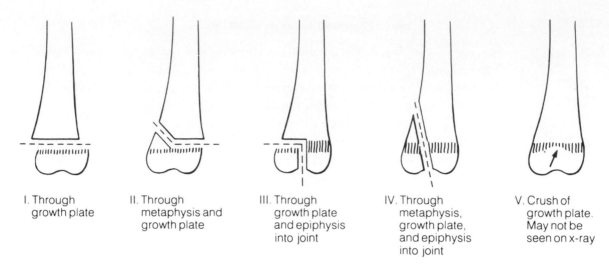

I. Through growth plate

II. Through metaphysis and growth plate

III. Through growth plate and epiphysis into joint

IV. Through metaphysis, growth plate, and epiphysis into joint

V. Crush of growth plate. May not be seen on x-ray

FIGURE 6.3. Salter-Harris classification of epiphyseal fractures.

Ask about the allergic triad: asthma, atopic dermatitis, and allergic rhinitis.

whereas those with an acute onset are associated with allergens. Patients or parents may report chest congestion, persistent or nighttime cough, exercise intolerance, dyspnea, recurrent bronchitis, pneumonia, irritability, or feeding difficulties in younger children. Keep in mind that asthma can occur without overt wheezing. Key asthma triggers include airway irritants (cigarettes, air pollution, ozone), allergies (pollens, dust mites, pets, cockroaches), exercise, cold weather, respiratory infections, drugs (aspirin, beta blockers), stress, foods, and food additives. Try to elicit a history of past severity, frequency of attacks, ER visits, hospitalizations, ICU admissions, courses of steroids per year, and number of school days missed as a result of asthma. Don't forget to ask about family history of asthma, allergies, and atopic disease. Associated conditions such as GERD and sinusitis can also make asthma worse.

Signs of asthma include wheezing, coughing, tachypnea, tachycardia, prolonged expiration, hyperresonance, intercostal and subcostal retraction, and nasal flaring. Patients may be unable to speak in full sentences owing to shortness of breath. Cyanosis, diminished breath sounds (due to poor air exchange), absence of wheezing, use of accessory muscles, and increasingly labored breathing should all raise red flags in your mind.

Differential. The differential diagnosis of asthma includes aspiration, foreign body, bronchiolitis, bronchopulmonary dysplasia, cystic fibrosis, GERD, vascular rings, acute bronchopulmonary aspergillosis, and pneumonia.

Workup. The diagnosis of asthma is based on an appropriate H&P and on pulmonary function studies demonstrating decreased vital capacity, increased functional residual capacity, increased residual volume, and reversal of pulmonary abnormalities by inhalation of aerosolized albuterol. CXR findings are often nonspecific, but may include hyperinflation. Helpful laboratory tests include:

- Spirometry demonstrating decreased one-second forced expiratory volume (FEV$_1$) and peak expiratory flow rate (PEF) in children six years or older
- Pulse oximetry
- Arterial blood gases (ABGs) demonstrating hypoxia and respiratory acidosis during acute exacerbations
- WBC count demonstrating eosinophilia
- CXR showing bilateral hyperinflation

Key indicators of asthma severity:

1. Frequent ER visits
2. History of intubation
3. Hospitalizations
4. Steroid use

BEWARE OF ASTHMA WITHOUT WHEEZING

During an asthma exacerbation, wheezes may actually be absent on lung exam. For wheezes to be produced, air must be moving through the lungs. In patients with a severe exacerbation, air movement may be so limited that wheezes are not heard. Once bronchodilator treatment is initiated and air movement increases, wheezes may appear, indicating clinical improvement. Conversely, the disappearance of wheezes is also important to note. While this may signal resolution of an exacerbation, it can also be an ominous sign that the patient's ability to move air through the lungs is decreasing. This exam finding indicates the need for more aggressive treatment.

KEY POINT

Treatment. A suggested algorithm for the emergent management of asthma is outlined in Figure 6.4. For pharmacologic treatment, the method of delivering medications will depend on the age of the child. For example, children under one year of age will often require nebulized medication. Children between one and four years of age may use a spacer with a face mask, and children over four years of age can use a metered dose inhaler (MDI) with a spacer.

- **Acute therapy:** Bronchodilators are the drug of choice in an acute attack (nebulized albuterol 0.15 mg/kg in 2–3 cc normal saline or MDI two puffs q 1–6 hours prn) as well as systemic steroids such as PO prednisone or IV methylprednisolone (Solu-Medrol). Treatment with corticosteroids for fewer than ten days does not require tapering.
- **Chronic therapy:** Educate patients to avoid allergens and triggers and to monitor peak flow each morning. Inhaled corticosteroids or cromolyn sodium (Intal), a mast-cell stabilizer, should be used for prevention. Leukotriene receptor antagonists may be added as another preventive measure.

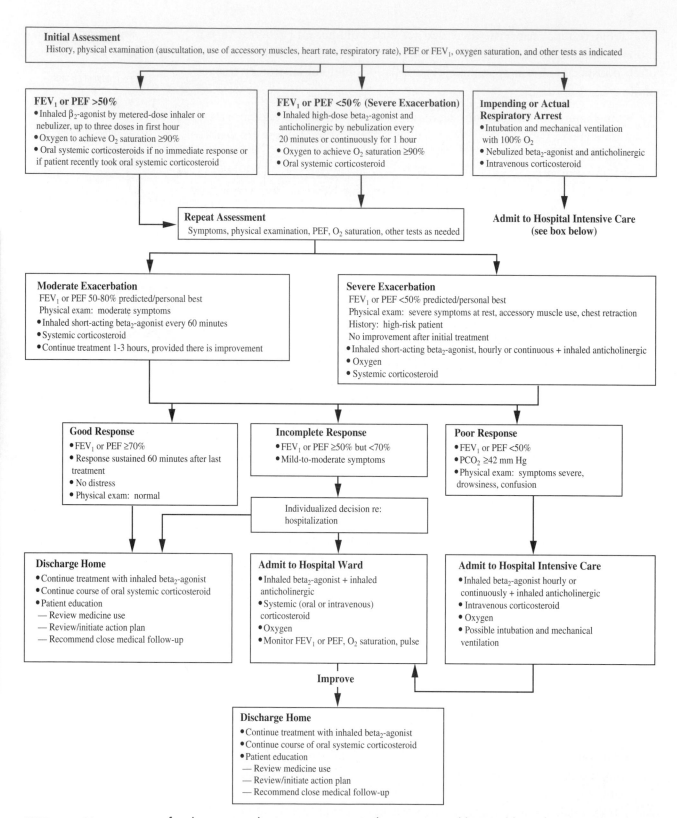

Initial Assessment
History, physical examination (auscultation, use of accessory muscles, heart rate, respiratory rate), PEF or FEV_1, oxygen saturation, and other tests as indicated

FEV_1 or PEF >50%
• Inhaled β_2-agonist by metered-dose inhaler or nebulizer, up to three doses in first hour
• Oxygen to achieve O_2 saturation ≥90%
• Oral systemic corticosteroids if no immediate response or if patient recently took oral systemic corticosteroid

FEV_1 or PEF <50% (Severe Exacerbation)
• Inhaled high-dose beta$_2$-agonist and anticholinergic by nebulization every 20 minutes or continuously for 1 hour
• Oxygen to achieve O_2 saturation ≥90%
• Oral systemic corticosteroid

Impending or Actual Respiratory Arrest
• Intubation and mechanical ventilation with 100% O_2
• Nebulized beta$_2$-agonist and anticholinergic
• Intravenous corticosteroid

Repeat Assessment
Symptoms, physical examination, PEF, O_2 saturation, other tests as needed

Admit to Hospital Intensive Care (see box below)

Moderate Exacerbation
FEV_1 or PEF 50-80% predicted/personal best
Physical exam: moderate symptoms
• Inhaled short-acting beta$_2$-agonist every 60 minutes
• Systemic corticosteroid
• Continue treatment 1-3 hours, provided there is improvement

Severe Exacerbation
FEV_1 or PEF <50% predicted/personal best
Physical exam: severe symptoms at rest, accessory muscle use, chest retraction
History: high-risk patient
No improvement after initial treatment
• Inhaled short-acting beta$_2$-agonist, hourly or continuous + inhaled anticholinergic
• Oxygen
• Systemic corticosteroid

Good Response
• FEV_1 or PEF ≥70%
• Response sustained 60 minutes after last treatment
• No distress
• Physical exam: normal

Incomplete Response
• FEV_1 or PEF ≥50% but <70%
• Mild-to-moderate symptoms

Poor Response
• FEV_1 or PEF <50%
• PCO_2 ≥42 mm Hg
• Physical exam: symptoms severe, drowsiness, confusion

Individualized decision re: hospitalization

Discharge Home
• Continue treatment with inhaled beta$_2$-agonist
• Continue course of oral systemic corticosteroid
• Patient education
— Review medicine use
— Review/initiate action plan
— Recommend close medical follow-up

Admit to Hospital Ward
• Inhaled beta$_2$-agonist + inhaled anticholinergic
• Systemic (oral or intravenous) corticosteroid
• Oxygen
• Monitor FEV_1 or PEF, O_2 saturation, pulse

Admit to Hospital Intensive Care
• Inhaled beta$_2$-agonist hourly or continuously + inhaled anticholinergic
• Intravenous corticosteroid
• Oxygen
• Possible intubation and mechanical ventilation

Improve

Discharge Home
• Continue treatment with inhaled beta$_2$-agonist
• Continue course of oral systemic corticosteroid
• Patient education
— Review medicine use
— Review/initiate action plan
— Recommend close medical follow-up

FIGURE 6.4. Management of asthma exacerbations: emergency department and hospital-based care. (Reprinted with permission, from *Guidelines for the Diagnosis and Management of Asthma.* Expert Panel Report 2. NIH Publication No. 97-4051, July 1997.)

Asthma is often classified by severity for the purpose of determining appropriate treatment (see Table 6.20). It is recommended that one begin with more aggressive therapy and then use a "stepdown" approach to treatment.

BRONCHIOLITIS

Bronchiolitis is an acute inflammatory illness of the small airways in children under the age of three. RSV is the primary agent, although PIV, adenovirus, influenza, and rhinovirus have also been implicated. Most cases occur in late fall to early spring.

TABLE 6.20. Classification of Asthma Severity.

	Symptoms	Nights with Symptoms	PEF or FEV$_1$ (% of Predicted)	Maintenance Medications[a]
Step 4: Severe persistent	Continual symptoms Limited physical activity Frequent exacerbations	Frequent	≤ 60%	Daily inhaled high-dose corticosteroids AND Long-acting bronchodilator AND PO steroids 2 mg/kg/day
Step 3: Moderate persistent	Daily symptoms Two or more exacerbations/week Exacerbations limit activity	More than one time/week	> 60 – < 80%	Medium-dose inhaled corticosteroids OR Low- to medium-dose inhaled steroid and long-acting bronchodilator; if needed, medium- to high-dose inhaled steroid and long-acting bronchodilator
Step 2: Mild persistent	Symptoms more than two times/week but less than one time/day. Exacerbations may affect activity	More than two times/month	≥ 80%	Low-dose inhaled steroid or cromolyn (or nedocromil). Zafirlukast or zileuton can be considered in children > 12 years.
Step 1: Mild intermittent	Symptoms fewer than two times/week, brief Asymptomatic between exacerbations	Less than two times/month	≥ 80%	No daily medication needed.

[a]All patients should use a short-acting bronchodilator (β_2 agonist) as needed for symptoms.

Signs and Symptoms. Patients often have rhinorrhea, sneezing, cough, and low-grade fever followed a few days later by tachypnea and wheezing. Examination may reveal signs of respiratory distress such as nasal flaring, rales, retractions, intermittent cyanosis, prolonged expiration, and diffuse wheezing. Apnea may be the presenting symptom in premature or young infants.

All that wheezes is not asthma.

Differential. The differential for wheezing includes asthma, pneumonia, heart failure, laryngomalacia, foreign body aspiration, GERD, and cystic fibrosis.

Workup. In addition to the H&P, CXR may reveal air trapping, peribronchial thickening, atelectasis, and infiltrates. The WBC count is typically normal. RSV can be identified in nasopharyngeal washes by direct fluorescent antigen (DFA) testing or culture.

Treatment. Mild cases can be treated at home with supportive measures such as oral hydration and antipyretics. Indications for hospitalization include marked respiratory distress (a resting respiratory rate of 50–60/min), hypoxemia, apnea, inability to tolerate oral feeding, chronic cardiopulmonary disease, or an unreliable home environment. Hospitalized children should be given supplemental oxygen and should be kept in contact isolation. Bronchodilators (beta agonists or racemic epinephrine) may be effective in some patients. Ribavirin aerosol has been shown to be mildly effective in severely affected or high-risk children. In the event of respiratory failure, intubation and mechanical ventilation may be necessary.

CROUP

Listen for a seal-like bark in croup.

Viral croup (laryngotracheobronchitis) is an acute inflammatory disease of the larynx, trachea, and bronchioles that especially affects the subglottic space (see Figure 6.5). Parainfluenza virus types 1 and 2 are the most common cause; other organisms include RSV, influenza virus, rubeola virus, adenovirus, and *M. pneumoniae*.

Signs and Symptoms. The clinical features of croup include low-grade fever, mild respiratory distress, stridor that worsens with agitation, a hoarse voice, and the characteristic barking cough resembling that of a dog or a seal (usually at night). The child prefers sitting upright, held by a parent in a calm, quiet atmosphere. Parents may note clinical improvement on the way to the hospital from the cool, crisp evening air.

Differential. A number of conditions may present with similar clinical features. These conditions include epiglottitis, foreign body aspiration, bacterial tracheitis, angioneurotic edema, and retropharyngeal abscess (see Table 6.21).

Croup has the "steeple sign."

Workup. The diagnosis is primarily clinical. Diminished breath sounds, restlessness, altered mental status, or cyanosis may indicate hypoxia. The PA radiograph will show subglottic narrowing, often referred to as the "steeple sign." The WBC is not very helpful, and the blood draw may actually worsen respiratory distress.

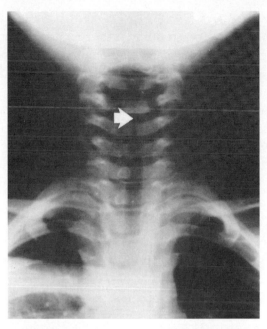

FIGURE 6.5. Croup. (Reprinted, with permission, from Saunders C. *Current Emergency Diagnosis & Treatment,* 4th ed. Stamford, CT: Appleton & Lange, 1992:448.)

TABLE 6.21. Characteristics of Croup, Epiglottitis, and Tracheitis.

Croup	Epiglottitis	Tracheitis
Age: three months to five years	Age: two to seven years	Age: older child, but may affect any age
Usually viral etiology, commonly parainfluenza	Usually group A streptococcus, S. *aureus*, or viral etiology	Often S. *aureus*
Develops over two to three days	Rapid onset over hours	Gradual onset over two to three days, followed by acute decompensation
Usually low-grade fever	High fever	High fever
Usually only mild to moderate respiratory distress	Commonly severe respiratory distress	Commonly severe respiratory distress
Prefers sitting up, leaning against parent's chest	Prefers "tripod" position with neck extended	May have position preference
Stridor improves with aerosolized racemic epinephrine	No response to racemic epinephrine	No response to racemic epinephrine
"Steeple sign" on AP neck films	"Thumb sign" on lateral neck films	Subglottic narrowing

Treatment

- Manage mild cases (no stridor at rest) supportively at home with cool mist therapy, oral hydration, and minimal handling.
- Moderate cases with stridor at rest may require oral corticosteroids (dexamethasone).
- More severe cases (respiratory distress at rest, hypoxia) require evaluation and treatment with cool mist therapy, IV hydration (if dehydration is present), and systemic steroids (oral or parenteral).
- Nebulized racemic epinephrine (0.5 mL of a 2.25% solution diluted with 2 mL sterile water) is reserved for patients showing signs of respiratory distress.
- Patients with impending respiratory failure require intubation. Use an endotracheal tube with a slightly smaller diameter than usual.
- In patients who do not respond to standard therapy for croup (cool mist, steroids, racemic epinephrine), consider other diagnoses. In particular, watch for bacterial tracheitis.

EPIGLOTTITIS

In comparison to viral croup, epiglottitis leads to inflammation and swelling of supraglottic structures (epiglottis and arytenoids) (see Figure 6.6). Epiglottitis can rapidly progress to life-threatening airway obstruction and is considered a true medical emergency. *H. influenzae*, type b was once the primary organism. With immunization, however, other organisms are now commonly found. These include *Streptococcus pneumoniae*, Group A streptococci, *Corynebacterium diphtheriae*, *Staphylococcus*, and viral agents.

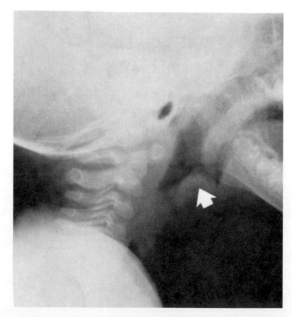

FIGURE 6.6. Epiglottitis. (Reprinted, with permission, from Saunders C. *Current Emergency Diagnosis & Treatment*, 4th ed. Stamford, CT: Appleton & Lange, 1992:47.)

Signs and Symptoms. Clinical features include sudden onset of high fever (39–40°C), dysphagia, anxiety, drooling, muffled voice, inspiratory retractions, cyanosis, and stridor. Patients sit with the neck hyperextended and the chin protruding ("sniffing dog" position) and lean forward in a "tripod" position. Respiratory arrest is possible upon progression to total airway obstruction.

Differential. See the differential diagnosis for croup.

Workup. Epiglottitis is a medical emergency and requires prompt diagnosis based on clinical suspicion. Definitive diagnosis is made by direct fiber-optic visualization of the cherry-red and swollen epiglottis and arytenoids. This procedure must be done under a controlled situation (i.e., in the OR in the presence of an anesthesiologist or ENT surgeon) in which the airway can be stabilized if needed. A lateral neck x-ray may assist in definitive diagnosis but should not delay airway stabilization. The classic x-ray finding is a swollen epiglottis obliterating the valleculae ("thumbprint sign"). The WBC count is usually elevated with a predominance of neutrophils.

Treatment. Once the diagnosis is made, intubation should be performed immediately (remember your ABCs). Next, blood cultures, a CBC with differential, and standard chemistries should be obtained. Start IV antibiotics that cover *H. influenzae* and *S. pneumoniae*, such as ceftriaxone (100 mg/kg/day).

Complications. The complications are related to the organism responsible for the disease. *H. influenzae* can result in bacteremia, pneumonia, cervical adenitis, and septic arthritis.

CYSTIC FIBROSIS

Cystic fibrosis is a multisystem autosomal-recessive disorder that results from a mutation in the cystic fibrosis transmembrane conductance regulator (CFTR) gene, which is involved in chloride conductance. It is the most common lethal genetic disease affecting Caucasians.

Signs and Symptoms. Patients present with respiratory, GI, reproductive, endocrine, and orthopedic signs and symptoms, which are outlined in Table 6.22.

Differential and Workup. The diagnosis of CF is made with a sweat chloride test result of > 60 mEq/L. Indications for performing the test are given in Table 6.22.

Treatment. Pulmonary disease is the most common cause of death (95%), so lung function must be carefully monitored with pulmonary function tests (in children over six years of age), sputum/throat cultures, and CXR. The pulmonary manifestations of CF are managed with aerosolized deoxyribonuclease (DNase), chest physiotherapy with postural drainage, bronchodilators, steroids, and antibiotics. Intermittent aerosolized tobramycin (bid for four weeks) for *Pseudomonas* has been shown to improve lung function and decrease infection. Patients are hospitalized for aggressive IV antibiotics whenever necessary.

Never use a tongue blade on a child with epiglottitis.

Epiglottitis has the "thumb print sign."

Table 6.22. Signs and Symptoms of CF.

Respiratory
- Asthma with clubbing of the digits
- Nasal polyps
- Chronic pansinusitis
- Recurrent pneumonia (especially staphylococcal)
- Chronic atelectasis, chronic pulmonary disease, pneumothorax, bronchiectasis, hemoptysis, or chronic cough
- Colonization with mucoid *Pseudomonas aeruginosa*
- X-rays showing persistent hyperaeration or atelectasis

Musculoskeletal
- Bone pain and joint effusion due to hypertrophic osteoarthropathy

Reproductive
- Infertility in men (due to obliteration of the vas deferens)
- Infertility in women (due to thick, spermicidal cervical mucus)

Genetic risk factors
- Sibling with CF
- Parent with CF

Gastrointestinal
- Meconium ileus (pathognomonic)
- Intestinal obstruction (meconium plug or recurrent intussusception)
- FTT
- Steatorrhea (foul-smelling, fatty stools) or chronic diarrhea
- Rectal prolapse
- Disaccharide intolerance or celiac disease in the differential diagnosis
- Prolonged jaundice
- Hepatic cirrhosis and portal hypertension

Miscellaneous
- Hypoproteinemia and edema
- Hypoprothrombinemia
- "Salty" taste or salt crystals on skin
- Unexplained hyponatremic-hypochloremic metabolic alkalosis
- Impaired glucose tolerance or type 1 diabetes

The GI manifestations of CF are managed with pancreatic enzyme supplements; H_2 blockers; antacids; a high-calorie, high-protein diet; and vitamin A, D, E, and K supplements.

Toxicology

LEAD POISONING

Lead toxicity is an important health issue in pediatrics. In recent decades, lead has been removed from gasoline and house paint, so most exposure comes from lead-containing paint remaining in buildings from before the 1970s. Other sources of exposure include industrial plants using lead, lead solder in pipes, lead-containing pottery (especially from Mexico and Central America), and some traditional herbal remedies. Lead poisoning requiring medical evaluation refers to levels > 20 μg/dL, but levels of 10–19 μg/dL can also be toxic. Lead levels > 70 μg/dL are considered severe and require chelation therapy.

Signs and Symptoms. Early symptoms of lead toxicity include irritability, anorexia, abdominal discomfort, vomiting, constipation, and hyperactivity or listlessness. Children may experience a decline in school performance and may have behavioral difficulties or even developmental delay. Lead encephalopathy is a more severe and acute presentation, with signs of increased ICP and risk of coma and death.

Signs include peripheral neuropathy (wrist and foot drops), Bruton's lines (purple lines on the gums), red-brown discoloration of the urine, and renal tubular acidosis. A child with pica (a desire to eat dirt) who lives in an old home with peeling paint should make you suspicious of lead poisoning.

Differential. Consider toxicity of other metals (arsenic, mercury), carbon monoxide exposure, ingestions, learning disabilities, attention-deficit hyperactivity disorder (ADHD), or medical causes of specific symptoms.

Workup. The CDC recommends screening lead levels for all children at 12 months and two years of age. If lead poisoning is suspected at any time, obtain a lead level. A peripheral blood smear may reveal basophilic stippling and a hypochromic microcytic anemia (often with concomitant iron deficiency). X-rays of bone can show lead lines.

Check lead levels at 12 and 24 months in all children.

Treatment. Patients with lead levels > 45 µg/dL should be started on succimer or, alternatively, calcium disodium EDTA. Children with levels > 70 µg/dL should be treated with EDTA and dimercaprol (BAL). Patients with encephalopathy should be managed in a pediatric ICU. Any iron deficiency should be corrected. In addition, the source of exposure must be removed, which may involve removing leaded paint and cleaning the surfaces while the inhabitants remain in a lead-free environment.

Trauma

CHILD ABUSE

Child abuse is an important medical issue, and most clinicians will encounter a case at some point in their careers. Child abuse includes physical and mental injury, sexual abuse, neglect, and, rarely, Munchausen's syndrome by proxy. Almost half of reported cases occur in children under one year of age. Children at increased risk for abuse include those with special needs or behavior problems, premature infants, and children of single, teenage, or substance-abusing parents. The presence of spousal abuse increases the risk of child abuse in the same household. Even after intervention, the abuse often continues, and the mortality rate for abused children is 5%.

Signs and Symptoms. Child abuse should be suspected when an injury is inconsistent with the description of events or when there is an unexplained delay in obtaining medical care. Signs of abuse include cuts and bruises in the pattern of an object (palm, belt buckle, bite) or those found on low-trauma areas such as the buttocks or lower back. Burn marks may be similarly distinctive and may take the form of burns on the buttocks or genitals without involvement of the hands or feet. Head injuries are the most common cause of death from abuse, and infants may present with apnea, seizures, subdural

Suspect child abuse if the story and the injuries don't match.

hematomas, retinal hemorrhages, or coma. Mandibular fractures, rib fractures, scapular fractures, and long bone spiral fractures in young children are commonly seen.

In cases of sexual abuse, there may be signs of genital trauma, sexually transmitted infections, or recurrent UTIs. Other complaints may include rectal or genital pain, discharge, or bleeding; constipation; and encopresis or enuresis. Signs and symptoms may also be subtler, such as sleeping and eating disorders, behavior and school difficulties, and sexualized behavior with peers or objects.

Neglect can result in nonorganic FTT. Signs of nutritional neglect include decreased subcutaneous fat in the cheeks, extremities, and buttocks. Neglected hygiene can result in diaper rash and impetigo, and children may have unwashed skin and clothing. Infants left on their backs can have flattening of the occiput and hair loss. Other signs include delayed social and speech development as well as behavior changes such as avoidance of eye contact, depressed affect, and absence of a cuddling response.

Workup. If abuse is suspected, children must have a skeletal survey and bone scan to check for occult and healing fractures. When appropriate, tests may be conducted to rule out medical conditions that can be confused with abuse, such as osteogenesis imperfecta (multiple fractures), bleeding disorders (bruising), and bullous skin disorders (blistering). If sexual abuse is suspected, specimens should be collected, and cultures should be taken from the mouth, rectum, and genitalia. In suspected abuse cases, laboratory and clinical studies may be conducted without parental permission. Photographs should be taken and injuries documented.

Treatment. Medical personnel are mandated to immediately report suspected abuse to state protection agencies before discharging the patient. Children may require hospitalization to stabilize injuries or for protection until an alternate placement has been secured. In order to avoid missing a case of abuse, it is essential to ask about abuse with every family.

HIGH-YIELD REFERENCES

WELL-CHILD CARE

General

Green M (ed.). *Bright Futures: Guidelines for Health Supervision of Infants, Children, and Adolescents.* Arlington, VA: National Center for Education in Maternal and Child Health, 2002. A great resource for information on well-child care.

Preventive Care

Recommendations for preventive pediatric health care. Committee on practice and Ambulatory Medicine, American Academy of Pediatrics. *Pediatrics*

2000;105:645. Available online at *http://www.aap.org/policy/re9939.html*. An outline of recommended preventive health measures throughout childhood.

Immunizations

National Immunization Program. Available online at *http://www.cdc.gov/nip*. This site contains the updated immunization schedule as well as other vaccine-related information and resources.

Growth Charts

National Center for Health Statistics: growth chart information. Available online at *http://www/cdc.gov.growthcharts*. This site contains CDC growth charts for different age groups and both genders.

CARDIOLOGY

Physical Exam

Rosenthal A. How to distinguish between innocent and pathological murmurs in childhood. *Pediatr Clin North Am* 1984;31:1229–1240. A very useful, concise discussion of the features of childhood murmurs.

Congenital Heart Disease

Saenz RB, Beebe DK, Triplett LC. Caring for infants with congenital heart disease and their families. *Am Fam Physician* 1999;59:1857–1868. A basic overview of congenital heart disease along with a discussion of medical and psychosocial treatment issues.

DERMATOLOGY

Diaper Dermatitis

Kazaks EL, Lane AT. Diaper dermatitis. *Pediatr Clin North Am* 2000;47: 909–919. A top-to-bottom review of a common outpatient topic.

Viral Exanthems

Gable EK, Liu G, Morrell DS. Pediatric exanthems. *Prim Care* 2000;27: 353–369. A good discussion of 12 major causes of viral exanthems in children.

GASTROENTEROLOGY

General

D'Agostino J. Common abdominal emergencies in children. *Emerg Med Clin North Am* 2002;20:139–153. Outlines a general approach toward abdominal pain in children and discusses common causes.

Appendicitis

Rothrock SG, Pagane J. Acute appendicitis in children: emergency department diagnosis and management. *Ann Emerg Med* 2000;36:39–51. Reviews the age-specific clinical presentation of pediatric appendicitis and outlines strategies to avoid misdiagnosis.

Failure to Thrive

Schwartz ID. Failure to thrive: an old nemesis in the new millennium. *Pediatr Rev* 2000;21:257–264. A well organized discussion of a complicated topic.

Intussusception

Harrington L et al. Ultrasonographic and clinical predictors of intussusception. *J Pediatr* 1998;132:836–839. A concise discussion of how to diagnose intussusception.

Pyloric Stenosis

Papadakis K et al. The changing presentation of pyloric stenosis. *Am J Emerg Med* 1999; 17:67–69. An interesting comparison of the presentation of pyloric stenosis over the past three decades.

GENETIC DISORDERS

General

"Online Mendelian Inheritance in Man" (OMIM™). Baltimore, MD: Johns Hopkins University. Available online at *http://www.ncbi.nlm.nih.gov/omim/*. A very useful database to help answer even the most obscure genetics questions that may arise during your rotation.

Down Syndrome

Health supervision for children with Down syndrome from the Committee on Genetics. *Pediatrics* 1994;93:855–859. Anticipatory care guidelines for children with Down syndrome, outlining preventive care measures throughout the life cycle.

HEMATOLOGY AND ONCOLOGY

Sickle Cell Disease

Wethers DL. Sickle cell disease in childhood: Part I. Laboratory diagnosis, pathophysiology, and health maintenance. *Am Fam Physician* 2000;62: 1013–1020.

Wethers DL. Sickle cell disease in childhood: Part II. Diagnosis and treatment of major complications and recent advances in treatment. *Am Fam Physician* 2000;62:1309–1314.

A comprehensive, easy-to-read, two-part series on sickle cell disease.

Childhood Cancers

Young G et al. Recognition of common childhood malignancies. *Am Fam Physician* 2000;61:2144–2154. A primary care–oriented discussion of the most common childhood cancers.

Acute Lymphoblastic Leukemia

Pui CH. Acute lymphoblastic leukemia. *Pediatr Clin North Am* 1997;44: 831–846. A review of the number one childhood cancer.

CNS Tumors

Robertson PL. Pediatric brain tumors. *Prim Care: Clin Off Prac* 1998;25:323–338. A useful discussion of brain tumors in children, including signs and symptoms by location.

Neuroblastoma

Alexander F. Neuroblastoma. *Urol Clin North Am* 2000;27:383–392. A review paper on neuroblastoma.

Wilms' Tumor

Neville HL, Ritchey ML. Wilms' tumor. Overview of National Wilms' Tumor Study Group results. *Urol Clin North Am* 2000;27:435–442. An easy-to-digest version of the recent Study Group conclusions.

IMMUNOLOGY

Juvenile Rheumatoid Arthritis

Ilowite NT. Current treatment of juvenile rheumatoid arthritis. *Pediatrics* 2002;109:109–115. A review of the state of the art in JRA.

Kawasaki Disease

Burns JC. Kawasaki disease. *Adv Pediatr* 2001;48:157–177. A good review paper on Kawasaki disease.

Shinohara M et al. Corticosteroids in the treatment of the acute phase of Kawasaki disease. *J Pediatr* 1999;135:465–469. A retrospective study evaluating the use of corticosteroids in the treatment of Kawasaki disease—a controversial topic that you will likely be asked about.

Immunodeficiencies

Woroniecka M. Office evaluation of children with recurrent infection. *Pediatr Clin North Am* 2000;47:1211–1224. Outlines a practical approach toward identifying primary and secondary immunodeficiencies on the basis of history and exam.

Laufer M, Scott GB. Medical management of HIV disease in children. *Pediatr Clin North Am* 2000;47:127–153. An overview of medical complications in children with HIV along with a pertinent discussion of ethics.

INFECTIOUS DISEASE

General

Pickering LK (ed.). *2000 Red Book: Report of the Committee on Infectious Diseases*, 25th ed. Elk Grove Village, IL: American Academy of Pediatrics, 2000. The classic resource for pediatric infectious disease information.

Fever Management

Baraff LJ. Management of fever without source in infants and children. *Ann Emerg Med* 2000;36:602–614. An update of the classic 1993 guidelines for management of fever without a source in children 0 to 36 months of age.

Meningitis

Wubbel L, McCracken GH Jr. Management of bacterial meningitis: 1998. *Pediatr Rev* 1998;19:78–84. A well organized review with recommended reading and a quiz.

Otitis Media

Bluestone CD. Clinical course, complications, and sequelae of acute otitis media. *Pediatr Infect Dis J* 2000;19:S37–S46. A good review paper on the course and outcome of AOM.

Glasziou PP et al. Antibiotics for acute otitis media in children. *Cochrane Database Syst Rev* 2000;4:CD000219. A meta-analysis of antibiotic use for pediatric AOM.

Pneumonia

McIntosh K. Community-acquired pneumonia in children. *NEJM* 2002;346:429–437. An excellent review article on a common topic.

Streptococcal Pharyngitis

Pichichero ME. Group A beta-hemolytic streptococcal infections. *Pediatr Rev* 1998;19:291–302. A well-organized review of the topic along with references and a quiz.

Urinary Tract Infection

The diagnosis, treatment, and evaluation of the initial urinary tract infection in febrile infants and young children (AC9830). Practice guideline from the American Academy of Pediatrics. *Pediatrics* 1999;103:843–852. A practice guideline from the AAP for initial UTIs in infants and children. Available online at *http://www.aap.org/policy/ac9830.htm*.

NEONATOLOGY

Apgar Score

Moster D et al. The association of Apgar score with subsequent death and cerebral palsy: a population-based study in term infants. *J Pediatr* 2001;138: 798–803. A population-based cohort study on the prognosis of infants with low Apgar scores.

Congenital Infections

Stamos JK, Rowley AH. Timely diagnosis of congenital infections. *Pediatr Clin North Am* 1994;41:1017–1033. A review article that places emphasis on differentiating the individual TORCHeS infections.

Neonatal Hyperbilirubinemia

Dennery PA, Seidman DS, Stevenson DK. Neonatal hyperbilirubinemia. *NEJM* 2001;344:581–590. A good review of a key neonatology topic.

Respiratory Distress Syndrome

Gnanaratnem J, Finer NN. Neonatal acute respiratory failure. *Curr Opin Pediatr* 2000;12:227–232. A practical review of neonatal RDS and its treatment.

Sudden Infant Death Syndrome

American Academy of Pediatrics Task Force on Infant Sleep Position and Sudden Infant Death Syndrome. Changing concepts of sudden infant death syndrome: implications for infant sleeping environment and sleep position. *Pediatrics* 2000;105:650–656. A review of the risk factors for SIDS and current recommendations for reducing risk.

NEUROLOGY

Febrile Seizures

The neurodiagnostic evaluation of the child with a first simple febrile seizure. Practice guideline from the American Academy of Pediatrics. *Pediatrics* 1996;97:770. Available online at *http://www.aap.org/policy/neuro.htm*. Practice guideline from the AAP for simple febrile seizures.

Nonfebrile Seizures

Hirtz D et al. Practice parameter: evaluating a first nonfebrile seizure in children. *Neurology* 2000;55:616–623. An approach toward evaluating a nonfebrile seizure in a child.

ORTHOPEDICS

Causes of Limp

Lawrence LL. The limping child. *Emerg Med Clin North Am* 1998;16:911–929. Outlines a thorough approach toward limp, including summaries of major causes and references for further reading.

Kocher MS, Zurankowski D, Kasser JR. Differentiating between septic arthritis and transient synovitis of the hip in children: an evidence-based clinical prediction algorithm. *J Bone Joint Surg Am* 1999;81:1662–1670. Addresses the difficulty in differentiating these two conditions; examines the evidence and provides a clinical algorithm.

Pediatric Fractures

England SP, Sundberg S. *Pediatr Clin North Am* 1996;43:991–1012. Reviews practical information regarding the initial evaluation and treatment of pediatric fractures.

PULMONOLOGY

Asthma

Emond SD, Camargo CA, Nowak RM. 1997 National Asthma Education and Prevention Program guidelines: a practical summary for emergency physicians. *Ann Emerg Med* 1998;31:579–589. A practical summary of the full 146-page practice guidelines for diagnosis and treatment of asthma. The full-text 1997 expert panel report can be viewed online at *http://www.nhlbi.nih.gov/nhlbi/lung/asthma/prof/asthgdln.htm*.

Bronchiolitis

Ngai P, Bye MR. Bronchiolitis. *Pediatr Ann* 2002;31:90–97. A good review of a common pediatric airway problem.

Croup, Epiglottitis, and Tracheitis

Stroud RH, Friedman NR. An update on inflammatory disorders of the pediatric airway: epiglottitis, croup, and tracheitis. *Am J Otolaryngol* 2001;22:268–275. A review paper that compares and contrasts three major pediatric airway disorders.

Cystic Fibrosis

Davis PB. Cystic fibrosis. *Pediatr Rev* 2001;22:257–264. A user-friendly and thorough review of the basic science and clinical aspects of cystic fibrosis.

TOXICOLOGY

Lead Poisoning

Markowitz M. Lead poisoning. *Pediatr Rev* 2000;21:327–335. An excellent and well-organized review of lead poisoning, including other suggested reading.

TRAUMA

Child Abuse

Kini N, Lazoritz S. Evaluation for possible physical or sexual abuse. *Pediatr Clin North Am* 1998;45:205–219. A review article with definitions, common injuries, and tips for the history and physical exam.

American Academy of Pediatrics Committee on Child Abuse and Neglect. Shaken baby syndrome: rotational cranial injuries—technical report. *Pediatrics* 2001;108:206–210. Discusses current knowledge about the "shaken baby syndrome."

MISCELLANEOUS

McCollough M, Sharieff GQ. Common complaints in the first 30 days of life. *Emerg Med Clin North Am* 2002;20:27–48. A concise discussion of common problems ranging from colic and constipation to altered mental status and apnea.

Clinical Handbook of Pediatrics $34.00
Schwartz

Lippincott Williams & Wilkins, 1999, 2nd edition, 975 pages, ISBN 0683304488

A spiral-bound pocket reference focusing on the diagnostic approach to a broad range of pediatric problems. Contains an extensive differential diagnosis list along with discussions of presenting symptoms, laboratory assessment, and treatment. Easy to read with good algorithms, tables, and figures. Also includes a useful chapter outlining the H&P along with many pearls.

 Practical Guide to the Care of the Pediatric Patient $39.95
Alario

Mosby, 1997, 1st edition, 830 pages, ISBN 0815101503

A spiral-bound, student-friendly pocket manual written in outline format with emphasis on high-yield clinical features, diagnostic evaluation, and management of pediatric diseases. Contains sections about the pediatric H&P, development, and routine health maintenance and preventive care. Offers more information on pathophysiology and differentials than *Harriet Lane*.

 Current Clinical Strategies: Pediatrics $9.95
Chan

Current Clinical Strategies, 2002 edition, 88 pages, ISBN 1929622082

A practical handbook detailing admit orders, specific pharmacologic treatment options, and management of common pediatric diseases. Includes useful charts on developmental milestones and immunization. Excellent value for its size and price. Will come in handy for subinterns, although a diagnosis must already be suspected in order for this book to be useful.

 Manual of Pediatric Therapeutics $39.95
Graef

Lippincott Williams & Wilkins, 1997, 6th edition, ISBN 0316141712

A relatively comprehensive spiral-bound manual that adequately covers the general principles, management, and treatment of common pediatric diseases, presented in a concise, outline format that makes good use of tables and charts. Includes brief discussions of pathophysiology, making it more appropriate for subinterns. Equivalent to the *Washington Manual* for pediatrics.

Nelson's Pocket Book Pediatric Antimicrobial Therapy, 2000–2001

$19.95

Nelson

Lippincott Williams & Wilkins, 2000, 14th edition, 140 pages, ISBN 0781725704

A specialized pediatric version of *Sanford* with a quick-reference guide to the selection and use of antimicrobials in children. Given that much of pediatrics is infectious disease, this text can serve as a good reference for students, especially subinterns. Format makes it easy to find pathogens, diseases, and recommended drugs of choice.

Pediatric Pearls: The Handbook of Practical Pediatrics

$39.95

Rosenstein

Mosby, 1997, 3rd edition, 492 pages, ISBN 0815186827

A quick-reference, easy-to-read pocket guide organized by organ system. Includes concise discussions of disease entities, treatment, and management. A useful supplement, but not a primary reference. Would benefit from more illustrations and figures.

Handbook of Pediatrics

$36.95

Merenstein

McGraw-Hill, 1996, 18th edition, 1029 pages, ISBN 0838536255

A useful handbook offering good coverage of a variety of diseases. Discusses etiology, pathophysiology, clinical findings, and treatment. Contains a limited drug formulary that is quite cumbersome, but makes excellent use of tables, charts, and algorithms. Sometimes lacking in practical wards information. May be good to read during breaks while on wards, but a bit bulky to carry around. Has not been updated in several years, so some information is out of date.

The Harriet Lane Handbook

$37.95

Siberry

Mosby, 2000, 15th edition, 1042 pages, ISBN 0323008127

The classic pocketbook designed for residents. Includes an extensive drug formulary section with pediatric dosing of common drugs. Numerous well-indexed tables and charts are interspersed throughout the text in an easy-to-read format. Roughly organized by system, including sections on pediatric subspecialties. Gives practical treatment and management information, but does not clearly discuss pathophysiology or include differential diagnoses. May be too technical for junior students, but good for subinterns and serious pediatric students.

On Call Pediatrics

$28.00

Lewis

W. B. Saunders, 2001, 2nd edition, 431 pages, ISBN 0721692230

A practical, portable guide to the pediatric problems one is likely to encounter on call. Takes a systematic approach that begins with the phone call and includes initial evaluation, differential diagnosis, workup, and initial management. Sections are well organized by common problems, but you will need to look elsewhere for more detail. Limited in breadth; cannot replace other pocket manuals in pediatrics. Not useful for beginning medical students.

TOP-RATED BOOKS

Review/Mini-Reference

 Nelson Essentials of Pediatrics $49.95

Nelson

W. B. Saunders, 2002, 4th edition, 958 pages, ISBN 0721694063

A condensed softcover version of *Nelson Textbook of Pediatrics* with concise explanations. Well organized into sections on clinical diagnosis, differential diagnosis, and treatment. Comparable to *Rudolph's Fundamentals of Pediatrics* in terms of quality. Recommend going to the bookstore and finding which style you like better, as both books are excellent texts for medical students rotating through pediatrics.

 Rudolph's Fundamentals of Pediatrics $64.95

Rudolph

McGraw-Hill, 2002, 3rd edition, 848 pages, ISBN 0838584500

An excellent, well organized, and readable softcover reference book written at an appropriate level for students on their pediatric clerkship. Includes useful algorithms summarizing approaches to common pediatric diseases. Suffices as a general home reference, but consider a more detailed textbook such as its parent book if you are going into pediatrics. A good companion book to *Rudolph's Pediatrics*.

 Blueprints in Pediatrics $34.95

Bradley

Blackwell Science, 2000, 2nd edition, 339 pages, ISBN 0632044861

A handy, concise, easy-to-read resource of high-yield information that is likely to appear on shelf and USMLE Step 2 exams. Presents an adequate amount of the basics, and includes good charts, diagrams, and key points. Not comprehensive enough to be a complete review book; some sections are too detailed while others are too simplistic. Offers a good overview of topics you are most likely to encounter while on rotation.

A⁻ Oski's Essential Pediatrics $39.95

Johnson

Lippincott Williams & Wilkins, 1997, 1st edition, 761 pages, ISBN 0397515146

Good, basic reference text organized by problem. Includes illustrations and tables. Easier to read than *Nelson* and gives a good overview of treatment and management, but lacks detail and depth. Sections vary in their coverage. Useful for the time-limited student. An interesting section at the end describes common syndromes with morphologic abnormalities, including line illustrations of distinctive facial phenotypes.

Underground Clinical Vignettes: Pediatrics $24.95

Bhushan

Blackwell Science, 2002, 2nd edition, 100 pages, ISBN 063204571X

A well-organized review of clinical vignettes commonly encountered on NBME shelf and USMLE Step 2 exams. Includes a focused, high-yield discussion of pathogenesis, epidemiology, management, and complications. Black-and-white images are included where relevant. Also contains several "mini-cases" in which only key facts related to each disease are presented. An excellent, entertaining, and easy-to-use supplement for studying during your clinical rotation. A color atlas supplement comes with the purchase of the full set of *Underground Clinical Vignettes*.

 Illustrated Textbook of Pediatrics $45.00

Lissauer

Mosby, 2001, 2nd edition, 410 pages, ISBN 0723431787

A solid, easy-to-understand textbook written at a good introductory level for medical students. Makes excellent use of numerous color photos, diagrams, case histories, and clinical tips. A good basic reference for learning and reviewing the fundamentals of pediatrics.

 Mosby's Color Atlas and Text of Pediatrics and Child Health $42.95

Chaudhry

Mosby, 2001, 1st edition, 414 pages, ISBN 0723424365

A highly visual reference with full-color photographs and radiographs throughout text. Slightly more dense with illustrations than the *Illustrated Textbook of Pediatrics*, but not as detailed in its coverage of pediatric disease manifestations, diagnosis, and treatment, making it less useful as a reference. Overall, a good book with nice images.

B **Clinical Paediatrics and Child Health** $45.00

Candy

W. B. Saunders, 2001, 1st edition, 398 pages, ISBN 0702017264

An introductory textbook designed for medical students on their pediatric clerkship. An excellent and comprehensive section is devoted to normal child development and approaching common illnesses. Also functions as a mini-encyclopedia of disorders, etiology, clinical findings, and management, although some of the diseases covered are a bit obscure. Overall, a good overview of general disease and pathophysiology, but lacking in detail of treatment and management.

TOP-RATED BOOKS

Review/Mini-Reference

B | **Lecture Notes on Paediatrics** | **$39.95**

Meadow

Blackwell Science, 2002, 7th edition, 256 pages, ISBN 0632050659

A portable review book on the core knowledge and fundamentals of pediatric disease. Offers a number of useful tables and figures. Unique sections are dedicated to describing the essentials of the pediatric clinical exam. Too superficial for practical wards use given its limited coverage of diagnostic approach and management, but useful as a supplement to other textbooks. Costly for the limited amount of material covered.

B | **Pediatric Secrets** | **$39.95**

Polin

Hanley & Belfus, 2001, 3rd edition, 729 pages, ISBN 1560534567

Presented in the question-and-answer format typical of the *Secrets* series. Organized by organ system and includes good use of tables, charts, and mnemonics. Designed to prepare students for pimping sessions, although these sessions are infrequent in pediatrics. Best used for quick self-testing during down time. Some questions are too specific and detailed. Too big to fit in coat pocket or carry around comfortably.

B | **Pediatrics** | **$37.95**

Bernstein

Lippincott Williams & Wilkins, 1996, 1st edition, 665 pages, ISBN 0683006401

An introductory softcover text geared toward junior medical students doing their pediatric clerkship. Divided into common primary care problems and pediatric subspecialty problems. Readable, although the text is a bit dry and not as comprehensive as similar texts. Some information is out of date, as the book has not been updated for several years. Few illustrations and tables.

B | **Pediatrics Recall** | **$29.95**

McGahren

Lippincott Williams & Wilkins, 2002, 2nd edition, 461 pages, ISBN 0781726115

Like *Secrets*, this book is meant for quick self-testing during your free time. Covers essential bare-bones issues of pediatric health and disease in a question-and-answer format. A bit too bulky to carry around in coat pocket.

B⁻ | **NMS Pediatrics** | **$33.00**

Dworkin

Lippincott Williams & Wilkins, 2001, 4th edition, 739 pages, ISBN 0683306375

A lengthy, detailed review book that covers most important pediatric disorders found on shelf and USMLE Step 2 exams. Although more comprehensive than *Blueprints*, its outline format is often not well organized and is occasionally too wordy. Few tables and figures are included to complement the text. Not particularly useful for management issues on the wards. Review questions are available at the end of each chapter, and a comprehensive test is included at the end of the book.

Pediatrics: A Primary Care Approach

$35.00

Berkowitz

W. B. Saunders, 2000, 2nd edition, 579 pages, ISBN 0721656234

A comprehensive review text with sections focusing on a key symptom or general disease category followed by step-by-step guidelines on diagnostic approach and treatment strategies. Case vignettes and questions relate to each disorder discussed. Readers may lose continuity in the discussion of particular diseases because of the format, which focuses only on the presenting complaint or category. Needs better use of illustrations and tables. Not applicable to exam review, but offers breadth of coverage sufficient to help one understand general pediatric issues. Specific treatment regimens must be found in another reference.

Essential Paediatrics

$47.00

Hull

Churchill Livingstone, 1999, 4th edition, 382 pages, ISBN 0443059586

A basic introductory textbook designed for medical students in their core clerkship rotation. Good tables and line illustrations are included in the margins. A bit over simplified for use on the wards, especially with respect to diagnostic approach and management.

TOP-RATED BOOKS

Review/Mini-Reference

Nelson Textbook of Pediatrics

$125.00

Behrman

W. B. Saunders, 2000, 16th edition, 2414 pages, ISBN 0721677673

An authoritative reference book that many consider the "gold standard" of pediatric textbooks. Well organized with clear explanations and comprehensive discussions on the diagnosis and treatment of pediatric disorders. Worth the investment for those pursuing pediatrics as a career; otherwise, best borrowed from the library. Great for preparing complete, detailed presentations.

Rudolph's Pediatrics

$130.00

Rudolph

McGraw-Hill, 1995, 20th edition, 2337 pages, ISBN 0838584926

A comprehensive hardcover reference book for serious pediatric students. Similar in price and scope to the *Nelson Textbook of Pediatrics*, although it may be a bit easier to read. An alternative worth considering. New edition is due in June 2002.

Current Pediatric Diagnosis and Treatment

$54.95

Hay

McGraw-Hill, 2000, 15th edition, 1272 pages, ISBN 0838516246

An up-to-date, comprehensive reference book with excellent organization of disease entities. Provides clinical information on ambulatory and inpatient medical care from birth to adolescence. Excellent use of tables, graphs, and illustrations. High-yield information is presented as essentials of diagnosis at the beginning of each section. Overall, a useful book for home reference. Easier to read than the "classic" texts, but not as detailed.

CHAPTER 7

Psychiatry

Ward Tips
High-Yield Topics
High-Yield References
Top-Rated Books

Psychiatry is the study and management of behavioral disorders. Given recent advances in the neurobiological understanding of major psychiatric disorders, as well as continuing additions to the psychiatrist's pharmacologic arsenal, many find psychiatry to be an increasingly exciting field in which to practice and conduct research. Even if you do not intend to enter psychiatry, the rotation will offer you valuable exposure to common psychiatric disorders (e.g., depression, schizophrenia, bipolar disorder, anxiety disorders, dementia, and delirium) that you will see for the rest of your career regardless of the specialty you choose.

WHAT IS THE ROTATION LIKE?

Psychiatry is more relaxed but can be emotionally intense.

In general, the psychiatry core rotation is one of the more relaxed and laid-back rotations that you will experience as a medical student. Thus, if you have the option of choosing the order in which to take your third-year medical-student core rotations, psychiatry would be a good rotation to take after surgery or OB/GYN to help you "catch your breath." On the other hand, the expectations and mechanics of this rotation are much different from those of the more conventional rotations. For example, medical students' exposure to the outpatient setting is often limited owing to the private nature of the activity. Consultation and liaison, as well as emergency crisis services, also play an important role for most psychiatric departments. Medical schools that are associated with a VA or children's hospital will allow students to focus on a unique psychiatric population, and students may rotate through any one or combination of these services.

Outpatient psychiatry encompasses a spectrum of activities ranging from one-time consultations and brief crisis intervention to medication management and long-term psychotherapy. Patients who require psychiatric hospitalization are admitted to an inpatient psychiatric service. Patients on other hospital services as well as those in the emergency room may develop or have a psychiatric illness; these services may consult psychiatry for advice.

WHO ARE THE PLAYERS?

Attending. As in every other specialty, the psychiatry attending bears ultimate responsibility for the patient. In contrast to most other specialties, however, the attending will not necessarily see all inpatients each day but will usually lead rounds. Many outpatients may never be seen by an attending at all.

Chief Resident. Each inpatient service usually has its own chief—a PGY-4 or PGY-5 who acts as a quasi-attending and who holds responsibility for the day-to-day organization of the ward, as well as for making decisions, supervising residents, and often leading rounds. Even more than is the case in other spe-

WARD TIPS

Psychiatry

cialties, your residents—especially the chief—will make or break your psychiatry rotation. A good chief will be your principal guide, teacher, judge, and jury during the rotation. Try to sit down with him or her on your first day (or even set up a meeting beforehand, if you are really interested in psychiatry) to discuss your goals for the rotation, the structure and rules of the ward/team, and your role on the team.

Resident. As a core member of the team, the resident may be the "primary clinician" (i.e., may bear full responsibility for all aspects of patient care), or he or she may act as "med backup" to non-MD primary clinicians, doing physicals and mental status exams, prescribing medications, and dealing with concurrent medical issues. PGY-1s, also known as "interns" in other specialties, are often called residents in psychiatry.

"Primary Clinician". Some psychiatry services use psychologists, social workers, or nurse clinicians to take care of admission interviews, paperwork, phone calls, and discharge dictations, with residents acting as "med backup." Although they may be skilled professionals and are often highly knowledgeable about community services, disposition, and other issues critical to managing psychiatric patients, these clinicians tend to have more limited knowledge about pharmacologic treatments.

Clinical Psychologist ("PhD" or "PsyD"). Psychologists perform assessments, conduct psychological testing (e.g., IQ tests, Rorschach inkblot tests), and perform psychotherapy. Some psychometric tests are dull, but try to observe a Rorschach (or have one done on you if you have a willing psychologist); they are fascinating and uncannily accurate.

Nurse. Nurses play a more central role on a psychiatric unit than is the case on other wards. They often know patients best and can therefore report on comments and behaviors that the MDs may have missed (psychiatric patients are often skilled at hiding their pathology during an interview but usually can't do so all day). As a result, nurses often speak first in rounds. Nurses may also have known patients for a decade or more over repeated hospitalizations and can thus give you a great deal of insight into a given patient's longitudinal course, usual baseline presentation, home and family situation, and so on. It is therefore critical to develop a good rapport with the nurses.

Social Worker. Social workers are experts on issues such as disposition, housing, finances, and transportation. Social workers are also involved in planning family meetings and helping educate family members about mental illness. Be nice to them, as they are highly effective in mobilizing your patients.

Psychiatry Assistant. Psychiatry assistants help the entire team with daily care tasks.

Recreational Therapist ("RT"). When patient stays were longer (i.e., months or even years), patients tended to have a lot of free time, which was principally filled by "therapeutic" games, crafts, cooking, and other activities organized by an RT. However, RTs have now been phased out in many hospitals, and patients often watch TV instead.

HOW IS THE DAY SET UP?

The day usually begins with a multidisciplinary-team meeting in which all the patients on the service are discussed. The team typically includes the attending, resident, nurse, and social worker together with the student. The nurse usually reports overnight events. If the student was on call, he or she presents the previous evening's admissions. During the discussion, plans are formulated for each patient (see below).

After the meeting, the student can complete as much work as he or she can before attending lectures and conferences; this includes checking labs and obtaining medical records. The student then has a chance to see the patient in the afternoon—a meeting that can vary in time and intensity depending on the specific circumstances. At the end of the workday, the student writes a progress note documenting both the overnight and day's events.

7:30–8:00 A.M.	Prerounds
8:00–10:00 A.M.	Morning rounds/new-patient presentation
10:00 A.M.–12:00 P.M.	Conferences/lectures/grand rounds
12:00 P.M.–1:00 P.M.	Lunch
1:00–4:00 P.M.	Clinic/floor work/scut time
4:00–5:00 P.M.	Afternoon rounds
OR	
1:00–5:00 P.M.	Consultation and liaison service
OR	
1:00–5:00 P.M.	Emergency crisis intervention

This is just a sample schedule; times and activities may vary depending on the structure of the rotation. In general, however, the afternoon on the inpatient psychiatry wards is generally scut time consisting of activities such as arranging medical, OB/GYN, and neurologic consultations on psychiatric patients, looking up articles on MEDLINE, and rounding up labs and x-rays (if necessary) for afternoon rounds.

WHAT DO I DO DURING PREROUNDS?

When prerounding, look for hours of sleep the night before, percentage of meals eaten the day before, vitals, medication compliance, and the type and amount of prn meds given. Also assess the patient for any change in target symptoms or the presence of medication side effects. Some of this information can be found in the nursing notes. Most importantly, perform a mental status exam.

HOW DO I DO WELL IN THIS ROTATION?

Emphasizing the biopsychosocial model, modern psychiatry incorporates biological, experiential, and sociocultural factors into a single paradigm. Doing well in psychiatry requires the development of interviewing skills, the study of psychopathology, and the acquisition of knowledge about psychopharmacology. Generally, psychiatry emphasizes the doctor-patient relationship in the healing process. Thus, the development of empathic skills and an ability to listen is critical to doing well in this rotation. The use of open-ended questions to acquire information about a patient's psychopathology is also a must.

Listening is an acquired skill that necessitates discipline and practice. Like a cardiologist who gathers much more information when listening to heart sounds than can a first-year medical student, a psychiatrist can distill a tremendous amount of information from an interview. What a patient tells a doctor extends beyond the content of his or her words; how the patient communicates and how the interviewer feels in response to that patient are just as important in assessing pathology.

In addition to developing interviewing skills, it is important to acquire a solid fund of psychiatric knowledge. Furthermore, observational skills need to be honed to monitor abnormalities in a patient's appearance, behavior, and affect. Specifically, this rotation provides an opportunity to learn the disorders of feeling, thinking, and behavior that interfere with the way a person functions and relates to others. You must also learn how to present a psychiatric history.

As a medical student, you often have the most recent experience on medicine wards of any member of the team. You can thus be a real asset in helping the team manage medical problems in psychiatric patients.

Many students find themselves initially disoriented by the unique organization and expectations of the psychiatry clerkship. Here are some tips from students and residents who've been there:

- Keep an open and inquiring mind. Psychiatric training benefits doctors in all fields.
- Be organized. Keep a card on every patient that includes a short history, a thorough medication list, and a checklist of things to do. Also make a card with the generic and trade names, common dosages, and side effects of the most frequently used psychiatric drugs, as well as a card with an outline of the mental status exam (MSE).
- When interviewing a patient, obtain a thorough medication history, including dates of use, effectiveness, and side effects.
- Get friendly with the support staff, especially the nurses! Psychiatry is highly multidisciplinary. Nurses know the patients well and often have great insight that can be shared with medical students.

Good listening and observational skills are a must.

Never let a labile patient get between you and the door.

- Remember—safety first. If you feel threatened, leave the room immediately and get help. While on this rotation, you may witness a "takedown" in which the staff physically pins down a violent, labile patient. This may look frightening and unpleasant, but it is often the safest and kindest option. When interviewing, especially in the inpatient setting, do not interview in the patient's room. Instead, try to interview in a location that respects the patient's confidentiality and allows for a nonobstructed departure from the room, if necessary. If the patient is potentially dangerous, leave the door to the interview room open. In such instances, a third person might be asked to stand inside or outside the room to be available if trouble arises.
- Take the initiative. When discussing your patient, think ahead and consider issues such as housing, finances, social supports, time of discharge, cultural issues, and community services.
- Try to pick up on how your patient makes you feel (e.g., depressed, anxious). You'll find that your patient often has similar feelings.
- In general, forget the white lab coat or any kind of uniform. Some institutions even ban ties and necklaces, as patients can use them to strangle the caretaker. However, bring your white coat on the first day of your rotation and wear it until you are told that you can leave it at home.
- Don't joke with your patients.
- Don't touch your patients. Touch is a powerful and volatile tool that should be used only after you have gained more experience.
- Don't share details of your life with your patients.
- Before you interview a patient, discuss the goals of diagnosis and treatment with your resident or attending. Is it to gather information or to treat? How deep do you want to go? Are there any sensitive topics from which you should steer clear?
- You will often experience a mix of feelings when dealing with psychiatric patients. Be willing to explore these feelings comfortably with your team. Having such feelings is not seen as a sign of weakness, but failing to deal with them can be detrimental.

WHAT IS DSM-IV?

DSM-IV, or the *Diagnostic and Statistical Manual, Fourth Edition,* is published by the American Psychiatric Association. The DSM is the standard diagnostic classification system used by all U.S. mental health workers (both clinicians and researchers) as well as by insurance companies and the federal government. The DSM, which is revised roughly once a decade to incorporate new research findings, consists of long lists of the criteria that are required to assign specific psychiatric diagnoses to patients. At first glance, the DSM may appear lengthy, complex, and confusing. However, you do not need to know the details of all the criteria. The more important criteria will be found here under the appropriate headings.

It is important to note that despite its precise and detailed diagnostic criteria, the DSM is not meant to be used by nonpsychiatrists in a "check the appropriate boxes" or "cookbook" fashion. To the contrary, the DSM merely offers guidelines for trained psychiatrists to apply using their experience and clinical judgment and is intended to ensure better diagnostic agreement among clinicians and researchers.

DSM-IV uses a "multiaxial classification," which is just a fancy way of saying that information is broken down into five categories (which should be used for presenting patients in rounds, write-ups, etc.):

1. **Axis I:** Psychiatric disorders
2. **Axis II:** Personality disorders and mental retardation
3. **Axis III:** Physical and medical problems
4. **Axis IV:** Social and environmental problems/stressors
5. **Axis V:** The Global Assessment of Functioning (GAF), which rates a patient's overall level of social, occupational, and psychological functioning (current and best in the past year) on a scale of 1 (completely nonfunctional) to 100 (extremely high level of functioning in a wide number of areas)

KEY NOTES

The psychiatric admit note is similar to its medicine counterpart except for the emphasis it places on past psychiatric history and the patient's personal history. Large portions of a psychiatric history often need to be obtained from other sources. At a minimum, you must talk to a family member and to the patient's regular doctor and review any old charts.

Chief complaint/reason for admission. Psychiatric patients often do not have a chief complaint, or they may voice a complaint that is incoherent, obscene, or irrelevant, so it is often necessary to briefly state how and why the patient ended up in the hospital or ER.

History of present illness (HPI). This includes symptoms, precipitants, time course, any medication changes or medication noncompliance, effects on function at home and work, and current treatment.

Past psychiatric history. This includes age of onset of symptoms, first psychiatric contact, first psychiatric hospitalization, number of hospitalizations, the date and duration of the most recent hospitalization, suicide attempts (when, how, seriousness), substance abuse (what, how much, how often, how long, any withdrawal, shared needles), and medications (what, how much, how long, what helped, side effects, why did patient stop taking them).

Past medical history. Past medical history should be obtained with the same thoroughness as in other specialties. However, a history of seizures, CNS infections, endocrine difficulties (e.g., thyroid), head trauma, allergies, and the presence of acute or chronic pain are particularly important to obtain.

Social history (SH). In psychiatry, heavy emphasis is placed on the social/personal history, as a patient's health, lifestyle, and social interactions may heavily influence his or her current psychiatric illness. It is therefore important to flesh out the details of a patient's birth, childhood, school performance, marriage, education, religious and cultural beliefs, occupational history, family and social relations, sexual history, hobbies and special interests, community supports, and current living arrangements. The patient's legal history, any history of violence, and a history of physical or sexual abuse should be documented. Attention should also be paid to family structure and significant interpersonal dynamics (e.g., divorced, adopted).

Family history (FH). Ask about any psychiatric illnesses that run in the family. Get details on diagnoses, severity, outcomes, and what medications helped. Ask about nonpsychiatric illnesses that run in the family as well.

A&O = Alert and oriented

AH = Auditory hallucinations

BAD = Bipolar affective disorder

CAD = Coronary artery disease

c/c/e = Clubbing, cyanosis, edema

CM = Caucasian male

CN = Cranial nerve

CTAB = Clear to auscultation bilaterally

d/o = Disorder

DTRs = Deep tendon reflexes

EOMI = Extraocular movements intact

FT = Fine touch

FTN = Finger to nose

HEENT = Head, eyes, ears, nose, and throat

HI = Homicidal ideation

h/o = History of

HSM = Hepatosplenomegaly

HTN = Hypertension

Sample Psychiatry Admit Note

ID/Chief complaint: TM is a 20-year-old CM college student brought in to the ER by his parents because he has been bedridden and increasingly isolative for 2 weeks.

Source of Information: Parents, who are reliable.

HPI: This is the patient's 1st inpatient admission for symptoms. Patient was in his USOH until 3 years ago, when he became depressed after failing a college class. Also at that time, he thought he was being "followed" and that "whispers were talking behind his back." A first diagnosis of schizophrenia of the paranoid type was made at that time by Dr. Jones, who started patient on Zyprexa (titrated up to 20 mg/day), which was effective. He has since seen four additional psychiatrists, and has tried Prozac for depressive symptoms with no success. Patient has been able to continue school part-time and function fairly well. However, for the last two weeks, his parents report that he has isolated himself in his room and does not leave except to use the restroom. He continually lies in bed with the sheets over his head and the blinds drawn. According to his parents, the patient was "mute and tearful, answering questions with single words and acting differently from his usual social self." At time of admission, patient endorses a running debate in his head from a single, unrecognized voice. The conversation revolves around daily activities and decisions such as choosing a seat. Patient denies VH/HI/SI. No prior h/o suicide attempts.

Patient reports that he currently has no appetite (eats only a small sandwich a day), sleeps four hours per night, and is not participating in any of his usual activities. He has been noncompliant with his Zyprexa for the past 3–4 months. He endorses a history of alcohol and cocaine use, but denies using for the last 3 months.

Past Psychiatric History: See HPI.

Substance use: Tobacco: 1/2 ppd × 4 years; EtOH: drinks approx. 12 beers/week × 6 years; Cocaine: intranasal cocaine 2 times/week × 5 years; Denies h/o IVDA.

PMH:

Childhood Illnesses: None.

Medical Illnesses: None.

Surgeries: None.

Hospitalizations: None.

Trauma: Head injury due to bicycle accident with brief LOC in 1995. No retrograde or anterograde amnesia. No hospitalization or treatment at that time.

Allergies: None.

Medications: Zyprexa 20 mg qd.

No herbs, supplements, or vitamins.

FH: H/o depression in all paternal male relatives, including father. One paternal uncle committed suicide at age 40. Mother with heavy EtOH use. No h/o schizophrenia or other psychiatric illnesses. No history of CAD, HTN, MI, or cancer.

SH: Pt was raised by his mother and father. Parents state that childhood development was normal, and he was a good student with A's and B's until his diagnosis 3 years ago. He currently lives at home with his parents in Los Angeles and attends a local junior college. He has been unemployed × 1 month and worked most recently at a grocery store. He has held multiple odd jobs over the past three years; his longest job was 6 months. No h/o arrests or legal problems. No current girlfriend, and patient is not sexually active. He has enjoyed playing the guitar since age 13.

ROS: Poor sleep, appetite, and energy. No recent weight change. Otherwise unremarkable except as above.

PE:

GEN: Disheveled 20-year-old male sitting in a chair in NAD.

VS: T 36.8 RR 18, orthostatic BP: sitting 150/82 P 104; standing 156/87, P 107.

SKIN: Tattoo on left shoulder; no rashes, scars, or lesions noted.

HEENT: NC/AT, PERRL, EOMI, no nystagmus, conjunctiva clear, OP clear with good dentition.

NECK: Supple, no LAD.

LUNGS: CTAB, no W/R/R.

CV: Tachycardic, regular rhythm, no M/R/G, normal S1/S2.

ABD: Soft, NT/ND, NABS, no masses or HSM.

EXT: Warm and well-perfused with cap refill < 2 sec. No c/c/e. Distal pulses 2+ bilaterally.

NEURO: MS: A&O × 4; CN: II–XII intact; Motor: Normal tone, bulk, and power throughout; Sensory: FT/PP/Temp intact & symmetric; cerebellar: FTN and HTS intact, Romberg negative; DTRs 2+ & symmetric; gait: normal, able to tandem gait.

MSE:

- Appearance: Clean-shaven, but hair and clothing are disheveled.

- Behavior: Marked psychomotor retardation with poor eye contact.

- Attitude: Cooperative with interview and questions, but somewhat withdrawn and guarded.

HTS = Heel to shin

IVDA = Intravenous drug abuse

LAD = Lymphadenopathy

LOC = Loss of consciousness

MDD = Major depressive disorder

MMSE = Mini-mental status exam

MS = Mental status

NABS = Normal active bowel sounds

NAD = No acute distress

NC/AT = Normocephalic, atraumatic

NT/ND = Nontender, nondistended

OP = Oropharynx

PE = Physical examination

PERRL = Pupils equal, round, reactive to light

PMH = Past medical history

PP = Pin prick

ppd = Pack per day

r/o = Rule out

RPR = Rapid plasma reagin

RUA = Routine urine analysis

SAD = Schizoaffective disorder

SI = Suicidal ideation

TH = Tactile hallucinations

TSH = Thyroid-stimulating hormone

USOH = Usual state of health

VH = Visual hallucinations

w/r/r = Wheezes, rales, rhonchi

- Speech: Slowed and hypophonic with prolonged speech latency. Coherent but with paucity of content.

- Mood: "Anxious".

- Affect: Blunted—patient tells stories with limited emotional expression.

- Thought process: Linear and goal-directed, without circumstantiality or tangentiality.

- Thought content: No SI/HI.

- Perception: Endorses AH "has voices inside that are debating about where to sit," making it difficult to make decisions. Denies VH/TH.

- Cognition: MMSE 28/30. Missed 2 points on WORLD backward.

- Judgment: Poor—patient wants to leave the hospital without treatment.

- Insight: Poor—patient does not feel that he is ill or that taking medication will help him.

Labs:

HIV Neg

RPR NR

TSH 1.6

RUA Neg

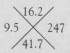

Assessment: TM is a 20-year-old male with a 3-year h/o depressive and paranoid symptoms, noncompliant with Zyprexa, now with 2 weeks of increasing isolation and auditory hallucinations.

Axis I: Schizophrenia of paranoid type with depressive features—Patient is exhibiting key features of schizophrenia of the paranoid type, including history of hallucinations and delusions for approximately 3 years. Patient is also showing concurrent features of a depressive episode, including lack of interest in normal activities, decreased appetite, and decreased sleep. At this time, it is unclear if there is concurrent schizophrenia and MDD; further information on concentration, level of energy, and overall mood (patient now denies being depressed) must be explored.

- r/o MDD with psychotic features.

- r/o BAD vs. SAD.

- r/o Substance-related/induced mood d/o.

Polysubstance abuse.

Axis II: Deferred.

Axis III: None.

Axis IV: Poor social support, substance dependence, lives at home, has difficulty holding jobs.

Axis V: GAF 35–40.

Plan:

- Risperidone 2 mg PO qam and qhs.

- Cogentin 1 mg PO BID.

- Wellbutrin SR 100 mg PO qam.

- Ativan 1 mg PO q4h prn anxiety.

- Tylenol 650 mg PO q6h prn headache, fever, or pain.

- Colace 100 mg PO BID, prn constipation.

- Monitor sleep, food intake, and activity level.

- Continue to explore and understand the patient's internal debate.

- Encourage milieu participation.

- Involve social work in planning outpatient rehab and a family meeting.

KEY PROCEDURES

The mental status exam is the single most important procedure medical students must learn. Like the physical exam, the MSE provides a way to objectively document mental function and behavior. Although most often used in psychiatry, some form of MSE should be a part of all medical exams. It is therefore helpful to create an MSE template that can be filled in during the interview. Always rule out organic causes of mental illness when evaluating psychiatric disorders.

WHAT DO I CARRY IN MY POCKETS?

You will want to carry a psychiatry handbook (see "Top-Rated Books") as well as your drug guide. You will rarely need a stethoscope. Female medical students may find themselves pocketless owing to the absence of a white coat.

Memorize the mental status exam.

ROTATION OBJECTIVES

Unlike other specialties, psychiatry has a more limited group of diagnoses. You should know the clinical characteristics, workup, and management of the following major psychiatric disorders. Disease entities and related issues discussed in this chapter are listed in italics.

Mental Status Exam

Mood Disorders
- *Major depressive disorder*
- *Dysthymic disorder*
- *Bipolar 1 disorder*
- *Bipolar 2 disorder*
- *Cyclothymia*

Psychotic Disorders
- *Schizophrenia*
- *Schizophreniform disorder*
- *Brief psychotic disorder*
- *Schizoaffective disorder*
- *Delusional disorder*

Anxiety Disorders
- *Generalized anxiety disorder*
- *Panic disorder*
- *Social phobia*
- *Specific phobia*
- *Obsessive-compulsive disorder*
- *Post-traumatic stress disorder*

Personality Disorders

Substance Abuse

Childhood and Adolescent Disorders
- *Attention-deficit hyperactivity disorder*
- *Autistic disorder*
- *Conduct disorder*
- *Mental retardation*
- *Learning disorders*

Miscellaneous
- *Adjustment disorder*
- *Anorexia nervosa*
- *Bulimia nervosa*

- *Somatoform and related disorders*
- *Suicidality*
- Dementia
- Delirium
- Pathologic grief
- Sleep disturbances
- Issues regarding the dying patient

Mental Status Exam

Table 7.1 offers a brief outline of the key components of an MSE. You may want to use this table as a guide in creating a template. One should, however, refer to a text or manual for a complete treatment of this subject.

TABLE 7.1. Mental Status Exam.

Component	Comments
Appearance and behavior	Grooming, appropriateness of dress, relatedness, and eye contact.
Attitude	The manner in which the patient interacts with the interviewer (e.g., cooperative, hostile).
Motor	Psychomotor agitation, psychomotor depression, tremor, posturing, and mannerisms.
Speech	Rate, rhythm, tone, fluency, enunciation, volume, clarity, amount, and abnormalities (e.g., aphasia).
Emotions	Mood: The patient's subjective, internal emotional state (e.g., dysthymic, euphoric, irritable, euthymic, and anxious). Affect: The outward expression, including facial expression, of a patient's internal emotional state (e.g., flat, blunted or restricted, labile, full, and expansive).
Thought process	The form of expression of a patient's thought, including quality, quantity, associations, and fluency of speech. Abnormalities include circumstantiality, tangentiality, flight of ideas, thought blocking, echolalia, neologisms, clanging, loosening of associations, and perseveration.
Thought content	The content of a patient's thoughts, including SI, HI, delusions, major themes, preoccupations, obsessions, ideas of reference, and poverty of thought.
Perception	Hallucinations (false sensory perceptions) and illusions (misinterpretations of actual stimuli).

Cognition	Evaluation of various brain functions and level of consciousness (e.g., alert, drowsy, stuporous, and comatose).
	 Includes the Folstein MMSE:
	 Orientation:
	   1. What is the year, month, date, day of the week, season? (5 points)
	   2. Where are we? Country, state, city, hospital, floor? (5 points)

TABLE 7.1 (continued). Mental Status Exam.

HIGH-YIELD TOPICS

Psychiatry

Component	Comments
	Registration:
	1. Name three objects and ask the patient to repeat the three objects. Repeat until the patient learns all three, and record the number of trials. (1 point each)
	Attention and calculation:
	1. Serial 7s: Stop after five answers. (1 point each)
	2. Spell "world" backward. (alternate)
	Recall:
	1. Recall the three objects that the patient repeated earlier. (1 point each)
	Language:
	1. Name two objects the interviewer points out. (naming, 2 points)
	2. Repeat the phrase "No ifs, ands, or buts." (repetition, 1 point)
	3. Follow a three-step command: "Take a paper in your right hand, fold it in half, and put it on the floor." (3 points)
	4. Read and obey the command "Close your eyes." (1 point)
	5. Write a sentence. (1 point)
	6. Copy a design (interlocking pentagons). (visual/spatial, 1 point)
Abstraction	Can the patient think abstractly? Ask the patient to explain the meaning of a proverb.
Judgment	Does the patient understand the consequences of his or her actions?
Insight	How aware is the patient of his or her illness, its etiology, and treatment options?

KEY POINT

DEFINITION OF KEY TERMS

- **Circumstantiality:** Indirect speech that is delayed in reaching the point but does eventually reach the desired goal (i.e., ability to get from point A to point B after some time).
- **Tangentiality:** Inability to have goal-directed thought (i.e., inability to get from point A to point B).
- **Flight of ideas:** Rapid, continuous use of words with constant shifting between connected ideas.
- **Pressured speech:** Rapid speech that is increased in amount and difficult to understand or interrupt.
- **Thought blocking:** Abrupt interruption in a train of thought before the thought or idea is completed.
- **Echolalia:** Persistent repetition of the words or phrases of one person by the patient.
- **Neologisms:** The creation of new words, often by combining syllables of other words.
- **Clanging:** Association of words with similar sounds but not meaning.
- **Loosening of associations:** Flow of thought with random shifting of ideas from one subject to another.
- **Perseveration:** Persistent response to a previous stimulus when a new stimulus is presented.
- **Ideas of reference:** A person's belief that an object (e.g., a radio or television) is speaking to him or about him.
- **Delusions:** Fixed, false beliefs that are not consistent with a patient's culture and cannot be corrected by reasoning.

Mood Disorders

Mood disorders are composed of mood episodes, each with a certain set of symptoms representing the patient's dominant mood state. The episodes—major depressive episode (MDE), mania, hypomania, and mixed—are not themselves diagnostic. However, they are used by psychiatrists to help make the diagnosis of a mood disorder.

MAJOR DEPRESSIVE DISORDER

Major depressive disorder is one of the most prevalent psychiatric disorders, carries a lifetime risk of 15–20%, and has an approximately twofold greater prevalence among females than among males. The average age of onset is in the third to fourth decades of life. Although socioeconomic status, culture, and race do not affect prevalence, chronic illness and stress increase the risk of having the disorder. MDD also complicates the diagnosis and treatment of chronic illnesses such as CAD and cerebrovascular accident (CVA). Recurrence rates are high, with a 50% recurrence after one episode, a 70% recurrence after two episodes, and a 90% recurrence after three episodes.

Numerous theories have been proposed regarding the etiology and pathophysiology of major depression. Although it has recently fallen into disfavor, perhaps the most widely known theory is the biogenic amine theory, which holds that depression is due to low levels of amine neurotransmitters (e.g., norepinephrine [NE] and serotonin [5HT]) in the synaptic cleft. Since antidepressants increase the functional amount of amine neurotransmitters in the CNS, they are said to increase the amount of biogenic amine that can bind to the receptor on the postsynaptic neuron.

Signs and Symptoms. The signs and symptoms of MDD are outlined in the mnemonic "SIG E CAPS."

Differential. The differential includes the following:
- **Psychiatric:** Mood disorder due to a general medical condition, substance-induced mood disorder, cocaine withdrawal, bereavement, schizoaffective disorder (SAD), dysthymia, dementia, bipolar disorder (depressed or mixed episode), and adjustment disorder with depressed mood.
- **Organic:** Hypothyroidism, AIDS, multiple sclerosis, Parkinson's disease, Addison's disease, Cushing's disease, anemia (especially pernicious anemia), infectious mononucleosis, neuroborreliosis, influenza, malnutrition, and malignancies (e.g., pancreatic cancer).
- **Drugs:** These include, among others, oral contraceptives, cimetidine, steroids, and some beta blockers.

Workup. According to DSM-IV, the criteria for diagnosis of an MDE include at least five symptoms of depression, at least one of which must be depressed mood or anhedonia. The symptoms must persist for at least two weeks, must

---

Symptoms of depression—

SIG E CAPS
Sleep—increased or decreased
Interest—anhedonia (loss of interest or pleasure)
Guilt or worthlessness
Energy—decreased energy or fatigue
Concentration—difficult or disturbed
Appetite—increased or decreased
Psychomotor retardation—more often than psychomotor agitation
Suicidal ideations

Hypothyroidism must be ruled out when evaluating a patient for depression.

cause significant social or occupational dysfunction, and must not be caused by drugs, medications, medical conditions, or bereavement. Normal bereavement begins immediately or a few months after the loss of a loved one. The symptoms are similar to those of MDD, but the latter is not diagnosed unless the symptoms of bereavement persist beyond two months or if excessive depressive symptoms (e.g., SI, excessive guilt, or preoccupation with worthlessness) are present. It is important to note, however, that bereavement may vary by culture. Thus, differentiating bereavement and MDD may be difficult in patients with a normal response lasting more than two months. It is also important to rule out organic causes of MDD, most significantly hypothyroidism; TSH should thus be checked.

When characteristic features are present, MDD can be further subdivided into the following categories:

- **MDD with psychotic features:** MDD associated with delusions and/or hallucinations that are commonly mood congruent. Psychotic symptoms must be present only during mood disturbances.
- **MDD with atypical features:** Patients have a pattern of chronic rejection sensitivity and are more likely to have hyperphagia and hypersomnia.
- **MDD with melancholic features:** Patients have severe anhedonia with the near-absence of pleasure and reactivity. They also experience early-morning awakening and severe weight loss.
- **MDD with postpartum onset:** MDE occurring within four weeks of parturition.
- **MDD with seasonal pattern:** Recurrent episodes of depression at the same time each year. There must be at least two seasonal episodes in the last two years, with the absence of episodes in the off-season.

SSRIs are the treatment of choice for major depressive disorder.

Treatment. A combination of psychotherapy and pharmacotherapy is the treatment of choice for MDD. Selective serotonin reuptake inhibitors (SSRIs) are relatively well tolerated and are considered first-line therapy for depression. However, tricyclic antidepressants (TCAs), monoamine oxidase inhibitors (MAOIs), and atypical antidepressants such as bupropion (Wellbutrin), venlafaxine (Effexor), and mirtazapine (Remeron) are also used. Electroconvulsive therapy (ECT) is generally reserved for refractory or catatonic depression. Several modes of psychotherapy have been used as well. Psychoanalytically oriented (psychodynamic) psychotherapy is perhaps the most commonly used therapy, but cognitive behavioral therapy (CBT) and interpersonal therapy are also effective.

DYSTHYMIC DISORDER

Dysthymic disorder has a 6% lifetime prevalence and shows a twofold greater incidence among females than among males. Patients with dysthymia exhibit a chronic depression of greater than two years' duration that is not severe enough to meet the criteria for MDD. The disorder lacks psychotic features, does not cause social or occupational dysfunction, and does not require hospi-

KEY ANTIDEPRESSANT MEDICATIONS

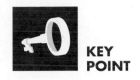

Selective Serotonin Reuptake Inhibitors

SSRIs include fluoxetine (Prozac), sertraline (Zoloft), paroxetine (Paxil), fluvoxamine (Luvox), and citalopram (Celexa).

- **Mechanism of action:** Serotonin (5HT)-specific reuptake inhibitors.
- **Clinical use:** Endogenous depression.
- **Side effects:** Agitation, anxiety, neuromuscular restlessness (similar to akathisia), insomnia, sexual dysfunction, GI distress, anorexia, and multiple drug interactions (always check in PDR), including the serotonin syndrome (restlessness, confusion, hyperthermia, muscle rigidity, cardiovascular collapse, death) when used with other serotonergic medications (e.g., MAOIs).
- **Pros:** Relatively well tolerated, so you can usually start at the therapeutic dose. Safe in overdose, with fewer side effects than TCAs. Citalopram is commonly used in patients who have multiple comorbid conditions, as it has very few drug interactions.
- **Cons:** Sexual dysfunction is very common and is often the cause of noncompliance. Like all antidepressants, they take two to three weeks to have an effect.

Tricyclic Antidepressants

TCAs include amitriptyline (Elavil), imipramine (Tofranil), desipramine (Norpramin), clomipramine (Anafranil), nortriptyline (Pamelor), and doxepin (Sinequan).

- **Mechanism of action:** Block reuptake of NE and 5HT.
- **Clinical use:** Endogenous depression, bedwetting (imipramine), obsessive-compulsive disorder (OCD) (clomipramine), and chronic pain.
- **Side effects:** Anticholinergic effects (dry mouth, blurred vision, constipation, urinary retention, delirium, worsening glaucoma), sedation, alpha blocking effects (orthostatic hypotension), cardiac arrhythmias (widened QRS, prolonged PR and QTc, potential for supraventricular tachycardia, ventricular tachycardia, and ventricular fibrillation), seizures, respiratory depression, hyperpyrexia, confusion, and hallucinations in the elderly. Tertiary TCAs (imipramine, amitriptyline) have more anticholinergic side effects and sedation than do secondary TCAs (nortriptyline). Desipramine is the least sedating.
- **Pros:** Cheap, well studied, and effective in severe depression.
- **Cons:** Poor compliance owing to side effects. Lethal in overdose, so must titrate slowly. The three Cs of TCA toxicity are **C**onvulsions, **C**oma, and **C**ardiotoxicity (arrhythmias).
- **Labs:** Check ECG before starting, after a few days, and at the therapeutic dose. Check blood levels if no response is obtained, excessive side effects occur, or there is suspected noncompliance.

Monoamine Oxidase Inhibitors

MAOIs include phenelzine (Nardil), tranylcypromine (Parnate), and isocarboxazid.

- **Mechanism of action:** Nonselective MAO inhibition.
- **Clinical use:** Atypical depressions, anxiety, and hypochondriasis.
- **Side effects:** Hypertensive crises ("tyramine reaction" or "cheese and wine reaction"; most foods are safe in moderation, but avoid aged cheeses, red wine, cured or pickled foods, yeast extracts, meperidine, and OTC sympathomimetic "cold and pain" drugs), headache, dizziness, insomnia, orthostatic hypotension, and weight gain.
- **Pros:** Cheap with a broad range of efficacy; the best drugs for atypical depression.
- **Cons:** Dietary restrictions and poor tolerability of side effects. Contraindicated for use with beta agonists, SSRIs, and meperidine.

Heterocyclic Antidepressants

- Second- and third-generation antidepressants with varied and mixed mechanisms of action. Expensive and rarely first line.
- **Bupropion (Wellbutrin):** The mechanism possibly involves dopamine reuptake inhibition. This medication is also used in smoking cessation (as Zyban). It is rarely lethal in overdose and has few sexual side effects, but other side effects include stimulation (tachycardia, agitation, constipation, tremors, diaphoresis), dry mouth, aggravation of psychosis, and tendency to cause seizures, especially in those with eating disorders.
- **Venlafaxine (Effexor):** Inhibits NE and 5HT reuptake. Can also be used in generalized anxiety disorder (GAD). Side effects include stimulant effects (insomnia, anxiety, agitation, headache, and nausea) and increased diastolic blood pressure. Blood pressure must be monitored.
- **Mirtazapine (Remeron):** An α_2-antagonist (increases NE and 5HT neurotransmission) and potent $5HT_2$ receptor antagonist. Has fewer sexual side effects, although it causes marked sedation, increased appetite, and weight gain (which could be of use in underweight patients with depression).
- **Nefazodone (Serzone) and trazodone (Desyrel):** Primarily inhibit serotonin reuptake by a mechanism different from that of the SSRIs. Both have short half-lives. Side effects are sedation (especially trazodone), postural hypotension, and priapism (trazodone only). Because of the side effect of sedation, trazodone in combination with another antidepressant may be effective in depressed patients with insomnia.

Electroconvulsive Therapy

- Despite its *One Flew over the Cuckoo's Nest* reputation, ECT is safe, simple, and one of the most effective treatments for depression. Patients usually require 6 to 12 treatments. ECT can be done on an outpatient basis and can be lifesaving for refractory or catatonic depression. It can also be used in bipolar disorder (for mania and depression) and acute psychosis.
- **Pre-ECT evaluation:** Conduct a history and physical (H&P); obtain an ECG, electrolytes, a CBC, liver function tests (LFTs), a routine urinalysis (UA), thyroid function tests (TFTs), a CXR, a spinal x-ray series, and

a brain CT; and alert anesthesiology in advance. Informed consent is required.

■ **Procedure:** The patient is kept NPO (nothing by mouth) for at least eight hours. Methohexital, a short-acting barbiturate, is given for anesthesia. Prior to inducing muscle paralysis with succinylcholine, a tourniquet is placed around an extremity to prevent paralysis in that area in order to monitor the seizure.

■ **Contraindications:** Recent MI, recent stroke, or intracranial mass. There is a relative contraindication in patients who are a high anesthesia risk.

■ **Side effects:** Postictal confusion, arrhythmias, headaches (resolves in hours), retrograde amnesia (usually no longer than six months), and sore muscles.

talization. If a patient has one or more episodes of major depression during a two-year period, a diagnosis of "double depression" is made. The differential diagnosis is similar to that of MDD.

Workup. To meet DSM-IV criteria for dysthymic disorder, in addition to depressed mood more days than not, a patient must exhibit two or more of the following six symptoms for more days than not over a period of at least two years:

■ Increased or decreased appetite
■ Increased or decreased sleep
■ Decreased energy or fatigue
■ Decreased self-esteem
■ Difficulty concentrating or disturbed concentration
■ Hopelessness

Dysthmia is the presence of at least two years of chronic depression that is not severe enough to meet the criteria for major depression.

BIPOLAR I DISORDER

Bipolar I disorder, or manic-depression, is an affective (mood) disorder with a 0.5–1.5% lifetime prevalence. Men and women are affected equally, and the average age of onset is 21 years. As in MDD, there is a strong genetic component, with a 70% concordance in monozygotic twins. The recurrence rate after one manic episode is 90%, and 10–15% of patients will commit suicide. Bipolar disorder is more commonly associated with substance abuse than other psychiatric disorders.

Signs and Symptoms. Although the disorder is termed *bipolar,* only a single manic episode is needed for a diagnosis of bipolar I. The signs and symptoms of a manic episode are outlined in the mnemonic "DIG FAST." In many cases, patients initially present with depression.

Signs and symptoms of mania—

DIG FAST
Distractibility
Insomnia—decreased need for sleep
Grandiosity—inflated self-esteem
Flight of ideas
Increase in goal-directed **A**ctivity and psychomotor **A**gitation
Pressured **S**peech
Thoughtlessness—seeks pleasure without regard for consequence (e.g., shopping sprees)

Differential. The differential includes the following:
- **Psychiatric:** Schizophrenia, SAD, cyclothymia, borderline personality disorder, and attention-deficit hyperactivity disorder (ADHD).
- **Organic:** Brain tumors, CNS syphilis, encephalitis, metabolic derangements, hyperthyroidism, and multiple sclerosis.
- **Drugs:** Cocaine, amphetamines, corticosteroids, anabolic steroids, phenylpropanolamine, isoniazid (INH), captopril, and antidepressants.

Workup. According to DSM-IV, the criteria for diagnosis of a manic episode include the presence of an elevated, expansive, or irritable mood with at least three (or four, if the mood is irritable) signs and symptoms from the "DIG FAST" mnemonic. The symptoms of a manic or mixed episode (i.e., one that meets the criteria for both an MDE and a manic episode) must be present for at least one week (or less if hospitalization was required). Like MDD, bipolar I has subtypes with characteristic features. Twenty percent of bipolar I patients suffer from rapid cycling in which there are at least four mood episodes (MDE, mania, hypomania, or mixed) in 12 months. This subtype carries a poorer prognosis. Bipolar I with psychotic features can feature mood-congruent or mood-incongruent delusions or hallucinations.

Treatment. Bipolar patients must initially be assessed for suicidal and homicidal ideation and the need for hospitalization. As in many psychiatric disorders, a combination of pharmacotherapy and psychotherapy is the treatment of choice. Psychotherapy focuses on helping patients understand and accept their illness, cope with its consequences, and maintain medication compliance. There are three targets for pharmacotherapy: acute mania, bipolar depression, and prophylaxis and maintenance:

1. **Acute mania:**
   - Mood control can be accomplished with lithium or with an anticonvulsant medication (e.g., valproic acid, carbamazepine).
   - Resolution of psychosis may require low-dose antipsychotics.
   - Anxiety can be managed with anxiolytic medications (e.g., benzodiazepines).
2. **Bipolar depression:** This is usually more difficult to treat than an MDE.
   - A mood stabilizer (e.g., lithium) is used with or without a short course of an antidepressant.
   - Patients must first be treated with a mood stabilizer to prevent the induction of mania ("manic switch") by an antidepressant. Antidepressants alone can also precipitate rapid cycling.
3. **Prophylaxis and maintenance:** The patient is usually given lifelong prophylaxis with a mood stabilizer after the second episode, after a first episode that is severe or life threatening, or if a strong family history exists. Lithium and valproic acid are considered first-line treatments; carbamazepine is a second-line agent if the first-line treatments fail. ECT is effective in bipolar disorder (for depressive and manic episodes) but is reserved for patients who are refractory to pharmacotherapy or when a more immediate treatment response is required.

KEY MOOD STABILIZERS

Lithium

- **Mechanism of action:** Not well established.
- **Clinical use:** The mainstay of treatment for bipolar disorder and mania (acute episodes and prophylaxis). It also has mild antidepressant effects.
- **Side effects:** Fine tremor, nausea, acne, weight gain, benign leukocytosis, arrhythmias, other ECG cardiac changes (flattened T waves or T-wave inversion), hypothyroidism, nephrogenic diabetes insipidus (lithium is an antidiuretic hormone [ADH] antagonist), chronic renal failure, and teratogenesis.
- **Pros:** Cheap and well studied in long-term use.
- **Cons:** Regular lab work is required in that long-term renal involvement is common. Dosage must be titrated owing to side effects. Lithium has a narrow therapeutic index—aim for a level of 0.8–1.2 in acute mania and a level of 0.6–1.0 for maintenance. Signs of toxicity (coarse tremor, arrhythmias, dysarthria, ataxia, nausea, and diarrhea) will first be seen at a level of 1.5, seizures and coma at around 2.5, and death at around 3–4. Treatment for toxicity may require dialysis. NSAIDs, ACE inhibitors (ACEIs), and diuretics (when first started) elevate the plasma lithium level.

Anticonvulsant Medications

- **Valproic acid (Depakote):** As effective as lithium in bipolar disorder and better in mixed mania, substance abuse, and rapid cycling. Can be used for acute episodes and prophylaxis. Side effects include GI distress, sedation, hepatotoxicity (e.g., rare hepatitis, elevated LFTs, and elevated ammonia), pancreatitis (rare), and thrombocytopenia (rare). Benefits of this medication include the fact that it is well tolerated, has a high therapeutic index, and is more benign in overdose. Patients can start at the therapeutic dose, and fewer blood tests are required once dosage is established. There is limited research on its long-term use in bipolar disorder. LFTs, platelets, and valproic acid levels should be checked at regular intervals.
- **Carbamazepine (Tegretol):** Probably less effective than the others, this is a second-line agent used in patients who do not respond to lithium. The most serious side effects are agranulocytosis (rare), aplastic anemia (rare), and Stevens-Johnson syndrome (surprisingly common) but also include hepatitis (rare) and ataxia, confusion, and tremors with toxicity. A CBC is needed before starting, on a monthly basis for three to six months, and then every three to six months.

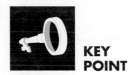

KEY POINT

HIGH-YIELD TOPICS

Psychiatry

Bipolar II disorder requires the presence of at least one major depressive episode and one hypomanic episode.

BIPOLAR II DISORDER

Bipolar II disorder, which was first outlined in DSM-IV, requires that patients have at least one MDE *and* one hypomanic episode; mixed and manic episodes are absent. According to DSM-IV, the criteria for diagnosing a hypomanic episode include at least four days of abnormally elevated, expansive, or irritable mood. During the mood disturbance, at least three signs and symptoms (or four, if the mood is irritable) from the "DIG FAST" mnemonic must be present. Unlike the manic patient, the hypomanic patient might show changes in baseline function, but these changes are not severe enough to require hospitalization, cause psychotic features, or lead to social or occupational dysfunction. At 0.5%, the lifetime prevalence is slightly lower in bipolar II than in bipolar I, and women are at a slightly greater risk. Bipolar II patients can show rapid cycling. Treatment is similar to that of bipolar I.

Cyclothymia requires the presence of dysthymia with intermittent hypomania lasting at least two years.

CYCLOTHYMIA

According to DSM-IV, the criteria for diagnosis of cyclothymia include dysthymia with intermittent hypomanic episodes. As in dysthymia, this condition is chronic, and its diagnosis requires two years of cycling hypomanic and dysthymic episodes without the presence of major depressive, manic, or mixed episodes. The patient must not be symptom free for more than two months at a time. Although the symptoms of cyclothymia are similar to those of bipolar I and II, they are not as severe and generally cycle more rapidly. The lifetime prevalence is approximately 1%, with a peak age of onset at 15 to 25 years. The female-to-male ratio is 3:2, and 30% of patients have a family history of bipolar disorder. Many cyclothymic patients also have borderline personality disorder, and approximately one-third to one-half will develop a mood disorder, most commonly bipolar II. The treatment of choice is a mood stabilizer, which has yielded high treatment success. Antidepressants may increase the rate of cycling and may precipitate manic episodes if the patient is not first treated with a mood stabilizer.

Psychotic Disorders

Psychotic disorders are defined by the presence of psychosis, which is a "gross impairment in reality testing."

SCHIZOPHRENIA

Schizophrenia is a psychotic disorder that is characterized by a disruption in thought, affect, volition, social behavior, and motor activity in which the patient becomes increasingly preoccupied with his internal environment. The lifetime prevalence is approximately 1%. Although men and women are equally at risk, men tend to develop the disease earlier (15 to 25 years as opposed to 25 to 35 years in women) and with greater severity than their female counterparts. There is an increased prevalence of the disease among lower socioeconomic classes in the United States, which has been explained by a "downward drift" of these patients into the lower classes owing to impairment from their disease. Overall, patients with this disease exhibit a chronic progressive course. Approximately 10–15% die by suicide, while nearly 50% of patients make a suicide attempt.

The cause of schizophrenia is unknown but likely involves a combination of polygenic and environmental factors. High rates of the disease have been found in families, and the likelihood of developing the disease increases with increasing relatedness. Dizygotic twins and children of a single schizophrenic parent have a 12% prevalence of schizophrenia; the prevalence increases to 40% and 47% with two schizophrenic patients or a monozygotic twin, respectively.

Various neurotransmitter abnormalities have also been identified in association with schizophrenia. Although high levels of 5HT and low levels of glutamate and GABA have been discussed, an imbalance of dopamine (the "dopamine hypothesis") is the most widely favored theory. The dopamine hypothesis postulates that increased dopamine activity and receptors in the limbic system correlate with the symptoms of disease. This hypothesis is supported by the fact that antipsychotic medications, which consist mainly of dopamine receptor antagonists, help alleviate psychotic symptoms, while dopamine agonists (e.g., cocaine and amphetamines) worsen or induce such symptoms. Abnormalities seen in the brains of schizophrenic patients both on CT and MRI scans, as well as on autopsy include enlargement of the third ventricle and lateral ventricles, diffuse cortical atrophy, atrophy of the cerebellar vermis, a thickened corpus callosum, and a smaller left parahippocampal gyrus.

Signs and Symptoms. According to DSM-IV, patients must present with at least two of the following signs and symptoms for at least six months:

- Hallucinations
- Delusions
- Disordered speech
- Grossly disorganized or catatonic behavior
- Negative symptoms

These symptoms must cause social and/or occupational dysfunction. Depression, if present, is brief in comparison to the duration of the illness. Symptoms are generally categorized and better understood as either positive or negative symptoms:

1. **Positive symptoms:** The presence of unusual thought, behaviors, or perceptions.
   - Hallucinations (most commonly auditory or visual, although any sensory modality is possible)
   - Bizarre delusions
   - Bizarre behavior (e.g., repetitive behavior, including echolalia, echopraxia, and odd dress)

- Thought-processing disorders (e.g., ideas of reference, tangentiality, neologisms, and loose associations)
2. **Negative symptoms:** Lack of normal social and/or mental function.
   - Alogia (lack of words)
   - Poverty of thought
   - Apathy
   - Anhedonia, avolition, asociality
   - Flattened affect

Differential. The differential includes the following:

- **Psychiatric:** Other psychotic disorders (e.g., schizoaffective, schizophreniform), mood disorders (e.g., bipolar, severe melancholia, mood disorder with psychotic features), delusional disorder, delirium, dementia, Cluster A personality type, and developmental disorders (e.g., Asperger's syndrome, autism).
- **Organic:** Early Huntington's disease, early Wilson's disease, complex partial seizures (e.g., temporal lobe epilepsy), frontal or temporal lobe tumors, early multiple sclerosis, early systemic lupus erythematosus (SLE), acute intermittent porphyria, electrolyte imbalances, hepatic encephalopathy, HIV encephalopathy, viral encephalitis, neurosyphilis, and endocrine abnormalities (e.g., Cushing's disease, calcium imbalance, thyroid dysfunction, and hypoglycemia).
- **Drugs:** Substance abuse (e.g., amphetamine, cocaine, or PCP) and medications (e.g., digoxin, adrenocorticotropic hormone [ACTH], INH, and L-dopa).

Workup. According to DSM-IV, the criteria for diagnosis of schizophrenia include the presence of two or more of the above signs and symptoms for a period of at least one month, with continuous evidence of social and/or occupational dysfunction secondary to psychiatric disturbance for at least six months. These symptoms cannot be due to a preexisting medical condition, a substance-related condition, or another psychiatric condition. Several subtypes of schizophrenia have been characterized (see Table 7.2).

Treatment. The treatment of schizophrenia consists primarily of antipsychotic (neuroleptic) medications as well as hospitalization and psychotherapy. Most neuroleptic medications work by blocking dopamine receptors. Psychosocial intervention includes supportive treatment such as vocational rehabilitation and arranged social support in the community.

SCHIZOPHRENIFORM DISORDER

Patients with schizophreniform disorder meet the criteria for schizophrenia, except that the duration of illness is one to six months. Social and/or occupational function may or may not be impaired. Males and females are equally affected, and prevalence is slightly less than that of schizophrenia (0.2%). Most patients will eventually develop schizophrenia, while others will develop a mood disorder.

TABLE 7.2. Types and Characteristics of Schizophrenia.

Subtype	Characteristics
Paranoid	Delusions or hallucinations (frequently auditory) Lacks disorganized speech, disorganized or catatonic behavior, and negative symptoms Relatively good self-care Best prognosis—relatively good preservation of thought, personality, and function over time
Disorganized	Prominent disorganized speech, disorganized behavior (poor personal appearance), and flat/inappropriate affect (e.g., disinhibited); does not involve catatonic behavior Worst prognosis
Catatonic	Requires two of five of the following symptoms: 1. Motor immobility (rigidity) 2. Excessive motor activity 3. Extreme negativism or mutism 4. Peculiar voluntary movement and bizarre posturing (waxy flexibility) 5. Echolalia or echopraxia
Undifferentiated	Has characteristics of more than one subtype
Residual	Patient met criteria for schizophrenia in the past but now lacks delusions and hallucinations Has residual negative symptoms or attenuated hallucinations, delusions, and other thought disorders

KEY POINT

KEY ANTIPSYCHOTIC MEDICATIONS

Antipsychotic medications are usually divided into "typical" and "atypical" medications. Atypicals cause fewer extrapyramidal symptoms (EPS), have a better side effect profile, and do not increase prolactin levels but are very expensive.

Typical Antipsychotics

Typical antipsychotics block dopamine receptors (mostly D_2 and D_4 subtypes) and are most effective in treating positive symptoms. These can be divided into high, medium, and low potency. Side effects are similar for all typical agents. Higher-potency drugs have more EPS, while lower-potency drugs have more anticholinergic, sedative, and orthostatic hypotensive effects. Examples are as follows:

- **High:** Haloperidol (Haldol), fluphenazine (Prolixin), thiothixene (Navane), and droperidol

BRIEF PSYCHOTIC DISORDER

This diagnosis carries a better prognosis than schizophrenia. Patients exhibit one or more of the following symptoms for one day to one month: delusions, hallucinations, disorganized speech, grossly disorganized behavior, and cata-

- **Medium:** Trifluoperazine (Stelazine) and perphenazine (Trilafon)
- **Low:** Thioridazine (Mellaril) and chlorpromazine (Thorazine)

Side effects include the following:

1. **Extrapyramidal symptoms:**

   - **Acute dystonia:** Early, sudden-onset twisting of the neck or rolling of the eyes (torticollis and oculogyric crisis, respectively), mainly in young men after roughly 10 to 14 days of treatment. Treat with IM anticholinergics such as benztropine (Cogentin), trihexyphenidyl (Artane), or diphenhydramine (Benadryl).
   - **Akathisia:** A subjective sense of inner restlessness in the legs, which may or may not result in objective manifestations of restlessness (e.g., walking around or difficulty remaining still). Treat with beta blockers (e.g., propranolol) or benzodiazepines (e.g., clonazepam, diazepam).
   - **Parkinsonism:** Resting tremor, cogwheel rigidity, bradykinesia, shuffling gait, and masklike facies. Treat with oral anticholinergics and possibly amantadine (a dopamine-releasing agent).
   - **Tardive dyskinesia (TD):** Involuntary, abnormal lip smacking, tongue protrusion, and writhing movements of the limbs or trunk. Occurs in 10–30% of long-term neuroleptic users, especially the elderly, women, and patients with mood disorders. Although treatment involves withdrawing neuroleptics or changing to clozapine, TD is often irreversible.

2. **Neuroleptic malignant syndrome (NMS):** Fever, rigidity, autonomic instability, and clouding of consciousness. Can give rise to rhabdomyolysis, myoglobinuria, and renal failure; in this case, creatine phosphokinase (CPK) is usually markedly elevated. The condition is uncommon but life threatening (20% mortality). Treat by withdrawing neuroleptics, initiating supportive measures, and sometimes by administering dantrolene, bromocriptine, or amantadine.

3. **Hyperprolactinemia:** Results in amenorrhea, galactorrhea, and gynecomastia. A pituitary tumor must be ruled out.

4. **Anticholinergic effects:** Include dry mouth, urinary retention, constipation, and orthostatic hypotension.

5. **Other effects:** Orthostatic hypotension, weight gain, sedation, seizures, and ECG changes or arrhythmias (e.g., conduction delays).

Atypical Antipsychotics

Atypical antipsychotics have fewer anticholinergic and extrapyramidal side effects. Because of this, they are currently used as first-line drugs in newly diagnosed schizophrenia. These agents are effective in treating patients with positive and negative symptoms as well as those who are refractory to typical antipsychotics. The first atypical antipsychotic was clozapine (Clozaril). Newer medications include ziprasidone (Geodon), risperidone (Risperdal), olanzapine (Zyprexa), and quetiapine (Seroquel). These medications do not cause agranulocytosis but may be less effective than clozapine in treatment-resistant patients. All medications of this class have some degree of 5-HT$_2$ receptor antagonism, but each has a different combination of receptor blockade. Key side effects of the atypicals as a whole include weight gain, type 2 diabetes mellitus, and QT prolongation.

- **Clozapine:** Thought to be more effective for treatment-resistant schizophrenia and negative symptoms. It causes agranulocytosis in 0.5–1.0% of patients, thus mandating a weekly CBC for the first six months of treatment and every other week thereafter. Side effects include severe sedation, anticholinergic effects, orthostatic hypotension, vertigo, dizziness, drooling, excessive salivation, weight gain, seizures, arrhythmias, and eosinophilia.

- **Risperidone:** The mechanism of action involves dopamine and serotonin receptor blockade. Risperidone does not cause agranulocytosis. Its side effects include a low incidence of EPS, hyperprolactinemia, fatigue, tachycardia, sedation, orthostatic hypotension, and weight gain.

- **Olanzapine:** Particularly effective in treating negative symptoms and in treating more agitated patients, olanzapine has a low incidence of EPS; its most common side effects are drowsiness, akathisia, weight gain, insomnia, and dry mouth. No hepatotoxicity has been reported.

- **Quetiapine:** This medication has a very low incidence of EPS. Side effects include somnolence and orthostasis. Usually dosed more than once daily.

- **Ziprasidone:** Side effects include QT prolongation, insomnia, and restlessness.

EVOLUTION OF EPS SYMPTOMS

- **4 hours:** Acute dystonia
- **4 days:** Akinesia
- **4 weeks:** Akathisia
- **4 months:** Tardive dyskinesia (often permanent)

KEY POINT

tonic behavior. Since the differential diagnosis of an acute psychotic episode is broad and this disorder is rare, the physician must rule out other causes. It should be noted that this disorder can occur with or without the presence of stressors, including parturition (episode within four weeks of giving birth). Treatment might include a brief hospitalization and possibly a short course of neuroleptics or benzodiazepines.

Timeline of psychotic disorders:

Schizophrenia: at least six months of psychotic features.

Schizophreniform disorder: one to six months of psychotic features.

Brief psychotic disorder: one day to one month of psychotic features.

SCHIZOAFFECTIVE DISORDER

Unlike schizophrenia and schizophreniform disorder, schizoaffective disorder is said to be present when a patient concurrently meets the criteria for schizophrenia and for MDE, manic episode, or mixed episode. Mood symptoms must be present for a significant portion of the disease, but acute psychotic symptoms (e.g., delusions, hallucinations) must be present for at least two weeks in the absence of mood symptoms. SAD also has bipolar and depressive subtypes. The lifetime prevalence is 0.5–0.8%, with a peak age of onset in the late teens and early 20s. Treatment involves a combination of an antipsychotic and a mood stabilizer; antidepressants and possibly ECT may be indicated for acute depressive types.

DELUSIONAL DISORDER

Like schizophrenia, delusional disorder is chronic. Unlike schizophrenia, however, its hallmark feature is nonbizarre (or plausible) delusions. To fulfill DSM-IV criteria, delusions must be present for at least one month in the absence of hallucinations, disorganized speech, disorganized behavior, or negative symptoms. The prevalence is 0.03%, with males and females equally affected. The age of onset is variable but generally peaks in the 40s.

The subtypes of delusional disorder are defined by the predominant delusional content as follows:

- **Persecutory:** Delusions that the individual is being harassed or malevolently treated.
- **Grandiose:** Delusions that the individual possesses exaggerated power, money, knowledge, and the like.
- **Erotomanic:** Delusions that another person, usually of higher status, is in love with the individual.
- **Somatic:** Delusions that the individual has a physical defect or medical condition.
- **Jealous:** Delusions that the individual's partner is unfaithful.
- **Mixed:** Delusions that are of more than one type.
- **Unspecified**

Treatment is difficult, as most patients are refractory to neuroleptics. Psychotherapy may provide some benefit.

Anxiety Disorders

Anxiety disorders are a group of disorders in which anxiety—the presence of a sense of impending doom or threat—is the prominent feature. The patient's anxiety is poorly based in reality, is out of proportion to actual threat, and is vague or poorly defined. The anxiety disorders are the most prevalent of all psychiatric disorders.

GENERALIZED ANXIETY DISORDER

Generalized anxiety disorder has a prevalence of nearly 5% in the United States, and females are affected twice as often as males. GAD commonly co-exists with other psychiatric disorders. Patients may report excessive worry as adolescents, but the disorder generally becomes prominent when patients reach their 20s. The etiology remains unclear, although it has been postulated that genetic and environmental factors as well as a number of neurotransmitter systems (including 5HT, NE, and GABA) may be involved.

Signs and Symptoms. The defining symptom of GAD is chronic, excessive anxiety or worry about a number of actual life events. In comparison to panic disorder, GAD does not involve discrete episodes of anxiety. Rather, patients consistently worry about nearly every aspect of their lives. Somatic manifestations are common and can include palpitations, light-headedness, dizziness, clammy hands, dry mouth, dysphagia, increased urinary frequency, difficulty breathing, abdominal pain, and diarrhea.

Differential. The differential includes the following:
- **Psychiatric:** Other anxiety disorders (e.g., panic disorder, obsessive compulsive disorder [OCD], social phobia, hypochondriasis), mood disorders (e.g., depression, dysthymia), and psychotic disorders.
- **Organic:** Hyperthyroidism, pheochromocytoma, and abnormalities of calcium, glucose, or phosphate.
- **Drugs:** Substance-induced anxiety disorder (e.g., intoxication with caffeine, cocaine, or amphetamines) and substance withdrawal (e.g., benzodiazepines, alcohol).

Workup. According to DSM-IV criteria, the patient must have excessive anxiety on more days than not for at least six months, along with at least three of the six following symptoms:
- Restlessness or a feeling of being "on edge"
- Easy fatigability
- Difficulty concentrating or "mind going blank"
- Irritability
- Muscle tension
- Sleep disturbance (insomnia)

Treatment. The most successful treatment is a combination of pharmacotherapy and psychotherapy. External causes of anxiety (e.g., caffeine, nicotine, sleep disturbances) should first be eliminated. First-line pharmacotherapy then includes the SSRIs, venlafaxine (Effexor), and buspirone (BuSpar). Like most psychiatric medications, these agents require several weeks to show a significant clinical effect. In the interim, patients may be given a benzodiazepine-buspirone combination. Benzodiazepines with longer half-lives are used, including clonazepam and diazepam. These medications take effect immediately but cause dependence and withdrawal with more than two or three weeks of use. Unlike many other medications, buspirone does not appear to cause tolerance, dependence, or withdrawal.

SSRIs and TCAs have been used for the treatment of GAD with depressive symptoms. CBT with a focus on relaxation techniques is a useful adjunct.

PANIC DISORDER

Panic disorder is characterized by unexpected, discrete periods of terror (panic attacks) as well as by anticipatory anxiety about future attacks. The lifetime prevalence is 1.5–3.5%, and women have a threefold increase in risk compared to males. The peak age of onset is in the mid-20s, and the disorder rarely presents after the age of 45. Although the cause of panic disorder remains unknown, researchers believe that it may be a conditioned response. The first episode is unexpected and sudden; thereafter, patients associate the panic with the situation in which the first attack occurred. They subsequently attempt to avoid any situation that might precipitate further attacks (anticipatory anxiety). As more attacks occur, more situations become associated with panic, and the patient's range of activities may become significantly limited. Fifty percent of patients with panic disorder have concurrent MDD.

Signs and Symptoms. According to DSM-IV, there are two criteria for the diagnosis of panic disorder. First, the patient must have recurrent, unexpected panic attacks that begin suddenly, peak in intensity within ten minutes, and include a sensation of intense fear along with at least four of the following symptoms:

- Palpitations or increased heart rate
- Sweating
- Trembling or shaking
- A sensation of shortness of breath or a feeling of choking
- Chest pain or discomfort
- Nausea or abdominal distress
- Dizziness or light-headedness
- Derealization or depersonalization
- Fear of losing control or going crazy
- Fear of dying
- Paresthesias
- Chills or hot flashes

Second, at least one attack must be followed by one month or more of one of the following:

- Persistent worry about additional attacks
- Worry about the implications of the attack
- Change in baseline function secondary to the attack

KEY ANTIANXIETY MEDICATIONS

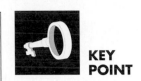

Benzodiazepines

- **Mechanism of action:** Bind to $GABA_A$ receptors to increase the affinity of GABA binding and to increase the frequency of chloride-channel opening.
- **Clinical use:** Used for a broad spectrum of anxiety disorders (e.g., GAD, social phobia, and panic disorder) and sleep disorders (e.g., insomnia) as well as for alcohol detoxification, seizures (e.g., status epilepticus), preanesthesia, catatonia, and mood, adjustment, or psychotic disorders with anxiety components. They are also used as muscle relaxants.
- **Duration of action:**
  - **Long $t_{1/2}$ (> 100 hours):** Clonazepam, clorazepate, chlordiazepoxide, diazepam, flurazepam, quazepam, prazepam, and halazepam
  - **Intermediate $t_{1/2}$ (10 to 20 hours):** Alprazolam, estrazolam, lorazepam, and temazepam
  - **Short $t_{1/2}$ (3 to 8 hours):** Oxazepam and triazolam
- **Side effects:** Sedation, slurred speech, ataxia, dizziness, anterograde amnesia, respiratory depression (especially in overdose with other sedative-hypnotics such as alcohol or in chronic obstructive pulmonary disease [COPD]), tolerance, cross-tolerance, and withdrawal due to dependence.

- **Pros:** Lorazepam, oxazepam, and temazepam are not metabolized by the liver and are safe in patients with hepatic dysfunction.
- **Cons:** Potentiation of alcohol and other CNS depressants increases the risk of sedation and respiratory depression. P_{450} inhibitors (e.g., cimetidine, fluoxetine, INH, and estrogen) increase benzodiazepine levels, while carbamazepine and rifampin decrease such levels. Benzodiazepines are most frequently abused in patients with a history of alcohol and/or drug abuse. The most commonly abused agents are lorazepam, alprazolam, and diazepam. Withdrawal symptoms are more severe and abrupt with shorter-acting agents.

Buspirone (BuSpar)

- **Mechanism of action:** Partial agonist at $5\text{-}HT_{1A}$ receptors.
- **Clinical use:** GAD. Not useful in panic disorder. Can augment antidepressant treatment in MDD or OCD.
- **Side effects:** The relatively few side effects of buspirone include infrequent sedation, dizziness, headache, and GI upset. There is no respiratory depression, tolerance, dependence, or withdrawal.
- **Pros:** Very safe and without the tolerance, dependence, and respiratory depression of benzodiazepines. Favored in patients with a history of substance abuse.
- **Cons:** Slow onset of action. Thus, not useful in panic disorder. Compared to benzodiazepines, there is less overall reliability in the treatment of anxiety.

Approximately 50% of patients will have associated agoraphobia, which is anxiety or fear of places or situations where escape might be embarrassing or difficult. Patients attempt to avoid such situations or endure them with extreme distress.

Differential. The differential includes the following:
- **Psychiatric:** GAD, social phobia, OCD, and post-traumatic stress disorder (PTSD).
- **Drugs:** Substance-induced anxiety disorder (e.g., caffeine, cocaine, or amphetamines).
- **Organic:** Pheochromocytoma, arrhythmia, pulmonary embolism, hypoxia, angina, and hyperthyroidism.

Treatment. Treatment involves a combination of pharmacotherapy and psychotherapy. The most effective psychotherapy is CBT with a focus on relaxation techniques and reversal of symptom misinterpretation. The mainstay of pharmacotherapy is antidepressants. SSRIs are first-line treatment, and TCAs and MAOIs are second-line choices. MAOIs are more efficacious than TCAs, although they are limited in use owing to their side effects. Benzodiazepines (e.g., alprazolam, clonazepam) may be used for immediate relief, but long-term use should be avoided owing to their addiction potential. Buspirone is not effective in panic disorder.

SOCIAL PHOBIA

Social phobia is characterized by at least six months of persistent, intermittent fear of a social or public situation in which the patient is exposed to unfamiliar persons or to situations in which his performance will be scrutinized. Phobias can be limited to specific situations (most commonly public speaking or meeting new people) or can be generalized (fear of nearly all social situations). Phobic situations usually provoke a panic attack and impair social or occupational functioning. Patients recognize that their fear is excessive and irrational. The disorder affects 3–13% of the population, with a female-to-male ratio of 1:1. Onset is usually in adolescence and is preceded by childhood shyness. The differential diagnosis is similar to that of other anxiety disorders. Treatment involves CBT with relaxation techniques. Pharmacotherapy consists of MAOIs, SSRIs, and occasionally beta blockers (e.g., for stage fright). Benzodiazepines are indicated if SSRIs are not effective.

SPECIFIC PHOBIA

Specific phobia is the most common psychiatric disorder among females and the second most common in men (after substance abuse disorder). Its lifetime prevalence is 10–25%, with females affected twice as often as males. Most cases do not cause significant impairment or distress, but comorbid anxiety disorders are common. Most phobias begin in childhood, although the age of onset is variable. Patients with specific phobia recognize that they have an excessive, irrational fear. Common specific phobias involve animals, blood, in-

Buspirone is not used to treat panic disorder.

jections (often with vasovagal syncope), or specific situations such as airplanes or heights. The differential diagnosis includes OCD, GAD, panic disorder, social phobia, avoidant personality disorder, normal shyness, or fear appropriate to the situation. Most childhood specific phobias resolve without treatment. For persistent phobias, the treatment of choice is behavioral therapy with flooding (sudden exposure to the feared object or situation) or gradual desensitization through incremental exposures. Relaxation and breathing techniques, hypnosis, insight-oriented psychotherapy, or CBT can also be used.

OBSESSIVE-COMPULSIVE DISORDER

Obsessive-compulsive disorder (OCD) has a lifetime prevalence of 2–3%. Although men and women are equally affected, men tend to develop OCD at an earlier age. The disorder usually begins during adolescence or early adulthood and shows a gradual progression. Issues complicating treatment and diagnosis are concomitant depression, reluctance to discuss symptoms, and substance abuse.

Signs and Symptoms. DSM-IV requires that the patient have either obsessions or compulsions and that the patient recognize them as excessive and irrational. Obsessions are defined as recurrent, intrusive thoughts, impulses, or images that cause anxiety and that the patient attempts to suppress or neutralize in order to decrease anxiety. The person recognizes that these thoughts, impulses, or images are a product of his own mind. Common obsessions include cleanliness, contamination, or a fear of harm to self or loved ones. Compulsions are defined as conscious, stereotyped behaviors or thoughts that the patient performs to prevent the distress or anxiety induced by the obsession. Compulsions might take the form of excessive cleaning (hands may be chafed secondary to frequent washing), elaborate rituals for conducting ordinary tasks (e.g., walking through the doorway), or excessive checking (e.g., multiple trips back home to check that the door is locked).

Differential. The differential includes the following:
- **Psychiatric:** GAD, specific phobia, trichotillomania, body dysmorphic disorder, obsessive-compulsive personality disorder (which, in comparison, is ego-syntonic and lacks separate obsessions and compulsions), Tourette's syndrome, schizophrenia (which can include obsessions and compulsions, but with hallucinations and delusions), and MDD (usually with obsessive rumination).
- **Organic:** Brain tumor or temporal lobe epilepsy.
- **Drugs:** Substance-induced anxiety disorder (e.g., cocaine, amphetamines, or caffeine).

Workup. In order for OCD to be diagnosed, a patient must have either obsessions or compulsions and must at some point recognize them as unreasonable and excessive. They must be time-consuming (take up more than one hour per day), cause marked distress, and interrupt normal social or occupational function.

Treatment. Pharmacotherapy is almost always indicated. Clomipramine is the treatment of choice. SSRIs are also effective, although usually at higher doses than those used for MDD. Behavioral therapy (e.g., exposure-response prevention, thought stopping, flooding) in combination with pharmacotherapy is most effective.

POST-TRAUMATIC STRESS DISORDER

Post-traumatic stress disorder (PTSD) can occur after an individual is exposed to a traumatic event that is associated with intense fear or horror and that involves actual or threatened harm. Its lifetime prevalence is about 8% and is highest in young adults. In populations exposed to combat or assault, however, prevalence approaches 60%.

Signs and Symptoms. Patients with PTSD persistently reexperience traumatic events through intrusive thoughts, flashbacks, and nightmares. In addition, patients must exhibit persistent avoidance of stimuli associated with the trauma and a numbing of responsiveness indicated by at least three of the following symptoms: anhedonia, amnesia, restricted affect, active avoidance of thoughts of the trauma or situations associated with the trauma, and "emotional numbing" or detachment. Patients with PTSD also experience symptoms of increased arousal as indicated by two of the following symptoms: hypervigilance, insomnia, increased startle response, poor concentration, and irritability. Additional associated symptoms include survivor guilt, personality change, dissociation, aggression, depression, substance abuse, or suicidality. Symptoms must be present for at least one month and are classified according to their duration:

- **Acute PTSD:** Symptoms present for less than three months.
- **Chronic PTSD:** Symptoms present for more than three months.
- **Delayed-onset PTSD:** Symptoms start more than six months after the traumatic event.

Differential. The differential diagnosis includes acute stress disorder (which is similar to PTSD, but symptoms occur within one month of the traumatic event and last two days to one month), MDD, OCD, anxiety disorder, adjustment disorder, malingering, and borderline personality disorder.

Treatment. SSRIs and mood stabilizers are first-line treatments, but adjunctive anxiolytics such as beta blockers, benzodiazepines, and α_2-agonists may be used if first-line treatment fails. Benzodiazepines are generally less effective but may be helpful in early stages. Patients with PTSD require higher-than-normal doses of antidepressants. CBT and support groups are also effective.

Personality Disorders

A personality is an enduring pattern of perceiving, relating to, and thinking about the environment, other people, and oneself that is exhibited in a wide range of important social and personal contexts. A personality disorder exists when an individual has a stable, enduring pattern of inner experience and behavior that deviates markedly from cultural expectations; is persistent, inflexible, and maladaptive; and causes significant impairment in social or occupational function or leads to subjective distress. Personality disorders are typically ego-syntonic, and as such, patients have little insight into their disorders. Personality disorders are coded on Axis II and affect the diagnosis and treatment of other comorbid conditions.

Personality disorders typically begin in childhood, crystallize by late adolescence, and affect all facets of the personality, including cognition, mood, behavior, and interpersonal style. Axis II disorders often coexist with, and affect the treatment of, acute psychiatric illnesses (Axis I).

Signs and Symptoms. Table 7.3 outlines the signs and symptoms of personality disorders. The mnemonic "MEDIC" summarizes the hallmark features of such disorders.

Differential. The differential diagnosis of personality disorders includes normal variants of an individual's personality, Axis I psychiatric disorders (e.g., schizophrenia, major depression, bipolar disorder, and anxiety disorders), delusional disorder, environmental stressors, and substance abuse.

Workup. The diagnosis of a personality disorder is made through identification of the persistent signs and symptoms discussed in Table 7.3, as well as through the presence of significant impairment in social or occupational functioning or subjective distress. Personality disorders are not diagnosed under the age of 18 and are difficult to diagnose in the face of an active Axis I disorder.

Treatment. Long-term psychotherapy is usually the treatment of choice for personality disorders. Behavioral therapy and pharmacotherapy have also been successful in specific contexts. Antianxiety medications and/or low-dose antipsychotics may be necessary for anxiety or agitation. Addressing the underlying personality disorder will assist in treating the major Axis I disorders.

Personality disorders are pervasive, persistent, maladaptive patterns of behavior.

Hallmark features of personality disorders—

MEDIC
Maladaptive
Enduring
Deviates from norm
Inflexible
Causes impaired social functioning

Substance Abuse

Substance abuse and dependence have a 13% lifetime prevalence in the United States, and alcohol is the most commonly abused substance (excluding tobacco and caffeine). Alcohol abuse and dependence have a lifetime prevalence of 6% in the general U.S. population. Males are affected nearly four times more frequently than females, but the incidence of alcoholism in women is increasing. The highest prevalence of alcoholism occurs in males between the ages of 21 and 34 years. Substance abusers are at increased risk for accidental and traumatic injuries, especially motor vehicle accidents. Intravenous (IV) drug abusers are at increased risk for acquiring HIV, hepatitis B, hepatitis C, endocarditis, cellulitis (especially among "skin poppers"), and STDs. Substance abusers are often exceptionally destructive both to themselves and to their families, and some—particularly opioid and crack addicts—will do almost anything to get

TABLE 7.3. Signs and Symptoms of Personality Disorders.

Cluster	Examples	Characteristics	Clinical Dilemma	Coping Strategy
Cluster A: "weird"	Paranoid	Persistent distrust and suspicion that others are harming or deceiving him; reluctant to confide in others and perceives attacks on character that are not apparent to others.	Patient is suspicious of physician and does not trust physician. Rarely visits physician.	Use a clear, honest attitude and a noncontrolling, nondefensive approach. Avoid humor and maintain distance. Patients' defense mechanisms are projection and fantasy.
	Schizoid	Social isolation and restricted emotional range (cold and detached); patients lack close friends, lack interest in sexual experiences, and are indifferent to praise.		
	Schizotypal	Odd beliefs, speech, behavior, or appearance; magical thinking, ideas of references, and unusual "out of body" perceptual experiences.		
Cluster B: "wild"	Borderline	Marked impulsivity, unstable sense of self and interpersonal relationships, and recurrent SI. Inability to control mood lability and chronic feelings of emptiness.	Patient will change the rules on the physician. The patient is clingy and demands attention. Feels that he/she is special. Will manipulate the physician and staff ("splitting").	Firm: Stick to the treatment plan and do not waffle. Fair: Do not be punitive or derogatory. Consistent: Do not change the rules. Patients' defense mechanisms are dissociation, denial, splitting, and acting out.
	Histrionic	Excess emotionality and attention seeking with a constant need to be the "center of attention." Inappropriate sexual or provocative behavior, self-dramatization, and suggestibility.		
	Narcissistic	Persistent grandiosity about self and accomplishments, need for excessive admiration, sense of entitlement, envy of others, and lack of empathy.		

TABLE 7.3 (continued). Signs and Symptoms of Personality Disorders.

Cluster	Examples	Characteristics	Clinical Dilemma	Coping Strategy
	Antisocial	Blatant disregard for the rights of others with failure to conform to social norms and lawful behavior. Impulsivity, deceitfulness, and lack of remorse. Disregard for the safety of self and others, aggression, and irresponsibility.		
Cluster C: "worried and wimpy"	Obsessive-compulsive	Preoccupation with details, cleanliness, order, and control over all aspects of life. Perfectionism is evident in excessive devotion to work over leisure. Patients have inflexibility in morals and values, inability to throw out worthless objects, miserly spending, and rigidity.	Patient may subtly sabotage his or her own treatment. Very controlling. Words are not necessarily consistent with actions.	Avoid power struggles. Passive wins over active. Give clear treatment recommendations, but do not push the patient into a decision. Patients' defense mechanisms: hypochondriasis, passive aggression, and isolation.
	Avoidant	Social inhibition, feelings of inadequacy, excessive shyness and hypersensitivity to rejection. Avoidance of activities and relationships for fear of being disliked and ridiculed.		
	Dependent	Submissive and clinging behavior, a need to be "taken care of," and difficulty making decisions, expressing disagreement, and initiating projects. Uncomfortable with being alone.		

money for drugs, including dealing, stealing, and prostituting themselves (and even their children). Always ask about the care of their children (you may need to contact child protection agencies) and how they obtain their drug money (this may give you clues to other potential medical and legal problems).

Signs and Symptoms. According to DSM-IV, substance dependence is characterized by at least three of the following signs and symptoms that last for at least one year:

- Tolerance
- Withdrawal
- Substance taken in larger amounts than intended
- Persistent desire or attempts to cut down
- Considerable time and energy spent trying to obtain substance, use substance, or recover from its effects
- Important social, occupational, or recreational activities given up or reduced because of substance use
- Continued use despite awareness of the problems that it causes

According to DSM-IV, substance abuse is a maladaptive pattern of substance use leading to clinically significant impairment or distress; symptoms have not met the criteria for substance dependence. DSM-IV criteria for substance abuse are met when at least one of the following symptoms is present for at least one year:

- Recurrent substance use resulting in failure to fulfill major obligations at work, school, or home
- Recurrent substance use in physically hazardous situations
- Recurrent substance-related legal problems
- Continued substance use despite persistent problems caused by use

Alcohol withdrawal syndromes consist of the following:

- **Uncomplicated withdrawal:** Occurs within several hours (usually six to eight hours) after cessation of drinking and is characterized by tremulousness, tachycardia, hypertension, diaphoresis, anxiety, nausea, insomnia, hypervigilance, hyperreflexia, weakness, tinnitus, blurred vision, paresthesias, and numbness.
- **Alcohol hallucinosis:** Occurs within two days after cessation of or decrease in drinking and is characterized by auditory hallucinations that persist after the withdrawal symptoms have disappeared. The sensorium is clear (no delirium). Delusions or paranoid ideation may be present.
- **Delirium tremens (DTs):** Occur approximately one to eight days after cessation of drinking (most often within 24 to 72 hours after cessation) and can be life threatening (untreated mortality of 15–20%). DTs are characterized by disorientation, fever, agitation, tremor, delusions, seizures, memory deficits, insomnia, visual and tactile hallucinations, and autonomic instability.

Table 7.4 outlines drug-specific signs and symptoms of substance abuse.

Differential. The differential diagnosis of substance abuse includes delirium and Axis I psychiatric disorders such as schizophrenia, MDD, bipolar depression, and anxiety disorders.

Workup. A complete history is necessary. The "CAGE" questions are a good screening test for identifying potential alcoholics. The evaluation of substance abuse and dependence should include a toxicology screen, CBC, electrolytes, LFTs, and a Breathalyzer or serum ethanol level. An elevated gamma-glutamyl

Identifying alcoholism—

CAGE

1. Have you ever felt the need to **C**ut down on your drinking?
2. Have you ever felt **A**nnoyed by criticism of your drinking?
3. Have you ever felt **G**uilty about drinking?
4. Have you ever had to take a morning **E**ye opener?

More than one "yes" answer makes alcoholism likely.

TABLE 7.4. Signs and Symptoms of Substance Abuse.

Drug	Intoxication	Withdrawal
Alcohol	Disinhibition, emotional lability, incoordination, slurred speech, ataxia, coma, blackouts (retrograde amnesia)	Tremor, tachycardia, hypertension, malaise, nausea, seizures, DTs, tremulousness, agitation, hallucinations
Opioids	CNS depression, nausea and vomiting, constipation, pupillary constriction, seizures, respiratory depression (overdose is life threatening)	Anxiety, insomnia, anorexia, sweating, fever, rhinorrhea, piloerection, nausea, stomach cramps, diarrhea
Amphetamines	Psychomotor agitation, impaired judgment, pupillary dilation, hypertension, tachycardia, euphoria, prolonged wakefulness and attention, cardiac arrhythmias, delusions, hallucinations, fever	Post-use "crash," including anxiety, lethargy, headache, stomach cramps, hunger, severe depression, dysphoric mood, fatigue, insomnia/hypersomnia
Cocaine	Euphoria, psychomotor agitation, impaired judgment, tachycardia, pupillary dilation, hypertension, hallucinations (including tactile), paranoid ideations, angina, and sudden cardiac death	Hypersomnolence, fatigue, depression, malaise, severe craving, suicidality
PCP	Belligerence, impulsiveness, fever, psychomotor agitation, vertical and horizontal nystagmus, tachycardia, ataxia, homicidality, psychosis, delirium	Recurrence of symptoms due to reabsorption from lipid stores; sudden onset of severe, random violence
LSD	Marked anxiety or depression, delusions, visual hallucinations, flashbacks	
Marijuana	Euphoria, anxiety, paranoid delusions, slowed sense of time, impaired judgment, social withdrawal, increased appetite, dry mouth, conjunctival injection, persecutory delusions, hallucinations, amotivational syndrome	
Barbiturates	Low safety margin, respiratory depression	Anxiety, seizures, delirium, life-threatening cardiovascular collapse
Benzodiazepines	Alcohol interactions, amnesia, ataxia, sleep, minor respiratory depression	Rebound anxiety, seizures, tremor, insomnia, hypertension, tachycardia
Caffeine	Restlessness, insomnia, diuresis, muscle twitching, cardiac arrhythmias	Headache, lethargy, depression, weight gain
Nicotine	Restlessness, insomnia, anxiety, arrhythmias	Irritability, headache, anxiety, weight gain, craving, tachycardia

Reprinted, with permission, from Le T et al. *First Aid for the USMLE Step 2*, 3rd ed. New York: McGraw-Hill, 2001:387.

TABLE 7.5. Management of Substance Intoxication.

Drug	Management
Hallucinogens (e.g., LSD)	If severe, benzodiazepines or traditional antipsychotics; otherwise, provide reassurance.
Cocaine/crack	Severe agitation is treated with haloperidol, benzodiazepines, antiemetics, antidiarrheals, and NSAIDs (for muscle cramps).
PCP	If severe, benzodiazepines; otherwise, provide reassurance.
Amphetamines	Same as with cocaine/crack.
Opioids	Naloxone/naltrexone block opioid receptors, reversing their effects. Beware of antagonist being cleared before opioid, particularly with longer-acting opioids such as methadone.

Reprinted, with permission, from Le T et al. *First Aid for the USMLE Step 2*, 3rd ed. New York: McGraw-Hill, 2001:387.

transferase (GGT) and mean corpuscular volume (MCV) suggest chronic alcohol abuse. Always offer HIV testing to substance abusers (especially IV drug abusers), as they often engage in high-risk behaviors.

Treatment. Treatment depends on the substance abused and the context in which it is used (see Table 7.5). The first goal is usually abstinence; treatment then targets the patient's physical, psychological, and social well-being. In other words, detoxification followed by rehabilitation is the model used to treat substance abuse. Treatment modalities vary widely because of the great variety of addictive substances.

The treatment of alcohol withdrawal includes the following:

- Rule out any medical complications (e.g., hepatic dysfunction, Wernicke's encephalopathy) by physical exam and laboratory tests.
- Start a benzodiazepine taper for withdrawal symptoms. Lorazepam, temazepam, or oxazepam should be used if the patient has liver dysfunction.
- Give multivitamins with thiamine (before glucose) and folate. Correct any electrolyte abnormalities.
- Check vital signs and give fluid replacement if necessary.
- For patients with an alcohol seizure history, give anticonvulsants and avoid neuroleptics, which decrease seizure threshold.
- Alcohol dependence can be treated with group therapy (Alcoholics Anonymous), disulfiram, and naltrexone.

Childhood and Adolescent Disorders

Childhood psychiatric disorders are complex, reflecting genetic as well as social factors. Many of these disorders are more common in boys, and they often coexist with other conditions. In addition, childhood disorders can persist into adulthood or parallel similar disorders in adults. In many cases, the combination of gender, maladaptive interactions between the child and the environment, and the unconscious or conscious prompting by parents can play a role in these disorders. Interviewing a child poses a unique dilemma; pictures, role playing, and storytelling are techniques used to facilitate the interview.

ATTENTION-DEFICIT HYPERACTIVITY DISORDER

Attention-deficit hyperactivity disorder (ADHD) is a disorder of inattention, hyperactivity, distractibility, and/or impulsivity that leads to significant impairment in academic and social function. It occurs almost nine times more often in boys than in girls. There is a genetic predisposition to this condition, so it is important to obtain a good family history when considering the diagnosis. ADHD generally presents in children between three and 13 years of age and typically manifests as poor performance in school. To make the diagnosis, at least some of the symptoms that cause impairment must have been present by age seven. Approximately one-third of patients will continue to have symptoms that require treatment as adults. Many children also have associated learning disabilities.

Signs and Symptoms. ADHD is classified as predominantly inattentive type, predominantly hyperactive-impulsive type (more common in boys), or combined type. Symptoms by subtype are as follows:

1. **Inattentive:**
   - Makes careless mistakes owing to inability to pay close attention to detail
   - Has difficulty maintaining attention in schoolwork or at play
   - Has difficulty listening even when spoken to directly
   - Fails to follow instructions or complete tasks or schoolwork
   - Has difficulty organizing tasks and activities
   - Avoids or dislikes tasks requiring concentration or sustained mental effort
   - Loses items necessary for completion of school tasks (e.g., pencils, paper, and books)
   - Is easily distracted by external stimuli
   - Is forgetful in daily activities
2. **Hyperactive/impulsive:**
   - Fidgety (e.g., squirms in seat)
   - Unexpectedly leaves desk in classroom
   - Runs about excessively in inappropriate situations
   - Has difficulty playing quietly
   - Is often "on the go" or acts as if "driven by a motor"
   - Talks excessively
   - Blurts out answers before questions have been completed
   - Has difficulty waiting his turn
   - Often interrupts or intrudes on others

Differential. The differential includes the following:

- **Psychiatric:** Learning disability, major depression, bipolar disorder, cyclothymic disorder, anxiety disorders, intermittent explosive disorder, and oppositional disorder.
- **Organic:** Head trauma.
- **Medications:** Bronchodilators and sedatives (sleeping pills may exhibit a paradoxic stimulant effect in children).
- **Normal active child.**

Workup. According to DSM-IV, the criteria for the diagnosis of ADHD include six or more of the above symptoms of inattention or six or more of the above symptoms of hyperactivity and impulsivity. These symptoms must be present before the age of seven and must cause clinically significant impairment in social and academic functioning. The signs and symptoms must be present for at least six months, cannot be accounted for by another Axis I disorder, and must be present in at least two spheres of the patient's life (e.g., school, home, and social life).

Treatment. First-line treatment for ADHD should be conservative and non-pharmacologic. The once-popular Feingold diet has been shown to be ineffective in the treatment of ADHD. Associated learning disabilities should be addressed along with maladaptive family behavior patterns. Behavioral modification techniques, such as holding children responsible for their behavior, are often useful and may be helpful in conjunction with pharmacotherapy. Pharmacologic treatment is used for cases in which impairment is significant and is not improved by conservative measures. It includes the following:

- **Psychostimulants:** Methylphenidate (Ritalin, Concerta), dextroamphetamine (Dexedrine), pemoline (Cylert), and dextroamphetamine + racemic amphetamine (Adderall)
- **Antidepressants:** Nortriptyline, imipramine, and bupropion
- **α_2-agonists:** Clonidine and guanfacine (better for hyperactivity/impulsivity symptoms than for inattention)

The adverse effects of stimulant medication include insomnia, decreased appetite, irritability, tachycardia, hypertension, exacerbation of tics, and reduced growth velocity. However, growth should return to normal when the medication is discontinued. Methylphenidate is a schedule II controlled substance with a significant potential for abuse, particularly by teenagers.

AUTISTIC DISORDER

Pervasive developmental disorders (PDDs) are severe, persistent impairments in developmental areas (e.g., communication, social interaction) or stereotypical, repetitive behaviors or interests. PDD encompasses multiple disorders, including autism, Asperger's syndrome, Rett's syndrome, and childhood disintegrative disorder.

Autistic disorder, like schizophrenia, involves a preoccupation with the internal world and generally presents with three hallmark features: deficiencies in communication, social interaction, and behavior. Autism has an incidence of 2–6/10,000 live births and frequently presents before the age of four. It is three to four times more common in males. Although autism was once attributed to a cold and distant mother, it is now believed that the disorder is organic in nature and that the emotional state of the parents is an adaptive response to the condition of the child. The etiology of autism remains largely unknown, although it has been associated with familial transmission, tuberous sclerosis, and fragile X syndrome. Nearly 75% of autistic children have comorbid mental retardation (MR), and approximately 25% have seizures.

Signs and Symptoms. Abnormal development is usually noted soon after birth. The first sign is often impaired social interaction, as the child fails to develop nonverbal communication skills such as a social smile. Later, the patient manifests an impaired ability or desire to create peer relationships and attach to parents and lacks the desire to show or share enjoyment. Communication deficiencies are marked and include impaired language development, inability to start or sustain a conversation, and use of repetitive or idiosyncratic language (e.g., echolalia, pronoun reversals, and abnormalities in speech quality). Finally, behavioral deficiencies are significant and are representative of the patient's fixation on the internal world to the exclusion of external reality. Patients may show ritualized behaviors (e.g., staring at the flushing toilet), stereotyped motor movements (e.g., body rocking), and preoccupation with a restricted interest or area of knowledge (e.g., sports trivia).

Differential. The differential includes the following:

- **Psychiatric:** MR, childhood psychosis, language disorders, OCD, Tourette's syndrome, and other pervasive developmental disorders (e.g., Rett's, Asperger's).
- **Organic:** Congenital deafness or blindness, congenital cytomegalovirus (CMV), hepatic encephalopathy, and fragile X.

Workup. All patients should receive a careful history, a complete MSE, monitoring of developmental milestones and delays, and evaluation of vision and hearing.

Treatment. This disorder is lifelong and, in most cases, prevents patients from living independently. A highly structured classroom setting helps patients learn communication and living skills, and behavioral management can help reduce stereotyped behaviors. Psychotherapy may be of benefit both to the parents and to the patient. Unless a comorbid disorder is present, medications are rarely useful. Neuroleptics may be given for aggressive and self-injurious behaviors, and anticonvulsants may be used for concurrent seizure disorder.

CONDUCT DISORDER

Conduct disorder is a repetitive and persistent pattern of inappropriate conduct for at least six months in which patients under 18 years of age ignore or violate the rights of others. Patients frequently have comorbid ADHD or learning disorders. The etiology is unknown, but it is likely that genetics and psychosocial elements (e.g., disrupted families, abuse, and delinquent peer groups) are involved.

Signs and Symptoms. Conduct disorder may be categorized as aggressive (e.g., violence, destruction, or theft) or nonaggressive (e.g., violation of rules, lying). Patients with this disorder may or may not form social bonds, but if they do, bonding with a loyal group often manifests in gang formation. Although similar, patients with oppositional defiant disorder do not show blatant disregard for the rights of others. Instead, such patients demonstrate disruptive, annoying behavior (e.g., loss of temper, defiance) in excess of that expected for their mental age.

Treatment. For both disorders, individual and family therapy is necessary to address emotional conflicts and sociocultural factors.

MENTAL RETARDATION

Mental retardation is intellectual functioning significantly below that expected for a child's developmental stage, with cognitive performance below the third percentile of the general population. MR has a prevalence of 1–2% and is two times more common in males than in females. There are many causes of MR, including genetic disorders, congenital infections, teratogens, and disease acquired after birth. Down syndrome and fragile X syndrome are common causes; the latter is the most common inheritable form of MR. Most children are born with physical malformations and fail to meet developmental milestones in a timely fashion. For diagnosis, a patient must have an IQ (defined as mental age divided by chronological age) ≤ 70, must have concurrent deficiencies in multiple areas of adaptive functioning (e.g., social skills, self-hygiene, and communication), and must have an onset of symptoms before the age of 18.

The differential diagnosis includes learning disorders, depression, seizure disorders, ADHD, and schizophrenia. Complete evaluation involves a physical exam that includes a neurologic exam, formal IQ testing, brain imaging, and an EEG if seizure disorder is suspected. There are various degrees of MR—mild, moderate, and severe—and management depends on severity (see Table 7.6). In general, patients with mild MR may be able to function in society and hold a job. Those with moderate MR should be able to perform activities of daily living and live in a group home. However, those with severe MR are unable to care for themselves and usually suffer a premature death.

LEARNING DISORDERS

Learning disorders are relatively common, affecting about 5% of school-aged children. Males are at a two- to fourfold greater risk than females. Diagnosis is

TABLE 7.6. Severity Levels of Mental Retardation.

Level of Retardation	IQ Score	Educational Potential
Mild	51–70	Educable
Moderate	36–50	Trainable
Severe	20–35	Limited
Profound	< 20	Very limited

usually made around the fourth or fifth grade. In comparison to MR, learning disorders are deficiencies in a particular area that place the child below the expected performance for his or her chronological age. There are three categories of learning disorders: reading, mathematics, and written expression. The differential diagnosis includes MR, communication disorders, ADHD, depression, anxiety disorders (e.g., school phobia), physical disorders (e.g., abnormal hearing or sight), cultural factors (e.g., language barriers), and poor teaching. Workup involves intelligence and subject-specific achievement testing. Management involves learning strategies to overcome deficits, academic remediation, and, if possible, teaching in environments that support patients.

Miscellaneous

ADJUSTMENT DISORDER

Adjustment disorder is a state in which emotional ideas and actions are the result of a particular stressor. The disorder must arise within three months of experiencing the stressor and, unless the stressor is chronic, must resolve within six months. To qualify as an adjustment disorder, Axis I or bereavement criteria must not be met.

ANOREXIA NERVOSA

Anorexia nervosa is an eating disorder with a prevalence of 0.5–1.0% of females and a female-to-male ratio of nearly 20:1. The peak ages of onset are ages 14 and 18, although the disorder has been diagnosed in much younger girls. The key feature of anorexia nervosa is a refusal to maintain a body weight over 85% of that expected for age and height. Patients also have a distorted body image (they perceive themselves, incorrectly, as fat) and an intense fear of gaining weight. They deny the potential medical consequences of starvation, and postmenarchal women develop amenorrhea (absence of three consecutive cycles) as a result of the disorder. Patterns of dieting include restricting (e.g., fasting, dieting, or exercising excessively) or engaging in binge-eating or purging behavior. Nearly two-thirds of patients have a history of an MDE. Mortality rates approach 10% for those patients who have been hospitalized for the disorder.

Signs and Symptoms. In addition to amenorrhea, patients exhibit involvement of all body systems, including lanugo (fine, soft body hair), scalp hair loss, peripheral edema, poor dentition, cold intolerance, lethargy or excessive energy, emaciation, bradycardia, hypotension, hypothermia, dry skin, electrolyte abnormalities (metabolic acidosis due to vomiting and/or metabolic alkalosis due to laxatives), leukopenia and anemia, diminished thyroid function, osteoporosis, encephalopathy, and hypercarotenemia. Psychologically, patients demonstrate decreased sexual activity, rigid personality, obsessive-compulsive features (e.g., counting calories), and a need to control the social environment.

Differential. The differential includes the following:

- **Psychiatric:** MDD, social phobia, OCD, bulimia nervosa, and body dysmorphic disorder.
- **Organic:** AIDS, malignancies, superior mesenteric ischemia (all of which cause vomiting or weight loss without a distorted body image), Addison's disease, diabetes mellitus, hyperthyroidism, and drug abuse.

Workup. Evaluation for eating disorders should include a complete H&P, height and weight measurements, CBC, serum albumin (decreased), electrolytes (hypocalcemia, hypokalemia, hyponatremia), endocrine tests, ECG, and a psychiatric evaluation.

Treatment. Early treatment involves monitoring caloric intake to stabilize weight and achieve weight gain. In severe cases, hospitalization may be required to restore nutritional status and/or to correct electrolyte imbalances. Later treatment includes individual, family, and/or group psychotherapy. SSRIs may help treat comorbid depression. Rapid refeeding can precipitate a refeeding syndrome.

BULIMIA NERVOSA

Bulimia nervosa has a prevalence of 1–3% in young females and 0.1–0.3% in males. It is characterized by recurrent episodes of binging (eating excessive amounts of food in a two-hour period) during which the patient feels a lack of self-control. Binge eating takes place rapidly and secretly. The patient then tries to compensate for the binge behaviors through vomiting, excessive exercise, or laxatives in order to prevent weight gain. Unlike patients with anorexia nervosa, bulimic patients maintain a normal or slightly elevated body weight despite their dysfunctional eating behaviors. Most patients have a history of dieting, and many have coexisting personality or impulse-control disorders.

Signs and Symptoms. Dental enamel erosion (from vomiting), enlarged parotid glands, scars on the dorsal surfaces of the hands (from inducing vomiting), menstrual irregularities, and electrolyte abnormalities (hypochloremic, hypokalemic metabolic alkalosis secondary to vomiting) are usually evident. Ipecac abuse can lead to cardiomyopathy.

Workup. To fulfill DSM-IV criteria, the binging and compensatory behavior must occur at least twice a week for three months. As is true with anorexic patients, bulimic patients' self-esteem is overly dependent on body weight, but bulimic patients tend to be more disturbed by and ashamed of their behavior. As a result, they often hide their behavior. However, they are more easily engaged in therapy.

Treatment. Psychotherapy and CBT are the most effective treatments and focus on behavior and body self-image modification. Antidepressants such as fluoxetine, imipramine, and desipramine are effective in both depressed and nondepressed patients.

SOMATOFORM AND RELATED DISORDERS

The principal characteristics of somatoform and related disorders are given in Table 7.7.

SUICIDALITY

Suicide is the eighth leading cause of death in the United States and is the second leading cause of death (after accidents) in people between the ages of 15 and 24. The incidence of suicide in America is increasing. In general, women are more likely to *attempt* suicide than men, but men are more likely to *complete* suicide. Men are also more likely to commit suicide by violent means such as firearms; women are more likely to commit suicide by drug ingestion. Although there are no signs or symptoms except for the act itself, certain risk factors predispose a person to commit suicide. Risk factors include a previous suicide attempt; male gender; increasing age; depression (depressed patients are 30 times more likely to commit suicide than the general population) or other psychiatric illness; recent recovery from suicidal depression (since patients have regained the energy to kill themselves) or recovery from a first episode of schizophrenia (since patients have developed insight); alcohol or substance abuse; the presence of rational thought or an organized plan; a family history of suicide; a recent severe stressor (e.g., bereavement, job loss, examinations); Protestant religion; chronic medical conditions or illnesses (e.g., terminal cancer, HIV); and divorced parents, unmarried status, and poor social support. Caucasians commit suicide more frequently than do African-Americans. Police officers and physicians are at an increased risk in comparison to the general population.

Workup. Ask the patient about a positive family history, a previous attempt, ambivalence about death, and feelings of hopelessness. Ask specifically about suicidal ideation, intent, and plan. Assess if the patient has an available means of committing suicide, and perform an MSE.

Treatment. Patients who express the desire to kill themselves, or who you believe may do so, require emergent inpatient hospitalization even if it is against their wishes. The actively suicidal patient needs intensive monitoring, close contact, and ongoing assessment. When the patient is stable, identification of

> **Suicide risk factors—**
>
> **SAD PERSONS**
> **S**ex (male)
> **A**ge
> **D**epression
> **P**revious attempt
> **E**thanol
> **R**ational thought
> **S**ickness
> **O**rganized plan
> **N**o spouse
> **S**ocial support lacking

Asking the patient about suicide will not plant the idea in the patient's head.

TABLE 7.7. Characteristics of Somatoform and Related Disorders.

Disorder	Characteristics
Somatization disorder	A history of many physical complaints beginning before age 30 and occurring over a period of several years. Individual symptoms must include four pain symptoms, two GI symptoms, one sexual symptom, and one pseudo-neurologic symptom. Symptoms cannot be explained by organic causes and are in excess of exam findings. Patients may have had multiple procedures or surgeries and often doctor-shop. Incidence is 5:1 female-to-male. Psychotherapy and regular, planned, brief primary care visits may be beneficial. Patients may have significant impairment in social, occupational, or other areas of functioning.
Conversion disorder	One or more neurologic complaints (e.g., paralysis, paresthesia, blindness, pseudoseizures) that cannot be explained by a medical disorder. Psychological factors must be associated with symptom onset in order for the diagnosis to be made. Patients often show a characteristic lack of concern ("la belle indifférence"). Conversion is most common in women, usually affecting adolescents and young adults. It can spontaneously remit, but anxiolytics may help. The symptoms are not intentionally produced or feigned.
Hypochondriasis	Preoccupation with and fear of having a serious disease resulting in significant psychological distress and/or impaired social or occupational functioning for more than six months. Based on misinterpretation of bodily symptoms. Men and women are equally affected. Onset is most common between the ages of 20 and 30. Group therapy and frequent reassurance from the physician are necessary for treatment.
Body dysmorphic disorder	Preoccupation with an imagined physical defect or abnormality (e.g., facial features, hair, body build) or, if a defect is present, excessive concern about that defect. The preoccupation must cause significant distress or impaired social and occupational functioning. Patients often present to dermatologists or plastic surgeons. Women are affected slightly more often than men, with an average onset at 15 to 20 years of age. May be associated with depression. Antidepressants such as SSRIs and clomipramine may be effective.
Malingering	This is not a somatoform disorder. It occurs when a patient intentionally feigns illness for secondary gain (e.g., financial compensation, avoiding work, or obtaining food or shelter). It differs from factitious disorder (defined below) in that what is sought is concrete and is usually related to material gain.
Factitious disorder (Munchausen syndrome)	This is not a somatoform disorder. It is the conscious simulation or creation of psychiatric or physical symptoms or illness for primary gain—in order to play the sick role and receive attention from medical personnel. It is most common in men and among health care personnel. Munchausen by proxy involves simulation of illness in another person, usually in a child by a parent.

KEY POINT

PRIMARY VS. SECONDARY GAIN

- **Primary gain:** Keeping unconscious psychological conflict outside of the patient's awareness (e.g., deriving psychological benefits from assuming the sick role)
- **Secondary gain:** Accruing obvious, tangible, external benefits from being sick (e.g., obtaining disability pay, avoiding jail time)

the underlying stressor or disorder is necessary, and appropriate treatment should be initiated. Patients frequently require intensive psychotherapy and inpatient hospitalization as well as antidepressant and antipsychotic medications. ECT may be used as a second-line treatment for an actively suicidal patient who is refractory to medications and psychotherapy. Severely depressed patients are often at greatest risk for suicide in the first few weeks after starting an antidepressant, as their energy may return before the depressed mood lifts.

HIGH-YIELD REFERENCES

MOOD DISORDERS

Major Depressive Disorder

Whooley MA, Simon GE. Managing depression in medical outpatients. *NEJM* 2000;343:1942–1950. An excellent, easy-to-read summary about the diagnosis (including suicide assessment) and treatment of depression. Includes excellent tables and flow chart.

Moore JD, Bona JR. Depression and dysthymia. *Med Clin North Am* 2001;85:631–644. A review of the diagnosis, pathophysiology, and treatment of depressive disorders. Also discusses management issues for special groups, including children, pregnant women, and the elderly.

Bipolar I Disorder

Keck PE et al. Bipolar disorder. *Med Clin North Am* 2001;85:645–661. An excellent review article that discusses subtypes within the bipolar spectrum, criteria for diagnosis, and currently available treatment options.

Maj M. Diagnosis and treatment of rapidly cycling bipolar disorder. *Eur Arch Psychiatry Clin Neurosci* 2001;251:Suppl. 2 II/62–II/65. Contrary to past belief that lithium was less effective than valproic acid for the treatment of rapid cycling bipolar disorder, this review shows recent evidence that lithium is actually an effective treatment.

Price LH, Heninger GR. Lithium in the treatment of mood disorders. *NEJM* 1994;331:591–598. An excellent paper summarizing the use of lithium in unipolar depression and bipolar disorder.

PSYCHOTIC DISORDERS

Schizophrenia

Goff DC et al. Schizophrenia. *Med Clin North Am* 2001;85:663–689. Review of the pathophysiology, diagnosis, and treatment of schizophrenia. Provides insight into the difficulty of treating the schizophrenic patient with comorbid conditions.

Tsuang MT et al. Towards reformulating the diagnosis of schizophrenia. *Am J*

Psychiatry 2000;157:1041–1050. An excellent overview of schizophrenia with a critical evaluation of DSM-IV diagnostic criteria. Also highlights the role of schizophrenia within the mood disorder spectrum.

ANXIETY DISORDERS

Generalized Anxiety Disorder

Gliatto MF. Generalized anxiety disorder. *Am Fam Physician* 2000;62: 1591–1600. A brief review of GAD.

Obsessive-Compulsive Disorder

Attiullah N et al. Clinical features of obsessive-compulsive disorder. *Psychiatr Clin North Am* 2000;23:469–491. A slightly long but comprehensive review of OCD.

Post-traumatic Stress Disorder

Yehuda R. Post-traumatic stress disorder. *NEJM* 2002;346:1081–1114. An excellent, brief review article about the epidemiology, pathophysiology, diagnosis, and treatment of PTSD in light of the September 11 tragedy.

SUBSTANCE ABUSE

McRae AL et al. Alcohol and substance abuse. *Med Clin North Am* 2001;85:779–801. An overview of the various drugs of abuse, associated symptoms of intoxication and withdrawal, and treatment options for individual substances.

CHILDHOOD AND ADOLESCENT DISORDERS

Attention-Deficit Hyperactivity Disorder

Smucker WD, Hedayat M. Evaluation and treatment of ADHD. *Am Fam Physician* 2001;64:817–830. A brief, easy-to-read review of the diagnosis and treatment of ADHD.

Herrerias CT et al. The child with ADHD: using the AAP Clinical Practice Guideline. *Am Fam Physician* 2001;63:1803–1810. A review article on the criteria for diagnosis of ADHD. Includes excellent flow charts.

Pervasive Developmental Disorders

Jankovic J. Tourette's syndrome. *NEJM* 2001;345:1184–1192. An overview of Tourette's syndrome that summarizes pathophysiology, diagnosis, and treatment and provides a comprehensive summary of associations with other psychiatric disorders (e.g., OCD and ADHD).

MISCELLANEOUS

Anorexia Nervosa and Bulimia Nervosa

Kreipe RE, Birndorf SA. Eating disorders in adolescents and young adults. *Med Clin North Am* 2000;84:1027–1049. An excellent overview of the various eating disorders, including diagnosis, management, impediments to treatment, and complications.

HANDBOOK/POCKETBOOK

Current Clinical Strategies: Psychiatry
Hahn

$12.95

Current Clinical Strategies, 2002 edition, 127 pages, ISBN 1929622023

A highly concise pocketbook designed for quick reference while on the wards. Contains DSM-IV diagnostic criteria, differential diagnoses, and updated treatment guidelines. An excellent psychopharmacology section at the end of the book contains tables comparing drugs and their side effects. Also included is a brief overview of the MSE and sample admitting orders for common psychiatric disorders. Good value for its size and price.

Kaplan & Sadock's Pocket Handbook of Clinical Psychiatry
Kaplan

$49.95

Lippincott Williams & Wilkins, 2001, 3rd edition, 479 pages, ISBN 0781725321

This staple quick-reference handbook discusses etiology, epidemiology, clinical features, and therapeutic measures in a well organized outline format. Contains up-to-date diagnostic criteria and treatment guidelines along with cross-references to its parent book, *Comprehensive Textbook of Psychiatry*. Useful tables and a general overview of the psychiatric examination are also included. Small print makes it difficult to read.

Practical Guide to the Care of the Psychiatric Patient
Goldberg

$36.95

Mosby, 1998, 2nd edition, 477 pages, ISBN 0815178921

A concise, easy-to-read, spiral-bound handbook patterned after the growing *Practical Care* series. Offers thorough coverage of all major psychiatric areas with DSM-IV criteria and numerous comparative charts and tables. Not comprehensive, but contains the basic information that a medical student needs. Also includes an interesting section on P-450 drug interactions. A drug formulary at the end of the book for commonly prescribed psychiatric medications includes some out-of-place drugs such as allopurinol, INH, and procainamide.

Psychiatry (House Officer Series)
Tomb

$29.95

Lippincott Williams & Wilkins, 1998, 6th edition, 291 pages, ISBN 0683306340

A compact pocketbook of commonly encountered psychiatric disorders, written in essay format with highlighted key words and phrases to help with rapid review. Contains good references for further in-depth study, a number of useful tables, and a color guide of psychiatric medications. A basic review book that is not comprehensive enough for primary study.

Manual of Psychiatric Therapeutics

$39.95

Shader

Little Brown and Company, 1994, 2nd edition, 378 pages, ISBN 0316782238

A spiral-bound pocketbook written in full text blocks, making it difficult to retrieve information. Provides concise reviews of basic definitions, the MSE, and drug treatments of major psychiatric disorders. Makes excellent use of tables. Targeted more toward psychiatric residents than toward junior medical students on their core rotations. An updated edition is due in August 2002.

On Call Psychiatry

$28.00

Bernstein

W. B. Saunders, 2001, 2nd edition, 308 pages, ISBN 0721692397

A compact guide with a format similar to that of the rest of the *On Call* series, addressing common problems the on-call physician will encounter in psychiatry. Not comprehensive enough for study, but reviews important concepts of clinical thinking. Geared more toward residents on call than toward medical students. Some sections are related less to psychiatry than to general inpatient care.

Quick Reference to the Diagnostic Criteria from DSM-IV-TR

$29.00

American Psychiatric Association

American Psychiatric Press, 2000, 4th edition, 496 pages, ISBN 0890420262

A pocketbook best used for review of diagnostic criteria rather than for general wards work or application to patient care. Offers comprehensive coverage of all DSM-IV-TR psychiatric diseases, but lacks a discussion of etiologies and therapies, thus negating its clinical usefulness. One should find the same diagnostic criteria for major disorders in other handbooks.

Psychiatric Pearls

$21.95

Lyness

F. A. Davis, 1997, 1st edition, 328 pages, ISBN 0803602804

A small pocketbook designed for medical students preparing for their psychiatric rotation. Key points are difficult to extract, as the book is written in essay form with few tables and other elements to highlight the text. Another reference is required for primary study for the rotation. A few highlighted "pearls" are provided.

Kaplan & Sadock's Concise Textbook of Clinical Psychiatry   **$39.95**

Kaplan

Lippincott Williams & Wilkins, 1996, 1st edition, 669 pages, ISBN 0683300091

An excellent, downsized version of *Kaplan's Synopsis* that retains all the clinical psychiatry you need to know minus the behavioral science. Based on DSM-IV and well organized with practical chapters on psychopharmacology and laboratory tests. A nice addition to the bookshelf of the non–psychiatry bound.

 Blueprints in Psychiatry   **$26.95**

Murphy

Blackwell Science, 2000, 2nd edition, 128 pages, ISBN 0632044888

A brief review text of psychiatry designed for shelf and USMLE Step 2 exams. Offers good coverage of high-yield topics with helpful tables. Short, compact, and easy to read within a few days. Lacks detail necessary for rounds and the clinical clerkship, but a great resource for rapid review. Limited discussion of psychopharmacology.

 BRS Psychiatry   **$29.95**

Shaner

Lippincott Williams & Wilkins, 2000, 2nd edition, 419 pages, ISBN 0683307665

A concise, easy-to-read, outline-format review book geared toward shelf and USMLE Step 2 exams. Covers a fairly comprehensive number of subjects for a psychiatry review book while highlighting the key points of each disorder, allowing for quick, focused learning. Questions are available after each chapter, and a comprehensive exam is given at the end of the book. More useful and readable than *NMS Psychiatry*.

 Psychiatry   **$36.00**

Cutler

W. B. Saunders, 1999, 1st edition, 351 pages, ISBN 072166721X

An excellent introductory text written at an appropriate level for medical students. Discusses all major psychiatric disorders with numerous clinical vignettes to illustrate how each disorder may present. Contains good quick-reference tables of DSM-IV criteria. Also includes chapters on the psychiatric interview, psychotherapy, and psychopharmacology.

B+ Clinical Psychiatry for Medical Students   **$39.95**

Stoudemire

Lippincott Williams & Wilkins, 1998, 3rd edition, 941 pages, ISBN 0397584601

A detailed review text for medical students that integrates biological, psychological, and sociological concepts into its discussion of psychiatric disease. Good tables and figures illustrate concepts. Discussions are lengthy but of interest to students considering a career in psychiatry. Would benefit from more information on general neurophysiologic processes within the brain, especially when the biological basis of psychiatric disease is discussed. Compare to *Concise Textbook of Clinical Psychiatry*.

DSM-IV-TR Casebook $48.95

Spitzer

American Psychiatric Press, 2001, 1st edition, 624 pages, ISBN 1585620599

This companion text to DSM-IV-TR consists of short clinical vignettes followed by a discussion of etiology, differentials, and treatment. Easy to read, but a long didactic tool for students interested in psychiatry. Geared more toward exam study than toward practical wards work. Useful as a supplement to a more comprehensive review book.

 Review of General Psychiatry $44.95

Goldman

McGraw-Hill, 2000, 5th edition, 583 pages, ISBN 0838584349

A lengthy but interesting introductory text for medical students interested in psychiatry. Includes a discussion of etiology, epidemiology, DSM-IV classification, differential diagnosis, and treatment modalities. Good clinical vignettes are interspersed throughout the text to help illustrate key principles. Another reference for specific drug therapy that includes drug dosing is needed to supplement this book for practical wards usage.

 Underground Clinical Vignettes: Psychiatry $24.95

Bhushan

Blackwell Science, 2002, 2nd edition, 53 pages, ISBN 0632045736

A well-organized review of clinical vignettes commonly encountered on shelf and USMLE Step 2 exams. Includes a focused, high-yield discussion of pathogenesis, epidemiology, management, complications, and associated diseases. Black-and-white images are included where relevant. Also contains several "mini-cases" in which only key facts related to each disease are presented. Offers a good discussion of differential diagnoses, but does not contain DSM-IV criteria. Overall, an entertaining, easy-to-use supplement for studying during your clinical rotation.

 NMS Psychiatry $32.00

Scully

Lippincott Williams & Wilkins, 2001, 4th edition, 320 pages, ISBN 0683307916

A highly detailed review book geared toward passing the shelf and USMLE Step 2 exams. Although comprehensive, its dull, dry outline form makes it difficult to read. Multiple-choice questions are located after each chapter and at the end of the book accompanied by lengthy explanations. Too detailed to be of use as a quick reference.

 Psychiatric Secrets $39.00

Jacobson

Lippincott Williams & Wilkins, 2000, 2nd edition, 500 pages, ISBN 1560534184

This book, written in the question-and-answer format typical of the *Secrets* series, offers detailed and clear explanations of important psychiatric concepts. Good for preparation for pimping sessions on rounds and for students interested in psychiatric trivia, but not a useful resource as a reference text. Can be interesting reading while waiting on the wards.

B **Psychiatry Recall** $28.00

Fadem

Lippincott Williams & Wilkins, 1997, 1st edition, 250 pages, ISBN 0683180045

Written in a quick question-and-answer format typical of the *Recall* series, this book reviews many high-yield facts that are covered on shelf and USMLE Step 2 exams. Lacks clinical vignettes, and some of the topics covered can be obscure while others are not given enough attention. Useful as a quick-review supplement for another more detailed text.

B⁻ **Clinical Psychopharmacology Made Ridiculously Simple** $13.95

Preston

MedMaster, 2001, 4th edition, 74 pages, ISBN 0940780445

A practical review of the pharmacologic treatment of psychiatric disease written with a patient-oriented perspective. Numerous algorithms are provided on when and how to treat a patient as well as on common errors to avoid and advice to give to patients. May be best suited for residents prescribing treatment. Includes limited discussion of mechanisms of action and adverse effects.

C⁺ **Psychiatry Made Ridiculously Simple** $12.95

Good

MedMaster, 1999, 3rd edition, 93 pages, ISBN 0940780224

A limited overview of psychiatry that is best read before the clinical clerkship. Its scant detail and superficial scope require that one find another reference text for a more in-depth review. Mnemonics and illustrations are entertaining but are not very useful.

C **Oklahoma Notes Psychiatry** $24.95

Shaffer

Springer-Verlag, 1996, 2nd edition, 249 pages, ISBN 0387946330

An outline-format review book geared toward the USMLE Step 2. Basic and incomplete; not useful for the wards.

Kaplan & Sadock's Synopsis of Psychiatry $75.00
Kaplan

Lippincott Williams & Wilkins, 1997, 8th edition, 1401 pages, ISBN 0683303309

A comprehensive reference text pared down from its parent version. Not a good exam review book, as it is too detailed for shelf and USMLE Step 2 study. Good tables, but occasionally difficult to find information on certain subjects. Good integration of information from basic science years and clinical years. A great reference for students going into psychiatry, although eventually you may want to consider the *Comprehensive Textbook* version during residency and practice. Compare with the *Concise Textbook* version for the amount of detail that you want.

Kaplan & Sadock's Comprehensive Textbook of Psychiatry $279.00
Kaplan

Lippincott William's & Wilkins, 1999, 7th edition, 3344 pages, ISBN 0683301284

The "gold standard" of psychiatric textbooks. Incredibly complete with interesting historical perspectives on psychiatric disease and treatment. Because of its size and hefty price, you should buy this only as a long-term investment if you know you are going to be a psychiatrist. Even then, you may wish to wait and consider its more compact alternatives, as the text may still be too detailed. Available as a two-volume set.

Current Psychiatric Diagnosis & Treatment in Psychiatry $54.95
Ebert

McGraw-Hill, 2000, 1st edition, 640 pages, ISBN 0838514626

A well-written text with a format consistent with that of the *Current* series. Offers a concise, easy-to-read reference with each discussion of a disease beginning with the corresponding DSM-IV diagnostic criteria. Includes a discussion of the psychological, biological, and sociological bases for disease. A good contender to *Kaplan & Sadock's Synopsis of Psychiatry*.

Psychiatry: Behavioral Science and Clinical Essentials $42.00
Kay

W. B. Saunders, 2000, 1st edition, 707 pages, ISBN 0721658466

A comprehensive review text that discusses the etiology, pathophysiology, clinical features, diagnosis (as per DSM-IV criteria), and treatment of major psychiatric disorders. Includes reviews of the fundamentals of neurobiology, genetics, sleep, and learning and memory. Long clinical vignettes are given at the end of each chapter. Overall, a good, detailed review text that is slightly less comprehensive than *Kaplan & Sadock's Synopsis of Psychiatry*.

DSM-IV-TR $57.95
American Psychiatric Association

American Psychiatric Press, 2000, 4th edition, 943 pages, ISBN 0890420254

A comprehensive reference for psychiatric diagnostic criteria. Includes all existing psychiatric diseases defined by the American Psychiatric Association. Lacks discussion of etiologic basis and treatment, detracting from its utility as a clinical resource. Not a worthwhile purchase unless you are considering psychiatry as a career.

TOP-RATED BOOKS

Textbook/Reference

HIGH-YIELD TOPICS

Psychiatry

Surgery

The general surgery rotation is among the most rigorous, challenging, and exhausting experiences to which students will be exposed in medical school. The large volume of clinical information that must be assimilated, the demands made on students' time and energy, and the accelerated pace of the work are generally considered to be unequaled among the core clerkships. Many students thus anticipate their surgery rotations with unbridled enthusiasm, extreme trepidation, or, more commonly, some combination of both. Your experiences in surgery, as with those of other services, will depend on your accumulation of knowledge, your performance of appropriate scut work, and your interactions with the clinical team, nursing staff, and ancillary personnel. Needless to say, the culture of surgery can color your experience and perceptions of the field, which is often described as regimented, hierarchical, unforgiving, and inverse-pyramidal (big and important at the top; small and abusable at the bottom). Most students, however, emerge from their surgery rotations with a vastly increased fund of knowledge, more confidence in their clinical skills, and, inevitably, a newfound appreciation for food and sleep.

WHAT IS THE ROTATION LIKE?

The surgery clerkship is designed to expose students to the principles of basic surgical management, including the evaluation of patients to determine the need for surgery; pre- and postoperative care; and hands-on experience in basic bedside procedures, sterile technique, and OR tasks (although such tasks are often limited to cutting sutures, retracting tissue, and suctioning). The structure of the rotation will vary from school to school, from hospital to hospital, and even from service to service at the same facility depending on the patient population served, the nature of the surgical illnesses managed, and the specific emphases of the attendings on a given service. As a rule, however, most core clerkships are structured to offer students inpatient and ambulatory experience in general surgery, with additional experience on a trauma/emergency service and, possibly, exposure to some of the surgical subspecialties, including otolaryngology, cardiothoracic, urology, orthopedics, neurosurgery, and plastic surgery. As with your other rotations, your experience in surgery will be heavily influenced by the team of residents and attendings with whom you work.

In addition to clinical experience on the surgery service, students often receive didactic instruction in the form of conferences and lectures on basic principles of patient management and surgical disease. These may include formal departmental grand rounds, weekly multidisciplinary conferences (e.g., gastroenterology, oncology), and lectures organized by the faculty for the students. You may also participate in weekly service conferences in which the house staff presents details of the patient census, operative and perioperative complications, and patient cases that illustrate interesting clinical issues. In addition to these didactic sessions, you may receive informal teaching sessions from the house staff as time permits. In what little time you have left over, of course, you will also be expected to read and assimilate as much material as possible throughout the course of your rotation.

HOW DO I DO WELL IN THIS ROTATION?

Your role on the surgery service will be a hodgepodge of scut work, reading, and simply being there with the team. The cardinal rule is that *you should always show up on time*. This may sound simple, but it is often difficult to remember where and when you were expected to meet with your team or attending, especially on postcall days. On the first day of the rotation, you should thus be sure to get the pager numbers of all the members of your team (keeping in mind that it is much more appropriate to page a sub-I or an intern to confirm the time and place for a meeting than to page your chief). Expect to stay late for evening rounds (unless excused by your chief), and make yourself visible to residents and attendings as often as possible without going overboard. Your residents may expect you to follow two to three patients closely and take primary responsibility for their management with direct supervision from the intern(s), or, alternatively, a "team approach" may be taken wherein the entire team shares responsibility for each patient (in which case you obviously won't be expected to know as much detail about every patient, but you may have more information to keep track of).

Work your butt off.

Work your butt off.

Work your butt off.

As is the case on most rotations, your primary role on surgery is that of "Highly Absorbent Information Sponge." Reading about perioperative care, the pathophysiology of surgical illness, the basics of trauma evaluation, and the like, will occupy a significant portion of your time, but necessarily so. The field of surgery is relevant to practitioners in all specialties, whether you want to go into primary care medicine, psychiatry, pathology, anesthesiology, or whatever.

It is wise to ask your attending or chief resident to sit down with you early in the clerkship in order to discuss the expectations they have for third-year students on their service. As stated above, you may be expected to participate in many intern-level tasks, which may include performing preoperative history and physicals (H&Ps) in clinic, checking labs and x-rays, following patients' intake and output (I/Os), taking out sutures and staples postoperatively, writing discharge paperwork, evaluating patients in the ER, placing and changing arterial and venous lines, assisting in the OR, writing medication orders, and giving presentations on rounds and in conferences. The balance of these activities will depend on your own initiative and on the demands of your service. Be willing to do a little extra scut work on other patients for some "quid pro quo" teaching from the interns; it will be well worth your while. You will discover that certain interns and residents are more "teaching friendly" than others; seek these individuals out. In general, you will have a successful surgery experience if you show interest, accept responsibility eagerly and fulfill it competently, make your interns' lives easier, laugh and smile a lot, follow your patients closely, be a team player, give crisp and succinct oral presentations, and make an extra effort to read and present interesting issues to the rest of the team. Do anything less and you will almost certainly pass the rotation but may get stepped on by overenthusiastic classmates or by solicitous sub-I's. Protect yourself by working hard. Hard work, after all, is what surgery is all about.

KEY POINT

TIPS FOR SUCCESS

The blueprint for survival and success on surgery focuses on several key factors:

- Enthusiasm
- Assertiveness
- Voracious reading
- Efficiency on rounds
- Efficiency at paperwork
- Efficiency in clinic
- Efficiency at eating
- Efficiency at sleeping
- Respect for authority
- Appropriate humility

WHO ARE THE PLAYERS?

Attendings. Every service is staffed by several attendings, each of whom has senior responsibility for the management of patients. Patients on the surgical service are either private patients followed by the attending in his or her private clinic or patients who were admitted to the service by the ward team (e.g., from the ER or from other services from which patients are referred for surgical management). In the latter cases, the attending who is "on call" for new admissions (i.e., for patients who are not admitted electively by their own attending physicians) will be responsible for patient management. The attendings on a given service will generally rotate call with one another on a weekly or monthly basis. Call is mostly from home, although some services, such as trauma, require that the attending be in-house.

The attending physicians bear ultimate responsibility for the perioperative management of their patients as well as for what takes place during the surgeries themselves. At most teaching institutions, much of the operating is done by the chief and senior residents under the guidance of the attending. The extent to which this is the case, however, depends on the nature of the service (i.e., on whether it is an elective general surgery service at a private hospital, a trauma surgery service at a county hospital, or a vascular service at a VA) as well as on the nature of the surgical disease and the complexity of the surgery. Simple procedures such as hernia repairs and appendectomies, for example, are frequently conducted by interns and junior residents, while complicated operations such as the Whipple procedure (pancreaticoduodenectomy for pancreatic cancer) are usually performed by the chief resident and attending. As a general rule, an attending is present for every surgery, although some procedures are done entirely by the residents under the attending's umbrella of guidance and responsibility.

Chief resident. If the attending acts as "chairman of the board" of the service, the chief resident functions as chief executive officer, assuming responsibility for the management of the entire service and for the day-to-day running of the ward team. All of the patients on the service are managed by the chief resident, regardless of their individual attendings. Hence, the chief resident must be aware of every important issue affecting each patient on the service, including lab and x-ray results, plans for wound/dressing/line care, plans for advancing patients' diets, and dispositions. Since each attending on a service may have specific preferences for certain management issues (e.g., staples out on day five, advance from NPO [nothing by mouth] to clear liquids versus soft diet), the chief must be well informed about these issues, as he or she must answer to the attendings if things go wrong.

Because culpability tends to roll downhill, it is in the best interests of all the residents and students to ensure that things function as smoothly as possible and that the chief is kept abreast of any problems that may arise. Chiefs spend most of their time in the OR, although they often have significant administrative and didactic responsibilities as well. They are generally in charge of arranging patient presentations for conferences and may schedule teaching sessions for the students on their service. They also arrange admissions and oversee consultations to other services. As a student, you may find that the chief resident has significant responsibility for your evaluation. The onus is therefore on you to ensure that your efforts do not go unnoticed by your chief.

Senior resident(s). On any given surgery service, there may be one or two senior residents (residents in their third or fourth clinical year) who assist the chief resident in the management of the service. Typically, the senior resident is responsible for running rounds in the morning and updating the service for the chief, since the chief may or may not walk on rounds with the team each morning. Also, when issues come up during the day that cannot easily be managed by the interns and junior residents, the senior resident may be called upon to assume responsibility, as the chief may be busy operating. Of course, senior residents do their fair share of operating as well, handling less complex cases such as bowel resections for cancer and mastectomies. You can expect to work more closely with your senior resident than with your chief on a daily basis. If this is the case, your senior(s) will play a critical role in your ultimate evaluation.

Interns and junior residents. These are the "scut monkeys" of the surgery service (as is the case on other services, although with surgery there is usually

Surgery fosters a more formal pecking order.

much more scut work to be done). Interns and second-year residents have responsibility for the minutiae of patient care (e.g., writing notes, checking labs, writing and dictating discharge summaries, checking wounds, and changing dressings). They respond to pages from the nursing staff when patients are crashing. They are harried, get little sleep, and often have no lives, so part of your job is to make their days easier.

Subinterns. Sub-I's include acting interns and fourth-year medical students. As a general rule, if there are sub-I's on your team, their goal will be to go into surgery. This means that sub-I's will be working hard to function at an intern level as well as to shine in the eyes of their chiefs and attendings. As a third-year student, you may be intimidated by the idea of working on a service with sub-I's and being compared to them. Bear in mind, however, that expectations of a third-year's performance differ from those of a sub-I. Also keep in mind that you are more than likely capable of performing most of the tasks that the sub-I's do; you're just on a steeper portion of the learning curve. A typical sub-I will be expected to take call on a schedule comparable to that of an intern (again, services vary in their expectations), will assume some responsibility for evaluating patients on consults or in the ER, will take on a fair amount of daily scut work, and will try to squeeze into the OR whenever possible. As acting interns, however, sub-I's should also assume some responsibility for the education of the service, particularly the third-year students. Use your sub-I's as a resource—they may have valuable advice to give you about performing well on surgery, not to mention more knowledge about surgical diseases.

HOW IS THE DAY SET UP?

Welcome to the 15-hour workday.

Typically, there are two to three OR days per week, during which the chief/senior residents and attendings will spend most of the day in surgery. Although some of the surgical cases may be simple outpatient "come-and-go" procedures such as breast biopsies and hernia repairs, most will be "come-and-stay" surgeries in which patients are admitted for postoperative care that lasts one to several days. The remainder of the work week will usually consist of clinic days on which new patients are seen for their referred problems, established patients are worked up for their preoperative evaluations, and postoperative patients are seen for follow-up. On both operative and clinic days, the entire inpatient service will need to be rounded on, and most teams will try to write all the progress notes on morning rounds before heading off to the OR or to clinic. This, of course, means that the workday starts especially early on a surgery service—usually anywhere from 5:00 to 6:00 AM. Here's the overall structure of a typical OR day on a general surgery service:

5:00–6:00 AM	Prerounds
6:00–7:30 AM	Morning rounds
7:30–8:00 AM	OR preoperative preparation of patients
8:00 AM–12:00 NOON	Surgery or work time
NOON–1:00 PM	Noon conference
1:00–6:00 PM	Surgery or work time
6:00–7:30 PM	"Afternoon" rounds
7:30 PM–?	Postrounds scut work

Note that the schedule given above is just a sample; times may vary depending on the number of patients on the service and the number and length of operative cases. On clinic days, the morning schedule is usually similar, as rounds must be completed before the start of clinic. The evening schedule may be lighter depending on whether clinic is scheduled in the afternoon and on how many patients need to be worked up or admitted for surgery the next day. On days in which there is not a great deal of scut work, the intern/residents on call that evening may offer to complete the work so that the rest of the team can leave for the day.

On operative days, the senior and chief residents will usually be tied up in the OR, so the responsibility for scut work, consults, and procedures will fall to the junior resident(s), intern(s), and students. You may thus find yourself shuttling around from the OR to the ward between cases to help the interns write orders, check labs, change dressings, see consults, get films read, and so on. Because your role in the OR is usually minimal, you may be expected to spend the bulk of your time doing scut work, especially if you are on a scut-heavy service with a high census (e.g., vascular surgery). In the OR, you may be able to participate in a case or may find yourself relegated to observing from outside the surgical field, depending on the attendings' and residents' preferences, your own interest in getting hands-on surgical experience, and the need for your help in taking care of patient issues on the floor. Overall, you should strive to create a balanced experience—one in which you spend enough time in the OR to understand sterile technique and get a basic handle on the issues of intraoperative care while devoting most of your time to helping residents take care of patients and reading relevant material.

WHAT DO I DO DURING PREROUNDS?

The daily tasks on a surgery service begin with prerounding. The team will expect you to preround on your patients (on average you will follow two to three patients; keep in mind that interns will also follow these patients in order to check your work, but you will have the responsibility to present them during rounds). On other services, the team may simply round as a group on every-

Balance your time between the OR and the wards.

WARD TIPS

Surgery

one and write the notes in transit from room to room. As a rule, each patient should be seen in the morning and the following information updated:

- **Basic information:** This includes diagnosis, surgical procedure, hospital day number, postoperative day number, antibiotic day number(s), and so on.
- **Events overnight:** Have there been any episodes of respiratory distress? Fever? Problems with pain management? Nausea or vomiting? Wound-site bleeding?
- **Subjective data:** How is the patient's pain control (on a scale of 1 to 10)? Has he/she passed gas or had a bowel movement? (This is relevant for postoperative feeding.) Is the patient tolerating POs?
- **Vitals:** This includes maximum and current temperature, blood pressure, HR, respiratory rate, O_2 saturation, and weight. Some chiefs may want the 24-hour ranges as well (use your discretion).
- **I/Os:** Record the total intake and output, and divide the input into PO intake (is the patient NPO, on clear liquids, or on solid food?) and IV fluids (type and rate of fluid repletion, boluses given). Divide output into urine output (including Foley status), stool output, emesis and nasogastric (NG) output, and output of indwelling drains.
- **Other data:** What kind and amount of pain medication is the patient getting? Is he/she on a patient-controlled analgesia (PCA) device or receiving boluses of pain meds from the nurses? What antibiotics is the patient on, and how many days remain in the regimen? Are any other significant medications being given (e.g., steroid taper, antiemetics, promotility agents)? Is the patient diabetic, and if so, how high has the blood glucose been running and how much insulin is the patient requiring?
- **Physical exam:** You should perform a focused, directed exam based on the patient's overall well-being and presenting problem. In general, all patients should receive a brief respiratory, cardiac, and abdominal exam in addition to a global assessment of mental status every morning. In addition, postop patients will require assessment of urinary status (look at the Foley bag), drain output, and wound healing. Look at the dressing/wound and ask yourself the following questions: Is there wound drainage? Purulent exudate? Excessive peri-incisional tenderness or erythema? Do the sutures or staples need to come out? Is there any sign of wound dehiscence?
- **Assessment/plan:** You should construct an assessment and plan for rounds even if it is incorrect. It shows that you have been thinking. Things to consider include diet, antibiotics, wound healing, and ultimate disposition.

KEY NOTES

After prerounds, you will need to complete brief SOAP progress notes on each patient. These will follow the typical format but will usually be significantly shorter on a surgery service, as seen below. Other types of chart notes you may encounter on the surgery rotation include the admission H&P, the operative note, the procedure note, and the postoperative check.

Admission H&P. If this is a preoperative H&P for an elective surgery, you should include a succinct history of present illness (HPI), a brief past medical history (PMH) with particular attention paid to illnesses that have significance for perioperative management (e.g., history of atrial fibrillation, chronic obstructive pulmonary disease [COPD], diabetes), and information on medications and allergies. Your exam should be comprehensive but should focus on the particular organ system in question (e.g., a thorough abdominal exam for GI cases and a detailed peripheral vascular exam for vascular cases) and should always include a rectal exam as well as a breast exam for women. In addition, the admit H&P should document that the attending/chief resident has discussed with the patient the risks, benefits, alternatives, and expectations of the surgical procedure, and that the patient understands these issues and grants consent.

SOAP note. This will serve as the daily progress note for each patient on the service unless they have been admitted or discharged that day, in which case a progress note is not necessary. SOAP notes should follow the following format:

SOAP Note

55 yo WM admitted for perforated peptic ulcer, HD#3, POD#2 s/p Graham patch, NPO, abx = Ancef D#1, Flagyl D#1, central line D#1.

S: Pt. ambulating, pain well controlled on PCA. c/o peri-incisional pain (3:10 this AM), no drainage. No flatus or bowel movements. Good use of incentive spirometer ($\uparrow$ 1500 cc). No other overnight issues.

O: VS T_m 38^3 / T_c 38^1 BP 110/63 P 86 R 16 O_2 sat 99% 2 L NC.

24 hr. I/O 2100/2000 (3000/2800—yesterday's I/O); UO 1500 (24 hr. total) = 2.3 cc/kg/hr.

$D_5$1/2 NS @ 80 cc/hr, JP output → 15 cc—12 hr. total. (If patient is in ICU, also document pulmonary artery catheter readings.)

PE: Gen: WD/WN male in NAD, A&O × 3.

CV: RRR, nl S1/S2, no M/R/G.

Chest: CTAB, no W/R/R, right chest tube suction intact with no air bubbles and moderate serosanguineous drainage.

Abd: Soft, NT/ND, hypoactive bowel sounds, no HSM, dressing C/D/I, staples intact, no induration/erythema.

Foley catheter in place; 300 cc of yellow fluid present in the Foley bag.

Labs:

136	101	14
4.2	22	0.9

< Hb/Hct 9.2/29 (10.1/30—i.e., yesterday's Hb/Hct)

A&O × 3 = Alert and oriented to person, place, and time

Abx = Antibiotics

C/D/I = Clean/dry/intact

c/o = Complains of

CTAB = Clear to auscultation bilaterally

Cx = Culture

D/C = Discontinue

HD = Hospital day

HSM = Hepatosplenomegaly

JP = Jackson-Pratt

M/R/G = Murmurs/rubs/gallops

NAD = No acute distress

NC = Nasal cannula

nl = Normal

NS = Normal saline

NT/ND = Nontender, nondistended

WARD TIPS

Surgery

N/V = Nausea, vomiting

OOB = Out of bed

POD = Postoperative day

RRR = Regular rate and rhythm

s/p = Status post

T_c = Current temperature

T_m = Maximum temperature

UO = Urine output

WD/WN = Well developed/well nourished

W/R/R = Wheezes/rhonchi/rales

CBD = Common bile duct

dx = Diagnosis

EBL = Estimated blood loss

GB = Gallbladder

GETA = General endotracheal anesthesia

IOC = Intraoperative cholangiogram

LR = Ringer's lactate

Wound Cx pending

CT scan, x-rays, etc.

A/P: 55 yo WM POD#2 s/p Graham patch for perforated peptic ulcer, doing well.

Low-grade temperature most likely secondary to atelectasis.

1. Continue antibiotic regimen.

2. Encourage OOB, ambulation, and incentive spirometry.

3. Consider D/C PCA; switch to oral analgesics.

4. Keep NPO for now; will advance to clear fluids when flatus passed.

5. D/C JP drain, D/C Foley.

Operative note. This is a note that is entered into the chart at the completion of a surgical procedure documenting the findings and events of the case. It is usually a brief summary and should include pertinent data regarding the participants, the pre- and postoperative diagnoses (which are usually the same but are sometimes different, particularly in exploratory cases), total fluid exchange, disposition, and any complications. A sample operative note is shown below.

Brief OP Note: Blue Surgery Team

Preop dx: Biliary colic.

Postop dx: Cholelithiasis.

Procedure: Laparoscopic cholecystectomy + intraoperative cholangiography.

Surgeons: Attending, resident (PGY-5), intern (PGY-1), med student (MS-3).

Anesthesia: GETA.

Fluids: 1400 cc LR.

Blood transfusions: None (no cell saver).

EBL: 200 cc.

Findings: Distended gallbladder with slightly thickened wall, multiple stones within GB, no CBD stones by IOC.

Specimens: GB to path (no cultures taken).

Drains: None.

Complications: None apparent.

Disposition: To recovery room in stable condition, awake and extubated.

Postoperative orders. Interns and sub-I's are normally responsible for writing postoperative orders. If you are comfortable writing postop orders, this is an area in which you can shine. A sample set of postoperative orders is shown below.

Postop Orders

Admit to: 3-West, General Surgery; attending: Dr. Jones; interns: Lee (x46789) & Smith (x97850); MS-3 Stone (x57689).

Diagnosis: Perforated peptic ulcer.

Condition: Stable.

Vitals: Per routine.

Allergies: NKDA.

Activity: As tolerated, OOB TID.

Nursing orders:

Strict I/Os.

DVT prophylaxis: Heparin 1000 units SC, SCDs.

Foley catheter to gravity.

Incentive spirometer 10 times/hr while awake.

Diet: NPO.

IV fluids: D5 1/2 NS + 20 KCl to run at 100 cc/hr.

Medications:

Abx: Cefotaxime 1 g IV q8 hours.

Analgesics: PCA.

(Do not forget to list all the patient's preoperative medications and prn medications.)

Studies: CXR in AM.

Labs: CBC, chem 7, UA in AM.

Call house officer if: HR > 100 or < 60; BP > 180/100 or < 90/60; RR > 25 or < 12; temp. > 39.5.

When considering the causes of fever in a postoperative patient, use the "5 Ws" mnemonic.

Postoperative check. Generally, patients will need to be seen two to four hours after surgery to be evaluated for immediate complications (e.g., hypotension, hemorrhage, dyspnea), adequacy of urine output, level of comfort, etc. A brief postoperative note—again in the standard SOAP format—should then be

---

Postoperative Fever Etiologies—

The "5 Ws"

Wind: atelectasis (the most common cause on the first postop day), pneumonia

Water: UTI

Wound: infection

Walking: pulmonary embolus arising from DVT

Wonder drug: drug fever due to meds such as aspirin

---

written. The subjective section of the note should primarily address the patient's postoperative pain control; the objective portion should include vital signs, intraoperative and postoperative blood loss and fluid intake, urinary output, wound drainage, appearance of the incision and dressings, postoperative lab results from the recovery room, and any significant abnormalities on physical exam. Always communicate abnormal findings and/or laboratory values to your team.

Don't forget to get and document informed consent.

Procedure note. Frequently, surgical patients will undergo other procedures, such as central line insertion, chest tube placement/removal, extubation, incision and drainage (I&D) of abscesses, thoracocentesis, paracentesis, lumbar puncture, and suturing of lacerations. When these are done as bedside procedures, they should be documented in the medical chart with an appropriate procedure note. The procedure note should follow the standard format. Remember to get informed consent and to document having done so in the chart.

KEY PROCEDURES

Because surgery is principally an intervention-oriented specialty, you should attempt to gain some hands-on experience with procedures that may be relevant to you in other specialties. These include suturing lacerations (including learning techniques of local anesthesia), knot tying and suture cutting, gowning and gloving in sterile fashion, arterial line placement, starting IVs, arterial blood gases (ABGs), paracentesis, thoracocentesis, chest tube placement, incision and drainage of abscesses, staple and suture removal, dressing changes, Foley catheterization, NG tube insertion, central venous cannulation, and drain pulling (see Tubes and Drains). You should also become familiar with the process of patient preparation and transfer to and from the operating suite. Surgical ties are best learned from a resident and then practiced at home. Of course, you'll get plenty of practice at retraction in the OR. Do not kill yourself trying to do all of these procedures, but make use of the opportunities that present themselves. Remember, if you fall in love with surgical procedures, you can always do a subinternship in your fourth year and go into surgery.

KEY POINT

TUBES AND DRAINS

- **JP drain:** Used to drain surgical wounds and keep bacteria and blood from building up; drains are usually attached to bulb suction. You will see the resident "strip" or milk these tubes, which means pulling along the length of the clear tube filled with blood to prevent clotting.
- **Penrose drain:** No suction—a yellow-colored tube used to drain large abscesses for cases in which a JP drain is ineffective.
- **NG tube:** A tube leading from the nasopharynx to the stomach; used preoperatively to drain the stomach of fluids (gastric decompression) and for the same purpose postoperatively. It can also be used for feeding when the patient's GI tract starts working after surgery.

- **G-tube or gastrostomy tube:** Goes from the stomach to the outside; resembles a permanent NG tube used for feeding patients with an obstruction above the stomach, or for decompression in patients with pyloric outlet obstruction. It is frequently used in older patients who are at risk for aspiration pneumonia from aspirating gastric contents.
- **J-tube or jejunostomy tube:** Primarily used for feeding.
- **GJ-tube/Moss tube:** Has two ports, which both enter the stomach; one stops there and the other goes to the jejunum. Acts like one G-tube and one J-tube.
- **T-tube:** A biliary tube shaped like a "T."

OPERATING ROOM ETIQUETTE

Interestingly enough, one of the most challenging (and often frustrating) concepts that a student must learn during his or her surgical ward rotations is the maintenance of a sterile field in the OR. This includes making sure you are not contaminating the operating field (or yourself) and staying out of the way of other team members in the OR (e.g., residents, scrub nurse, circulating nurse, x-ray technicians). Since you will probably be the least experienced member of the group, it is important to know some of the points of etiquette associated with working in the OR. These include the following:

- When you first enter the OR and before you scrub in, introduce yourself both to the OR circulating nurse and to the scrub nurse, and tell them that you will be scrubbing in on the case. Tell the circulating nurse what size gown and gloves you will need. If you don't know your glove size, follow this general guideline: size 6 = small; size 7 = medium; size 8 = large.
- Remember to double-glove to protect yourself against needlesticks. In double-gloving, many people prefer that the outer set of gloves be one-half size larger than the inner set so that they aren't too tight.
- Ask the circulating nurse or resident if he or she needs any help in moving or positioning the patient on the operating table or "prepping" the patient for surgery. In some hospitals, the nurses will prep the patient; in other facilities it may be up to you (ask your resident or sub-I prior to your first OR case).
- Before scrubbing, place your beeper on one of the nonsterile side tables with a piece of paper attached to it giving your name. This will not only allow the circulating nurse to return your pages but also help you find the beeper if you accidentally leave it in the OR after the case is over.
- Remember to take off any jewelry (e.g., rings, bracelets, watches) and put on your mask, cap, and safety eyewear before you start scrubbing.
- Although there is no specific rule on how long to scrub, a good rule of thumb is to scrub for five minutes prior to the first case of the day. For subsequent cases, be sure to scrub one to two minutes longer than your

The OR affords third-year students opportunities to perform certain procedures, such as insertion of Foley catheters and NG tubes.

attending so that he or she won't be able to criticize you for not scrubbing thoroughly enough.

- Offer to help with the draping of the patient after you are gowned. If no help is needed, quietly stand out of the way of others who are doing so.
- Do not reach over or pass any instrument unless you are specifically instructed to do so.
- When the surgeon is using the bovie (electrocautery device) to incise fat, muscle tissue, and fascia, use the suction device to suck up the smoke and noxious odor associated with it.
- When you return needles or blades back to the scrub nurse, always announce out loud the presence of any sharps on the field that are returned to the instrument tray (e.g., "needle down," "knife back"). It is also helpful to announce to the anesthesiologist when the initial incision is made so that he or she knows when the surgery has started and can document the time of incision. At the end of the case, ask the anesthesiologist for the estimated blood loss and how much fluid the patient received intraoperatively (this information is then recorded on the operative note).
- Try to make yourself helpful by paying attention to minor details such as providing adequate retraction, adjusting the overhead lights, and suctioning excess blood from the area of dissection. These measures will allow the surgeon to have good visualization of the operative field.
- Those of you who wear glasses should be aware that the easiest way to contaminate yourself is to accidentally adjust your glasses with your sterile glove. Work to avoid that habit in the OR.
- If you do end up contaminating your gown, glove, or sleeve, step out of the operating field and let the scrub nurse know so that he or she can replace the contaminated parts and help ensure that you do not end up contaminating anything else.

If you follow these basic principles of OR etiquette, you are likely to find your OR experience to be more enjoyable and less stressful. One last thing: Don't forget to carry a pen in the pocket of your scrubs so that you can write the operative note and postoperative orders when the case is complete.

HOW TO SUTURE LIKE A PRO

One way to get more out of your OR experience is to become proficient at suturing and surgical knot tying. Unfortunately, the only way to become proficient at these skills is to practice, practice, practice! The best way to sharpen your suturing technique is to go to the ER and obtain the following:

- **Sutures of different types and sizes:** The most common sutures with which to practice surgical knot tying are 3–0 silk suture ties. Ideally, however, you should try to become proficient in suturing with many different types of sutures, such as 5–0 nylon (most commonly used when suturing up the skin), 1–0 Vicryl (most commonly used when suturing up deep fascia and muscle layers), and 4–0 Vicryl (most commonly used when closing up the subcutaneous layer). It is also helpful to remember which sutures are absorbable (e.g., Vicryl, PDS, Dexon, chromic catgut) as opposed to nonabsorbable (e.g., nylon and silk); which are natural (e.g., silk, catgut) as opposed to synthetic (e.g., nylon, PDS); and which are monofilament (e.g., nylon) as opposed to braided (e.g., silk, Dexon, Vicryl).

- **A "laceration tray" from the ER:** Specific instruments you will need include a needle holder, a pair of pickups, and a pair of suture scissors. Laceration trays usually have many of these instruments in varying sizes.
- **A box of gloves:** Remember that when you are suturing on a patient, you should be double-gloved to protect against needlesticks. It would thus make sense to practice suturing and surgical knot tying with two sets of gloves on so that it won't prove to be too awkward when you work on a real patient.
- **A suture removal kit:** This should include a pair of forceps as well as a fine-pointed pair of scissors for taking out sutures.

The next step is to find a fourth-year medical student (e.g., a sub-I) or an intern (ideally one who is not very busy) who is willing to show you how to suture and tie surgical knots. The types of suture methods that you should learn include:

- Simple interrupted sutures (most commonly used to close up skin lacerations)
- Vertical mattress sutures (used to close skin that is under tension)
- Horizontal mattress sutures (also used to close skin that is under tension)
- "Buried" (subcutaneous) sutures
- Figure-of-eight sutures (used to tie off a bleeding vessel)
- Running sutures (used to quickly close deep fascial layers)

As for surgical knot tying, focus on learning how to tie surgical knots by the "instrument tie" and the two-handed free knot tie before progressing to the more advanced one-handed surgical knot tie. Good materials to practice suturing on include pigs' feet (for the classic diehard surgeon-to-be), orange peels, and two-sided sponges.

WHAT DO I CARRY IN MY POCKETS?

Like any rotation, surgery has its necessary gear. Unlike most residents, however, surgery residents try to carry little extraneous material with them, as they tend to shift rapidly from OR to clinic to ward to cafeteria and must therefore be as unencumbered as possible. As a student, you too are usually allowed to adopt this minimalist stance. This means not carrying around too many handbooks and not wearing a fanny pack laden with tuning forks, otoscopes, and the like. The main requirements for the surgery rotation include:

Checklist

❏ **White coat:** Always wear one on the first day. Find out if you're expected to wear it daily or just in clinic.

❏ **Stethoscope:** Essential on any rotation. However, beware of the fact that many surgeons frown on wearing the stethoscope as a necklace ("dog collar"), as this is a sign of an internal medicine resident. To be safe, carry your stethoscope in the pocket of your white coat.

❏ **Penlight:** Critical for its common uses (checking pupils) and for examining wounds and the like.

❏ **Trauma scissors:** "Trauma scissors" or surgical shears are a pair of heavy-duty scissors that are used primarily to cut through a patient's clothing during an acute trauma situation or to cut through bulky dressings on rounds. These handy, all-purpose scissors will prove useful during both your general surgery and inpatient OB/GYN rotations. To score points with your chief/senior resident, cut your patients' dressings open when you preround so they are easy and quick to remove on rounds.

❏ **Index cards/clipboard/patient data sheets:** You will need something portable to manage the information (e.g., lab data) on each patient. Figure out which method works most effectively and efficiently for you, and then stick with it and abandon extraneous gear. Keep in mind that clipboards can and often do get lost.

❏ **Drug guide:** A must-have throughout your medical training (until you get to the level where you don't have to look up drug doses—which won't come for several years).

❏ **Antimicrobial guide:** *Sanford's Guide to Antimicrobial Therapy* is an excellent pocket resource for bacterial susceptibilities and drug dosing for common scenarios.

❏ **Surgery handbook:** There are a number of useful, concise pocket guidebooks for surgery students and residents. It is advisable to spend some time evaluating these books before purchasing one, as they differ markedly in style and organization (but are mostly consistent in content). Some of the more popular handbooks are reviewed in this chapter.

You should probably purchase the above items if you don't already own them. Most will come in handy for other rotations, and a good pocket handbook is great to have as a quick reference before conferences or teaching (pimping) rounds. Sometimes it is also helpful to carry spare gauze (Kerlix rolls and 4 × 4 cotton gauze pads), surgical tape, and other wound care accessories for rapid dispensing at the request of your chief resident on rounds. Many students use a bucket or tray stocked full of the items the team may conceivably need for wound checks and dressing changes on morning rounds.

ROTATION OBJECTIVES

The third-year surgery clerkship often involves time not only in general surgery but also in some of the surgical specialties. The following three questions can help you focus on the specific topics at hand:

- What is the natural history and appropriate evaluation of the present surgical problem?
- How do surgeons make the decision to intervene and prioritize the various therapeutic options?
- How do surgeons evaluate the risks and benefits of those therapeutic options in the context of a patient's problems, overall status, and life expectancy?

Given these considerations, the following list outlines common diseases and key topics that you are likely to encounter in the course of your surgery rotation. Disease entities further discussed in this chapter are listed in italics.

Gastroenterology

- *Acute abdomen*
- *Appendicitis*
- *Biliary disease (cholelithiasis and biliary colic, acute cholecystitis, choledocholithiasis, acute cholangitis)*
- *GI bleeding (upper vs. lower GI)*
- *Hernias (inguinal, femoral, hiatal, other)*
- *Inflammatory bowel disease (Crohn's disease, ulcerative colitis)*
- Liver disease (portal hypertension [see Chapter 3, Internal Medicine], hepatocellular carcinoma, liver metastases)
- *Diseases of the lower GI tract* (volvulus, intussusception, *diverticular disease [diverticulosis, diverticulitis]*, polyps, *colorectal cancer*, colitis, constipation, hemorrhoids, fistulas, fissures)
- *Diseases of the upper GI tract* (achalasia, gastroesophageal reflux [see Chapter 3, Internal Medicine], peptic ulcer disease [see Chapter 3, Internal Medicine], gastritis, gastric cancer, gastroenteritis, *small bowel obstruction*)
- *Diseases of the pancreas* (*acute pancreatitis, chronic pancreatitis*, pancreatic pseudocysts, *pancreatic cancer*)
- Splenic rupture, ascites

Breast

- *Breast cancer*
- Other breast disorders (fibrocystic disease, fibroadenoma)

Cardiothoracic Surgery

- Coronary artery disease
- Congenital and valvular heart disease
- Lung cancer (see Chapter 3, Internal Medicine)

- Pulmonary emboli (see Chapter 3, Internal Medicine)
- Potentially life-threatening injuries and their treatment (pneumothorax, tamponade [see Chapter 3, Internal Medicine], etc.)

Otolaryngology
- Head and neck tumors
- Hyperthyroidism
- Hyperparathyroidism

Urology/Nephrology
- Incontinence
- Benign prostatic hypertrophy
- Prostatic cancer
- Renal and ureteral stones

Vascular Surgery
- *Abdominal aortic aneurysm*
- Carotid vascular disease, diabetic vascular disease
- *Peripheral vascular disease, acute arterial occlusion*, deep venous thrombosis, varicose veins, lymphedema

Other
- Anesthesiology (intubation)
- Burns
- Fluids and acid-base balance (also see Chapter 2)
- Wound healing/surgical infection
- Trauma and shock (see Chapter 2, Practical Information for All Clerkships)

Gastroenterology

ACUTE ABDOMEN

The workup of a patient with an acute abdomen is one of the most interesting diagnostic challenges you will face and is a key component of the surgical rotation. Early diagnosis of the acute abdomen is critical, as many of the disease processes involved require early intervention if one is to prevent significant morbidity and mortality.

Signs and Symptoms. The differential diagnosis of the acute abdomen is usually made after the following history has been assessed:

- Onset, duration, and progression of pain (e.g., maximal at onset, intermittent, constant, worsening)
- The location and distribution of pain at onset and at presentation
- The nature of the pain (burning, cramping, sharp, aching)
- Aggravating and mitigating factors

- Associated nausea, vomiting, anorexia, or change in bowel function
- Associated hematemesis, hematochezia, or melena
- Associated gynecologic complaints and last menstrual period
- Any similar episodes in the past
- Underlying metabolic or endocrine disease processes (e.g., diabetes, Addison's disease, porphyria)
- Other past medical history (e.g., coronary artery disease [CAD], heart failure, abdominal surgery, hernias, gallstones, EtOH-abuse, peptic ulcer disease [PUD])
- Current and past medications

The physical exam is indispensable in making the diagnosis of acute abdomen. Pertinent aspects of the exam include the following:

- Begin with general observation. How ill is the patient? Is he or she writhing in pain? Lying motionless in the fetal position?
- Evaluate vital signs for hypotension, fever, tachycardia, tachypnea, inflammation, and/or sepsis.
- On abdominal exam:
  - **Inspect:** Look for distention, symmetry, scars, trauma, and obesity. Ask the patient to point to the location of maximal pain.
  - **Auscultate:** Absent or hypoactive bowel sounds may mean ileus (remember that you must listen for three full minutes to make this diagnosis). Listen for high-pitched sounds or tinkles (obstruction) and bruits (aneurysm).
  - **Palpate:** Start at the quadrant farthest from maximal pain. First touch lightly, and then gradually increase to deep palpation. Assess for tenderness to palpation, rebound tenderness, referred pain, guarding (voluntary or involuntary), masses, and hernia (inguinal, femoral, incisional).
  - **Percuss:** Shifting dullness or a fluid wave indicates ascites. Percuss the liver and spleen to assess for hepatosplenomegaly.
- Assess the patient for flank tenderness (indicative of renal inflammation or a retrocecal appendix).
- Perform a rectal exam for occult blood, mass lesions, tenderness, sphincter tone, and the presence or absence of stool in the rectal vault.
- Perform a pelvic exam to check for adnexal tenderness, masses, cervical discharge, cervical motion tenderness, and uterine size and consistency.
- Assess the patient for additional findings suggestive of jaundice, urinary tract abnormalities, and dehydration (dry mucous membranes, sunken eyes, tenting of the skin).

Differential. Because the differential diagnosis for acute abdomen is broad, it is useful to categorize the etiologies according to abdominal quadrants. Although these disease processes may present atypically in terms of the location and nature of abdominal complaints, Figure 8.1 provides a rough guide to formulating your differential (see also Figure 8.2).

All female patients with an acute abdomen need a pelvic exam and a pregnancy test to rule out pelvic inflammatory disease (PID), ectopic pregnancy, ovarian torsion, etc.

An excellent review of the workup and basic management of the acute abdomen is Cope's Early Diagnosis of the Acute Abdomen.

Right upper quadrant (RUQ)	Left upper quadrant (LUQ)
Acute cholecystitis/biliary colic	Acute pancreatitis
PUD	Perforated viscus
Gastritis	Myocardial infarction
Cholangitis	Splenic rupture/infarction
Hepatitis	Gastroesophageal reflux disease
Pneumonia	(GERD)/gastritis
	PUD

Epigastrium

GERD	Pancreatitis (acute/chronic)
PUD	Angina, myocardial infarction
Gastroenteritis	Perforated viscus
Esophagitis	Abdominal aortic aneurysm (AAA)
Gastritis	

Right lower quadrant (RLQ)	Left lower quadrant (LLQ)
Acute appendicitis	Diverticulitis
Inflammatory bowel disease (IBD)	Sigmoid volvulus
Meckel's diverticulum	Colorectal cancer
Acute cholecystitis	Mesenteric ischemia
Pyelonephritis, nephrolithiasis	Colitis
Diverticulitis	Pyelonephritis, nephrolithiasis
Ovarian torsion, cyst, ruptured	Ovarian torsion, cyst, ruptured
ectopic pregnancy, PID	ectopic pregnancy, PID
Intussusception	
Colon cancer	

FIGURE 8.1. Quick differential of acute abdomen by quadrant.

Additional disorders to consider in the differential diagnosis of acute abdomen, which are often difficult to localize, include small bowel obstruction (SBO), paralytic ileus, diabetic ketoacidosis, addisonian crisis, acute intermittent porphyria, uremic crisis, sickle cell crisis, toxins (lead, venom), pericarditis, obstructive uropathy, and ischemic bowel disease.

Workup. The standard initial workup includes CBC with differential; chem-7; liver function tests (LFTs); amylase; lipase; kidneys, ureters, and bladder (KUB); and urine pregnancy test in women. Further workup is driven by the history, physical exam findings, and symptoms.

Treatment. The key to managing an acute abdomen is to determine through the H&P whether the condition represents a surgical abdomen (i.e., an abdomen in need of emergent surgical treatment) or whether it can be treated with expectant management. For unstable patients in whom a surgically correctable or identifiable cause is suspected, exploratory laparotomy is the appropriate management. Mainstays of expectant management include the following:

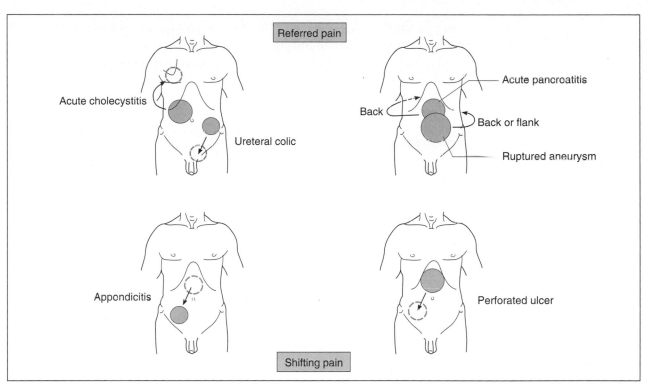

FIGURE 8.2. Referred pain and shifting pain in the acute abdomen. Solid circles indicate the site of maximum pain; broken lines indicate sites of lesser pain. (Reprinted, with permission, from Way L, Doherty G. *Current Surgical Diagnosis & Treatment,* 11th ed. New York: McGraw-Hill, 2003.)

- NPO
- NG suction in cases of nausea and vomiting, hematemesis, or suspected GI tract obstruction
- Aggressive IV fluid hydration and correction of electrolyte abnormalities
- Monitoring of vital signs with telemetry or frequent manual measurements
- Serial abdominal exams to evaluate the patient for the progression or resolution of peritonitis
- Foley catheterization to evaluate fluid status and response to rehydration therapy
- Serial laboratory exams, including CBC and electrolytes

APPENDICITIS

Acute appendicitis should *always* be near the top of your differential diagnosis for an acute abdomen (approximately 7% of people in the United States will develop appendicitis at some point in their lifetime). The incidence peaks in the teens to the mid-20s. Keep in mind that appendicitis is more likely to present atypically and to progress to perforation in young children and the elderly than in the general population (as many as 75% of elderly pa-

In cases of abdominal pain, acute appendicitis must always be in the differential.

tients perforate). Appendicitis may also present atypically in patients with retrocecal appendices or during pregnancy. If untreated, appendicitis can progress to perforation (which carries a 5% mortality rate), peritonitis, or abscess formation.

Etiology. Luminal obstruction of the appendix may be caused by hyperplasia of lymphoid tissue (55–65%), a fecalith (35%), a foreign body such as food, a carcinoid tumor, or a parasite. This results in accumulation of fluid and mucus behind the obstruction, distention of the appendix, inflammation, and, in many cases, secondary bacterial overgrowth. As this process continues, overdistention of the appendix can result in high intraluminal pressure, compression of the capillary blood supply, and resulting appendiceal ischemia. The inflammatory process may also become contained by the omentum or peritoneum, resulting in a periappendiceal abscess. Both can result in perforation of the appendix with subsequent peritonitis due to leaked intestinal contents. The mainstay of treatment for acute appendicitis is early diagnosis and operative intervention before perforation has occurred.

Signs and Symptoms. A classic description of the progression of acute appendicitis is as follows:

- Pain begins around the umbilicus as a dull, vague discomfort and may last anywhere from one to twelve hours. The pain is caused by irritation of visceral peritoneum due to stretching/distention of the appendix.
- Nausea, vomiting, and anorexia follow the pain. Hunger is rare in these patients, and its absence is known as a positive "hamburger sign" (meaning that patients have no desire to eat a hamburger).
- Pain may wane slightly for a brief period, and a low-grade fever may be seen.
- Pain then localizes to the RLQ at McBurney's point (two-thirds of the distance from the umbilicus to the right anterior superior iliac spine). Pain is now sharper owing to the irritation of parietal peritoneum from the progressively distended appendix.
- If perforation occurs, there may be a transient decrease in the pain. Ultimately, diffuse tenderness develops (maximal at McBurney's point) along with rebound, guarding, high fever, hypotension, and a high WBC count. The patient is most comfortable lying completely still and may report pain on the drive to the ER as a result of "bumps" in the road.
- **Rovsing's sign:** Referred pain in the RLQ is elicited by deep palpation in the LLQ. This sign is specific but fairly insensitive.
- **Psoas sign:** RLQ pain is elicited by passive extension of the hip (this is caused by stretching the iliopsoas tendon, which overlies the appendix). This sign is not sensitive (see Figure 8.3).
- **Obturator sign:** RLQ pain is elicited by passive internal rotation of the hip. This sign is also insensitive (see Figure 8.3).
- A palpable RLQ mass may indicate an abscess.
- Rectal exam generally elicits pain on right side.

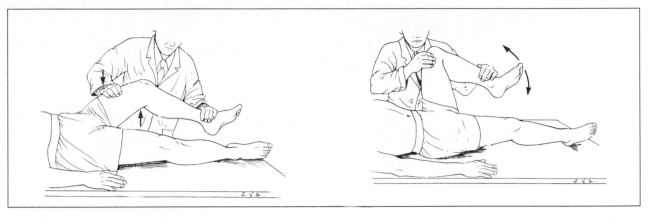

FIGURE 8.3. Psoas test and obturator test. (Reprinted, with permission, from Saunders CE, Ho MT. *Current Emergency Diagnosis & Treatment,* 4th ed. Stamford, CT: Appleton & Lange, 1992:114.)

Differential. The differential should include the following:

- Gastroenteritis (nausea and vomiting are reported *before* the pain, the pain is poorly localized, and there is no leukocytosis)
- Intussusception (seen mainly in patients under the age of two)
- IBD
- Gynecologic disorders such as PID (cervical motion tenderness, discharge, bilateral lower abdominal tenderness, high fever), ovarian cyst torsion, ectopic pregnancy, and mittelschmerz (due to a ruptured ovarian follicle in the middle of the menstrual cycle)
- Testicular torsion, epididymitis
- Diverticulitis
- SBO
- Mesenteric ischemia
- AAA
- Pancreatitis (atypical presentation)
- Acute cholecystitis (atypical presentation)
- Perforated peptic ulcer
- Pyelonephritis, nephrolithiasis
- Diabetic ketoacidosis

Workup. The diagnosis of acute appendicitis is based largely on the H&P. Laboratory and radiographic findings may be of some use in confirming the diagnosis, but their absence does not rule out appendicitis. Laboratory and radiographic findings include the following:

- Mild leukocytosis (11,000–15,000) with a left shift (> 75% PMNs is seen in 75% of patients). Keep in mind that leukocytosis is often present with gastroenteritis.
- UA may show a few RBCs or WBCs.
- KUB is often not helpful, although it may demonstrate a fecalith, an absent bowel gas pattern in the RLQ, a loss of the psoas shadow, and/or free air (indicative of perforation).

- Abdominal CT may be useful in establishing a diagnosis of appendiceal abscess.
- Ultrasound is useful in female patients owing to its ability to rule out gynecologic abnormalities. It can also detect an enlarged appendix or an appendiceal abscess.

Patients in whom appendicitis is strongly suspected should be taken to the OR immediately for exploratory laparotomy and appendectomy.

Treatment. The treatment of acute appendicitis is early appendectomy along with the institution of NPO status, IV fluids, and NG suction if indicated. In simple acute appendicitis, patients are treated with antibiotics for 24 hours. In cases of perforation, antibiotics are often continued until the patient is afebrile and the WBC count normalizes. Open appendectomy via RLQ incision has been the standard for many years, but laparoscopic procedures are becoming more common because of the benefits of shorter hospital stays and decreased postoperative complication rates. Laparoscopy confers the additional advantage of allowing definitive diagnosis to rule out gynecologic diseases or other processes before the appendix is removed ("diagnostic laparoscopy"). Normal appendices are removed approximately 15–20% of the time (this rate is higher in women owing to gynecologic disease), and this is considered acceptable by virtue of the life-threatening potential of this disease. As diagnostic accuracy continues to improve, this proportion will decrease.

Treatment of a walled-off periappendiceal abscess often consists of conservative therapy that includes broad-spectrum antibiotics along with ultrasound- or CT-guided percutaneous abscess drainage. An elective "interval" appendectomy should then be performed approximately six to eight weeks after the acute episode has resolved.

BILIARY DISEASE

The four major disease processes to be aware of in the biliary system (see Figure 8.4) are:

- **Cholelithiasis and biliary colic:** Transient obstruction of the cystic duct without acute inflammation or infection, resulting in recurrent bouts of postprandial abdominal pain.
- **Acute cholecystitis:** Acute inflammation of the gallbladder caused by stone impaction in the cystic duct. This may be accompanied by sepsis, gallbladder necrosis, or abscess formation.
- **Choledocholithiasis:** The presence of gallstones in the common bile duct produces symptoms of cholangitis, pancreatitis, biliary colic, and/or jaundice.
- **Acute cholangitis:** This is a potentially life-threatening infection caused by gallstone or biliary sludge blockage of the common bile duct, and can lead to severe septic shock without early intervention.

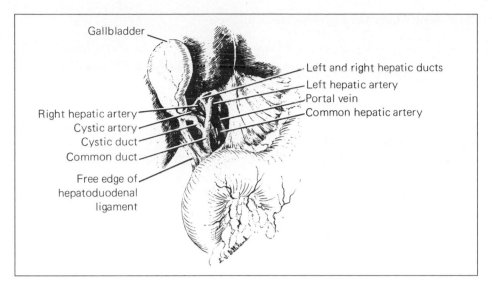

FIGURE 8.4. Anatomy of the gallbladder. (Reprinted, with permission, from Way L, Doherty G. *Current Surgical Diagnosis & Treatment,* 11th ed. New York: McGraw-Hill, 2003.)

Cholelithiasis and Biliary Colic

Gallstones may be asymptomatic in up to 80% of patients. When symptoms are present, they result from transient cystic duct blockage due to impacted stones. Risk factors for cholelithiasis include the classic "5 Fs"—**F**emale, **F**orty, **F**ertile, **F**at, and **F**latulent—along with oral contraceptive (OCP) use, rapid weight loss, total parenteral nutrition (TPN), advanced age, cirrhosis, infection, chronic hemolysis, Native American heritage, hyperlipidemia, and somatostatin therapy.

Signs and Symptoms. Signs and symptoms of gallstones include the following:

- Postprandial abdominal pain (usually in the RUQ) radiating to the right subscapular area or epigastrium. The pain is typically abrupt in onset with gradual relief.
- Nausea and vomiting are commonly seen.
- Fatty food intolerance, dyspepsia, and flatulence are also common.
- The patient may have RUQ tenderness and a palpable gallbladder.
- Patients generally do not present with fever or peritoneal signs.

Differential. Acute cholecystitis, PUD, acute pancreatitis, GERD, MI, and hepatitis must be considered.

Workup

- RUQ ultrasound may show gallstones (this imaging modality is 95% sensitive).
- ECG and CXR are performed in order to rule out cardiopulmonary processes.
- In certain cases, it is worth considering an upper GI series to rule out hiatal hernia or ulcer.

Treatment. Treatment options are as follows:

- Dietary modification (avoid triggering substances like fatty foods).
- Pharmacologic dissolution of cholesterol stones with ursodiol (Actigall), which desaturates the bile, impairing cholesterol nidus formation. This drug is effective in only approximately 50% of patients, and there is frequent recurrence.
- Lithotripsy uses extracorporeal shock waves to break up stones and is followed by dissolution therapy of the small fragments.
- Cholecystectomy (usually laparoscopic) represents definitive and curative therapy.

ESSENTIALS OF GALLSTONES

- Stone formation requires (1) imbalance of the ratio of cholesterol/lecithin/bile salts, (2) a nucleating nidus, and (3) stasis.
- Cholesterol stones constitute 75% of all stones, are radiolucent, and arise when bile becomes supersaturated with cholesterol, leading to cholesterol precipitation.
- Pigmented stones make up 25% of all stones and are radiopaque; black stones contain calcium bilirubinate and are caused by hyperbilirubinemia due to chronic hemolysis or cirrhosis. Brown stones are associated with biliary tract infection and may have gram-negative bacteria in their core.
- Only 15% of gallstones are visible on KUB.

Acute Cholecystitis

Acute cholecystitis is an inflammation of the gallbladder caused by prolonged blockage of the cystic duct, typically by an impacted stone (cholelithiasis). The obstruction results in distention, inflammation, infection, and, in extreme cases, gangrene of the gallbladder. Some cases of acute cholecystitis occur in the absence of cholelithiasis. This condition, known as acalculous cholecystitis, is often seen in chronically debilitated patients, in patients receiving TPN, and in trauma or burn victims.

Signs and Symptoms. Patients present with nausea, vomiting, and RUQ pain that is similar to that of biliary colic but is more severe, is of longer duration, and is often associated with guarding and/or rebound tenderness. Patients will often have fever as well as Murphy's sign—i.e., inspiratory arrest during deep palpation of the RUQ due to gallbladder inflammation (a positive Murphy's sign is pathognomonic for acute cholecystitis). Patients may also present with Boas' sign, or pain referred from the gallbladder to the right scapular region. Finally, the gallbladder is palpable in up to one-third of cases of acute cholecystitis.

Differential. Biliary colic, cholangitis, acute appendicitis, acute pancreatitis, GERD, perforated peptic ulcer, hepatitis, MI, pneumonia, and renal colic should be considered.

Workup

- Leukocytosis (12,000–15,000) is commonly seen.
- Mild hyperbilirubinemia (1–2 mg/dL) is often present; serum amylase and alkaline phosphatase may also be elevated. Bilirubin levels > 2 mg/dL suggest the presence of a concomitant common bile duct stone.
- Ultrasound is a key component of the workup and often shows stones, biliary sludge, pericholecystic fluid, a thickened gallbladder wall, and/or a sonographic Murphy's sign. Abdominal x-rays are far less useful.
- The HIDA scan (a nuclear medicine test of gallbladder function) is considered the gold standard for diagnosing acute cholecystitis, although it is rarely used. A positive scan shows nonfilling of the gallbladder, which indicates cystic duct obstruction.

Treatment

- Initiate NPO, IV fluids, and IV antibiotics (often cefazolin).
- For patients without significant operative risk factors, the ideal plan is early cholecystectomy within 72 hours of onset of symptoms (laparoscopic vs. open). An intraoperative cholangiogram should be carried out during this procedure in order to rule out common bile duct stones (choledocholithiasis).
- Expectant management is acceptable if the patient has significant medical problems. Since 60% of cases resolve spontaneously, clinically stable patients can be treated medically until resolution of the acute inflammation, with a four- to six-week delay until cholecystectomy if their medical condition improves. Keep in mind that acalculous cholecystitis is treated with emergency cholecystectomy owing to the increased risk of gangrene and perforation.

Complications. The progression of acute cholecystitis most commonly results in abscess formation (15–20% of cases). Other complications include sepsis, gallbladder gangrene, perforation, fistula formation, and empyema.

Choledocholithiasis

Choledocholithiasis is simply the presence of gallstones in the common bile duct. Although it is sometimes asymptomatic, presenting symptoms often include biliary pain, jaundice, episodic cholangitis, and pancreatitis. Symptoms vary according to the degree of obstruction, the duration of the obstruction, and the extent of bacterial infection. Choledocholithiasis should be considered in patients with a history of fever, jaundice, and biliary colic. Its hallmark is an elevated level of alkaline phosphatase, and this can be the only abnormal laboratory value in patients without jaundice. Management generally

Ultrasound is the gold standard for gallstones; ultrasound and physical examination are the gold standards for cholecystitis; HIDA is used when equivocation exists.

HIGH-YIELD TOPICS

Surgery

453

consists of operative stone removal by common bile duct exploration or endoscopic retrograde cholangiopancreatography (ERCP) with sphincterotomy.

Acute Cholangitis

Acute cholangitis is a bacterial, parasitic, or chemical infection of the biliary duct system caused by obstruction of the common bile duct by stones, strictures, or neoplasms. The organisms most commonly responsible for acute cholangitis are gram-negative bacteria such as *Escherichia coli*, *Klebsiella*, *Pseudomonas*, *Enterobacter*, *Proteus*, and *Serratia*.

Signs and Symptoms. The signs and symptoms of acute cholangitis include the following:

- **Charcot's triad:** RUQ pain, fever/chills, and jaundice (the complete triad is present in only ⅓ of patients).
- **Reynold's pentad:** Charcot's triad plus shock and altered mental status. The presence of these symptoms indicates ascending cholangitis.

Differential. The differential diagnosis includes acute cholecystitis, acute pancreatitis/pancreatic sepsis, and acute hepatitis.

Workup

- Ultrasound may show dilated ducts, stones, or masses.
- Blood cultures are positive in roughly 50% of cases.
- Patients may have elevated WBC counts, hyperamylasemia, elevated alkaline phosphatase, elevated transaminases, or increased gamma-glutamyl transferase (GGT).

Treatment

- IV antibiotics should be initiated along with aggressive IV fluid management. Most patients require admission to an ICU or a step-down unit.
- Patients with acute toxic cholangitis require emergent bile duct decompression via endoscopic sphincterotomy, percutaneous transhepatic drainage, or operative decompression.
- After the acute episode has been managed in routine cases, ERCP should be performed to locate the obstruction and possibly to treat the cause with stone extraction, stent placement, or sphincterotomy.

GI BLEEDING

Upper GI Tract Bleeding

Upper GI bleeding (UGIB) is defined as bleeding proximal to the ligament of Treitz, which includes the esophagus, stomach, and duodenum.

Etiology. The most common cause of UGIB is duodenal ulcers (25% of cases). Other causes include gastric ulcers, acute gastritis, esophageal varices, and Mallory-Weiss tear (a gastroesophageal junction tear following violent vomiting or retching). Risk factors for UGIB include alcohol consumption, smoking, chronic aspirin/NSAID use, PUD, severe vomiting, anticoagulation, bleeding disorders, steroid use, burn injuries, and trauma.

Signs and Symptoms. The signs and symptoms of UGIB include the following:

- **Hematemesis:** Vomiting bright red blood or coffee-ground emesis (blood exposed to gastric acid).
- **Melena:** Black, tarry stools due to an upper GI bleeding source.
- **Hematochezia:** Bright red blood per rectum (BRBPR) may be seen in cases of vigorous upper GI bleeding.
- Dehydration (pallor, tachycardia, orthostasis, syncope), shock, epigastric discomfort, and guaiac-positive stools are commonly seen.

Differential. In addition to the causes listed above, the clinician must consider gastric cancer, esophagitis, splenic vein thrombosis, epistaxis, and hemoptysis.

Workup. The workup of UGIB is often concomitant with treatment and involves a thorough history, NG tube aspirate, KUB, endoscopy, and laboratory tests.

Treatment. Treatment consists of the following measures:

- **Resuscitate:**
  - Using two large-bore IVs (16–18 gauge), resuscitate the patient with lactated Ringer's (2 L) followed by packed RBCs until he or she is hemodynamically stable. Insert a Foley catheter to assess fluid status.
  - Type and cross six units of blood, and order a CBC, chem-7, LFTs, and prothrombin time/partial thromboplastin time (PT/PTT) (the initial HCT lags behind actual blood loss in the acute setting).
  - Assess the magnitude of the hemorrhage using vital signs, serial HCTs, oxygen saturation, and evidence of active bleeding.
  - Correct any underlying coagulopathy with fresh frozen plasma (FFP)/vitamin K, give supplemental O_2, and give platelets for severe thrombocytopenia.
- **Identify the bleeding source:**
  - **NG tube:** If aspiration yields bright red blood or coffee grounds, perform saline lavage of the GI tract to remove blood clots until clear fluid returns. A nonbloody bilious aspirate suggests a source distal to the ligament of Treitz, or lower GI bleeding (LGIB).
  - **Endoscopy (EGD):** Identify the site of bleeding and coagulate the bleeding vessels.
  - **Angiography:** In order to identify GI bleeding with angiography, the rate of bleeding must be > 0.5 cc/min. If a source is identified, perform selective sclerotherapy or embolization.
- **Control bleeding:**
  - Sclerotherapy or embolization should be used during the localization procedure.
  - Vasopressin is often used to improve hemodynamic stability. It is used specifically in the presence of varices to decrease mesenteric

circulation and ultimately decrease flow to the varices. Keep in mind that vasopressin leads to vasoconstriction of the enteric circulation but also causes coronary vasoconstriction. Therefore, it is commonly given with nitroglycerin to reduce the risk of MI. Somatostatin is also being used.

- Balloon tamponade (with a Levine tube) can be used as a temporary measure (< 48 hours) in cases of refractory variceal hemorrhage.

KEY POINT

SURGICAL INDICATIONS FOR UGIB

- **General:** In 80–85% of cases, bleeding will stop spontaneously; approximately 20% will require surgery.
- **PUD:** Surgery is indicated if patients require six or more units of blood in the first 24 hours or if they rebleed while receiving maximal medical therapy.
- **Esophageal varices:** If bleeding continues despite medical measures, consider performing a transjugular intrahepatic portosystemic shunt (TIPS) procedure. In this case, interventional radiology staff pass a stent via the jugular vein and the inferior vena cava (IVC) to bridge the liver into the portal venous system and decompress the portal hypertension.

Lower GI Tract Bleeding

Lower GI bleeding is defined as bleeding distal to the ligament of Treitz, including the jejunum, ileum, colon, and rectum. Most cases of LGIB occur in the colon.

Etiology. The etiologies of LGIB include diverticulosis, angiodysplasia, colon cancer, hemorrhoids, IBD, intussusception/volvulus, and use of NSAIDs, anticoagulants, or steroids.

The number one cause of LGIB in adults is diverticulosis; the number one cause in children is Meckel's diverticulum.

Signs and Symptoms. Signs and symptoms of LGIB include:

- Hematochezia (BRBPR), melena, anorexia, fatigue, and in some cases abdominal pain.
- A history of change in bowel habits or in stool caliber.

Differential. The differential should consider the following:

- **Acute:** Diverticulosis, angiodysplasia, IBD, intussusception, volvulus, UGIB, and ischemic colitis.
- **Chronic:** Colorectal cancer, hemorrhoids, and fissures.

Workup. The workup generally occurs with treatment but can include CBC, chem-7, and type and cross.

Treatment

- **Resuscitate:** The procedure is the same as that for UGIB. Bleeding stops spontaneously after two units of transfusion in 90% of cases.

- **Identify the bleeding source:**
  - NG tube aspiration yields bilious GI contents in the case of LGIB.
  - Digital rectal exam, anoscopy, and/or sigmoidoscopy are performed to rule out hemorrhoids or polyps.
  - Colonoscopy.
  - A technetium-labeled RBC scan is sensitive for slow bleeds but is less specific than angiography.
  - **Angiography:** As with UGIB, this requires brisk bleeding (> 0.5 cc/min) to make the diagnosis.
- **Control the bleeding source (may be difficult):**
  - Vasopressin injection is often performed during angiography.
  - Laser coagulation or electrocoagulation.
- **Surgical indications are as follows:**
  - Persistent bleeding despite angiographic or endoscopic therapy.
  - Segmental colectomy if the bleeding site is well localized.
  - If it is not possible to localize the bleeding site, consider total colectomy with ileorectal anastomosis or a temporary ileostomy and a Hartmann pouch (in which the distal rectal stump is sutured closed).

HERNIAS

A hernia is defined as an abnormal protrusion of a structure through the tissues that normally contain it (see Figure 8.5). Hernia is the most common surgical disease in men and is eight to nine times more common in males than in females.

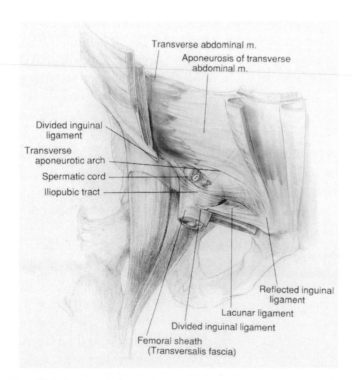

FIGURE 8.5. Hesselbach's triangle. (Reprinted, with permission, from Schwartz SI et al (eds). *Principles of Surgery,* 7th ed. New York: McGraw-Hill, 1999:1588.)

Inguinal Hernia

Inguinal hernias represent an abnormal protrusion of abdominal contents (usually the small intestine) into the inguinal region through a weakness or defect in the abdominal wall. These hernias are defined as direct or indirect according to their relationship to the inguinal canal. A review of the anatomy of this region is relevant to the discussion of inguinal hernias.

- **Direct inguinal hernia:** A herniation of abdominal contents through the floor of Hesselbach's triangle. This is most often due to an acquired defect in the transversalis fascia from mechanical breakdown, and thus the risk increases with age. The contents of the hernia sac do not traverse the internal inguinal ring; they herniate directly through the abdominal wall and are contained within the aponeurosis of the external oblique muscle.
- **Indirect inguinal hernia:** Herniation of abdominal contents through the internal inguinal ring of the inguinal canal. The contents often traverse the external inguinal ring as well and end up in the scrotum. This type of hernia is generally due to a congenital patent processus vaginalis and is the most common hernia in both men and women.

Treatment. Surgical management is indicated unless specific contraindications are evident. Surgery is warranted because of the possibility of incarceration and strangulation. The repair of a direct inguinal hernia involves correcting the defect in the transversalis fascia that allowed protrusion of the herniated bowel loop or omental segment. Many surgical strategies exist (high ligation of the hernia sac, Bassini repair, McVay repair, and mesh repair), but these differ with respect to the structures that are sutured, the number of abdominal wall layers involved in closure, and the like. Indirect inguinal hernias are repaired by isolating and ligating the hernia sac and reducing the size of the internal inguinal ring to allow only the spermatic cord structures to pass through.

Recurrence after repair of inguinal hernias occurs in 1–3% of patients. Risk factors for recurrence include excessive suture line tension, use of an absorbable suture, failure to properly identify the hernia sac, postoperative wound infection, and chronic conditions that increase intra-abdominal pressure, such as constipation, morbid obesity, prostatism, and chronic cough.

Femoral Hernia

A femoral hernia is caused by the protrusion of abdominal contents through the femoral canal medial to the femoral vein. Eighty-five percent of femoral hernias are seen in women. This type of hernia has the highest risk of incarceration and strangulation owing to the narrow and unforgiving femoral canal, which is bordered superiorly by the inguinal ligament.

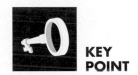

INGUINAL HERNIA ANATOMY AND KEY TERMS

Anatomy

- **Layers of abdominal wall:** Skin, subcutaneous fat, Scarpa's fascia, external oblique muscle, internal oblique muscle, transversus abdominis muscle, transversalis fascia, and peritoneum.
- **Inguinal (Poupart's) ligament:** The thickened lower border of the aponeurosis of the external oblique muscle, which runs from the anterior superior iliac spine to the pubic tubercle on each side.
- **Inferior epigastric artery:** The branch of the external iliac artery that supplies the lower portion of the abdominal wall.
- **Hesselbach's triangle:** An area formed by the inguinal ligament inferiorly, the lateral border of rectus abdominis muscle medially, and the inferior epigastric vessels laterally (see Figure 8.5).
- **Superficial (external) inguinal ring:** A defect in the external oblique aponeurosis through which the spermatic cord or round ligament passes en route to the scrotum/labia majora.
- **Deep (internal) inguinal ring:** A defect in the transversalis fascia lateral to Hesselbach's triangle through which the spermatic cord emerges from the peritoneal cavity.

Key Terms

- **Reducible hernia:** The contents of the hernia sac return to the abdomen with manual pressure.
- **Incarceration:** The hernia cannot be reduced by external manipulation.
- **Strangulation:** The blood supply to the contents of an incarcerated hernia is compromised, resulting in ischemia.

Hiatal Hernia

Hiatal hernias are present in 80% of patients with GERD. There are two types of hiatal hernias:

- **Type I:** Sliding hiatal hernias constitute > 90% of cases. In this type of hernia, the gastroesophageal junction and the fundus of the stomach are displaced into the mediastinum. Patients can be asymptomatic, although reflux, dysphagia, and esophagitis are commonly seen. Treatment consists largely of antacid use, small meals, and head elevation.
- **Type II:** Paraesophageal hernias constitute < 5% of cases. In this type of hernia, the fundus herniates alongside the esophagus while the gastroesophageal junction remains in normal position. Incarceration and strangulation are common complications, and surgical repair is therefore indicated.

Other Hernias

- **Sliding hernia:** One wall of the hernia sac is formed by a viscus (cecum or sigmoid colon).
- **Pantaloon hernia:** A combination of a direct and an indirect hernia.
- **Richter's hernia:** Only one wall of the viscus lies within the hernia sac.
- **Spigelian hernia:** A ventral hernia occurring at the semilunar line at the lateral edge of the rectus muscle.

INFLAMMATORY BOWEL DISEASE

Inflammatory bowel disease is the name that is given to the chronic, often progressive inflammatory disease processes that affect the small bowel, colon, and rectum to varying degrees. The two principal disorders, Crohn's disease and ulcerative colitis, differ in their histologic and clinical manifestations, their natural course, and their modes of therapy. The etiologies of both diseases are still unknown.

CROHN'S DISEASE (REGIONAL ENTERITIS)

Crohn's disease is a chronic, progressive granulomatous disease of the GI tract. Its peak incidence occurs between the ages of 20 and 40. Crohn's disease is characterized by:

- Segmental involvement ("skip lesions") from the mouth to the anus, most commonly at the terminal ileum and cecum
- Transmural involvement of the bowel wall with stricture formation
- Cobblestone mucosa, creeping mesenteric fat, fissures, linear ulcers, and granulomas

Look for extraintestinal manifestations in suspected IBD.

Signs and Symptoms. Signs and symptoms of Crohn's disease include:

- Diarrhea (usually nonbloody), fever, and malaise
- Recurrent abdominal pain and distention
- Anorectal lesions (fissures and fistulae)
- Malnutrition and weight loss
- Extraintestinal manifestations, including polyarticular arthritis, uveitis, stomatitis, erythema nodosum, pyoderma, cutaneous ulcers, and hepatobiliary disease

Differential. Ulcerative colitis, acute appendicitis, infectious colitis, irritable bowel syndrome, diverticular disease, colon cancer, TB, and lymphoma must be included in the differential.

Workup. Workup should include the following:

- **Lab studies:** Anemia (patients are generally B_{12}, folate, and iron deficient), hypoalbuminemia, and an abnormal D-xylose test.
- **Barium enema:** Strictures ("string sign"), cobblestones, and transverse fissures (see Figure 8.6).

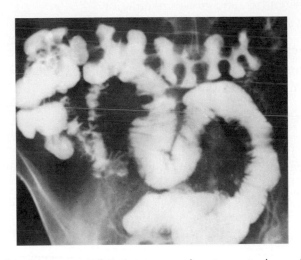

FIGURE 8.6. Crohn's disease on barium x-ray, showing spicules, edema, and ulcers. (Reprinted, with permission, from Way L, Doherty G. *Current Surgical Diagnosis & Treatment,* 11th ed. New York: McGraw-Hill, 2003.)

- **Sigmoidoscopy:** Patchy involvement, mucosal ulceration, cobblestoning, and fissures.

Treatment

- **Medical management** consists of supportive care, including NPO, IV fluids, and TPN for severe flare-ups. Steroids, sulfasalazine (for acute flare-ups), azathioprine, 6-mercaptopurine, and metronidazole are also useful.
- **Operative management** is generally reserved for complicated cases; multiple surgeries are often required, and resections are noncurative (there is a 50% recurrence rate). Therefore, surgery should be avoided at all costs. Indications for surgery include obstruction, fistula, abscess, and intractable disease; consider stricturoplasty or bypass whenever possible.

SBO is the number-one indication for surgery in Crohn's disease.

ULCERATIVE COLITIS

Ulcerative colitis is a chronic inflammatory disease of the rectum and colon. It exhibits a bimodal age distribution from ages 15 to 30 and 50 to 70 and is more prevalent among Ashkenazi Jews. Ulcerative colitis is characterized by the following:

- Involvement of the colon and rectum only
- Continuous proximal progression beginning in the rectum
- Mucosal involvement only
- Pseudopolypoid mucosal appearance, crypt abscesses, and multiple superficial ulcers

Signs and Symptoms. Signs and symptoms include the following:

- Diarrhea (usually bloody)
- Abdominal pain, tenesmus, and rectal urgency

Surgery

- Fever, weight loss, and growth retardation
- Extraintestinal manifestations similar to Crohn's

Differential. Ulcerative colitis, acute appendicitis, infectious colitis, irritable bowel syndrome, diverticular disease, colon cancer, TB, and lymphoma must be considered in the differential.

Workup

- Anemia, leukocytosis, increased erythrocyte sedimentation rate (ESR), hypoalbuminemia, and fluid/electrolyte abnormalities are commonly seen.
- Bacterial stool cultures are obtained in order to rule out an infectious etiology.
- Barium enema demonstrates contiguous mucosal irregularity, multiple small ulcers, pseudopolyp filling defects, and a "lead pipe" colon (see Figure 8.7).
- Sigmoidoscopy shows friable, edematous, and hyperemic mucosa in a contiguous pattern and can be used to take a biopsy.

Treatment

- **Medical management** consists of maintenance on sulfasalazine (prolongs remission) and supportive care, including NPO, IV fluids, NG suction, IV steroids, antibiotics, and TPN.

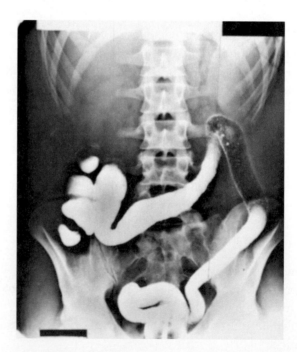

FIGURE 8.7. Ulcerative colitis on barium enema x-ray of the colon. Note the shortened colon, the "lead pipe" appearance due to loss of haustral markings, and the fine serrations at the edge of the bowel wall, which represent multiple small ulcers. (Reprinted, with permission, from Way L, Doherty G. *Current Surgical Diagnosis & Treatment,* 11th ed. New York: McGraw-Hill, 2003.)

- **Surgical management** is indicated in the presence of massive hemorrhage, toxic megacolon, colorectal cancer, obstruction, or medically refractory disease.
- A colectomy can be performed with an ileoanal anastomosis and ileal pouch.
- Proctocolectomy with ileostomy is curative, but patients with ileostomy have a high incidence of impotence and bladder dysfunction.

Complications. Complications include toxic megacolon, increased risk of colon cancer, and primary sclerosing cholangitis.

DISEASES OF THE LOWER GI TRACT

Diverticular Disease

Diverticulosis is a condition in which diverticula (outpouchings of the GI tract) are found within the colon, most commonly in the sigmoid portion (95% of cases), with sparing of the rectum. The mucosa and submucosa herniate through the muscular layer, forming false, or pulsion, diverticula. This is caused by weakness in the bowel wall related to areas where blood vessels enter and leave the colon as well as by increased intraluminal pressure. Diverticulosis is more common in Western and industrialized countries, and risk factors include low-fiber diets, chronic constipation, and family history. Patients are often asymptomatic, although massive bleeding is not uncommon. A crucial component of the workup for diverticulosis is colonoscopy and barium enema to rule out colon cancer. Treatment consists of conservative measures, including a high-fiber diet.

Diverticulitis results from perforation of a diverticulum and typically results in peritonitis. Signs and symptoms include LLQ pain, constipation or diarrhea, fever, chills, anorexia, nausea, and vomiting. There is generally leukocytosis, and radiology demonstrates air-fluid levels and/or free air under the diaphragm. It should be borne in mind that barium enema should not be performed in cases of suspected diverticulitis owing to the risk of further perforation and extravasation of contrast into the peritoneum. Initial management consists of IV fluids and broad-spectrum antibiotics. Surgery is performed if there is evidence of obstruction, fistula, free air, sepsis, or worsening clinical condition. If surgery is emergent (i.e., there is no time to "prep" the bowel), the surgeon resects the involved bowel segment(s) and creates a colostomy and a Hartmann's pouch. If the surgery is elective, the surgeon removes the involved portion(s) of bowel and performs a primary anastomosis.

Massive lower GI bleeding is common with diverticulosis but rare with diverticulitis.

Colorectal Cancer

Colorectal cancer is the second leading cause of cancer mortality in the United States after lung cancer. It affects approximately 150,000 new patients per year and accounts for 50,000 to 60,000 deaths annually. There is an increasing incidence with age, with a peak incidence at 70 to 80 years.

Signs and Symptoms. In the absence of screening, colorectal cancer typically presents symptomatically only after a prolonged period of silent growth (see Figure 8.8). Abdominal pain is the most common presenting complaint. Further distinguishing features are as follows:

- **Right-sided lesions:** Cancers are often bulky, fungating, and ulcerating masses that most commonly present with anemia from chronic occult blood loss. Patients may complain of weight loss, anorexia, weakness, or vague abdominal pain. Obstructive symptoms are rare, since feces in the right colon is fluid and the cecal wall is distensible.
- **Left-sided lesions:** Cancers are typically "apple-core" obstructing masses (see Figure 8.9). Patients typically present with a change of bowel habits (decreasing stool caliber, constipation, or obstipation). Blood-streaked stools are common with mild lesions. Obstruction is often present, since feces in the left colon are more solid, and the wall is less distensible.
- **Rectal lesions:** Patients usually present with BRBPR and may have tenesmus and/or rectal pain. Rectal lesions can coexist with hemorrhoids, so rectal cancer must be ruled out in all patients with rectal bleeding.

Differential. IBD, diverticulitis, ischemic colitis, hemorrhoids, PUD, and other intra-abdominal malignancies should be considered in the differential.

Workup

- Obtain a CBC (which often shows microcytic anemia), stool occult blood, and a baseline carcinoembryonic antigen (CEA) (nonspecific, but useful for follow-up after treatment to screen for recurrence).
- Sigmoidoscopy should be performed and all suspicious lesions biopsied.
- Transrectal ultrasound is used to determine the depth of invasion for rectal cancer.

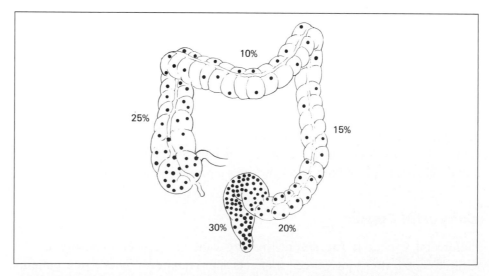

FIGURE 8.8. Distribution of cancer of the colon and rectum. (Reprinted, with permission, from Way L, Doherty G. *Current Surgical Diagnosis & Treatment,* 11th ed. New York: McGraw-Hill, 2003.)

RISK FACTORS AND SCREENING FOR COLORECTAL CANCER

Risk Factors

- Age.
- **Hereditary syndromes:** Familial adenomatous polyposis (100% risk), Gardner's disease, hereditary nonpolyposis colorectal cancer (HNPCC).
- Family history.
- **Inflammatory bowel disease:** Ulcerative colitis carries a higher risk of progression to colon cancer than does Crohn's disease.
- **Adenomatous polyps:** Villous polyps progress more often than tubular polyps; sessile more than pedunculated. Lesions > 2 cm carry an increased risk.
- Past history of colorectal cancer.
- High-fat, low-fiber diet.

Screening

- A digital rectal exam (DRE) should be performed yearly after age 55. Up to 10% of lesions are palpable with a finger.
- Stool guaiac for occult blood should be performed every year for patients over 55. Up to 50% of positive guaiac tests are due to colorectal cancer.
- It is possible to visualize and biopsy 50–75% of lesions with sigmoidoscopy, which should be carried out every three to five years for those over 55.
- Colonoscopy is indicated every ten years beginning at age 40 in patients with a family history of colon cancer or polyps.

- Visualize the entire colon via colonoscopy to rule out synchronous proximal lesions.
- Order a barium enema (air contrast) to rule out missed lesions after incomplete colonoscopy (see Figure 8.9).
- Abdominal CT/MRI are used for staging colon cancer.
- Metastatic workup should include CXR, LFTs, and an abdominal CT. Metastasis may arise from:
    - **Hematogenous spread:** Blood-borne metastases commonly go to the liver (40–50% of cases), lungs, bone, and brain.
    - **Lymphatic spread:** Pelvic lymph nodes are often affected (primary method of extension).
    - **Direct extension:** Local viscera.
    - **Peritoneal spread.**

Treatment

- **Preoperative bowel prep:** Preparation should consist of mechanical cleaning (e.g., GoLytely) and oral antibiotics.

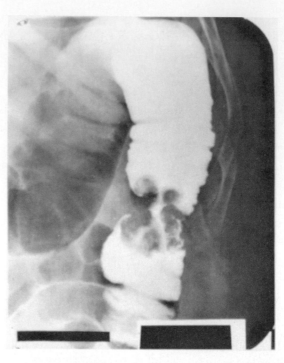

FIGURE 8.9. Barium enema x-ray showing the classic "apple core" lesion of an encircling carcinoma in the descending colon. Note the loss of mucosal pattern and the "hooks" at the margins of the lesion due to undermining. (Reprinted, with permission, from Way L, Doherty G. *Current Surgical Diagnosis & Treatment,* 11th ed. New York: McGraw-Hill, 2003.)

- **Colonic lesions:** Surgical resection of the lesion is carried out with bowel margins of 3–5 cm. The lymphatic drainage and mesentery at the origin of the arterial supply are also resected. Primary anastomosis of bowel can usually be performed.
- **Rectal lesions:** The resection technique depends on the proximity of the lesion to the anal verge.
  - **Abdominoperineal resection (APR):** For low-lying lesions near the anal verge, remove the rectum and anus and provide a permanent colostomy.
  - **Low anterior resection (LAR):** For proximal lesions, perform a primary anastomosis of the colon to the rectum.
  - **Wide local excision:** This technique is used for small, low-stage, well-differentiated tumors in the lower one-third of the rectum.
- Ileoanal anastomosis spares the patient an abdominal ileostomy; pouch procedures ("continent ileostomy") provide a reservoir to maintain fecal continence.
- Consider adjuvant chemotherapy in cases of colon cancer with positive nodes. Radiation has proven ineffective for colon cancer, although it can be used effectively to treat rectal cancer.
- Follow up with serial CEA levels, colonoscopy, LFTs, CXR, and abdominal CT (for metastasis).

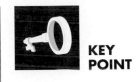
DUKES' STAGING (ASTLER-COLLER MODIFICATION)

		Five-Year Survival
A	Tumor limited to submucosa	> 90%
B1	Tumor invades into muscularis propria	70–80%
B2	Tumor invades through muscularis propria	50–65%
C1	B1 plus nodes	40–55%
C2	B2 plus nodes	20–30%
D	Distant metastasis/unresectable local spread	< 5%

DISEASES OF THE UPPER GI TRACT

Small Bowel Obstruction

Small bowel obstruction represents blocked passage of bowel contents through the duodenum, jejunum, or ileum. Fluid and gas can build up proximal to the obstruction, resulting in fluid and electrolyte imbalances and significant abdominal discomfort. The obstruction can be complete or partial and may be very dangerous if strangulation of the bowel occurs.

Etiology. SBO may arise from:

- Adhesions (60% of cases) from a prior abdominal surgery
- Hernias (10–20% of cases)
- Neoplasm (10–20% of cases)
- Intussusception
- Gallstone ileus
- Stricture from IBD
- Volvulus

The number-one cause of SBO in adults: adhesions; the number-one cause in children: hernias.

Signs and Symptoms. Signs and symptoms may include:

- **Cramping abdominal pain:** Pain follows a recurrent crescendo-decrescendo pattern at intervals of five to ten minutes (see Figure 8.10).
- **Vomiting:** Early emesis is nonfeculent if the obstruction is proximal. In distal obstruction, vomiting typically follows the pain and is feculent in nature. Keep in mind that feculence is due to secondary bacterial overgrowth, not actual emesis of feces.
- **Obstipation.**
- **Complete obstruction:** No flatus or stool is passed.
- **Partial obstruction:** There is continued passage of flatus but no stool.
- Fever, hypotension, and tachycardia (due to dehydration) are not uncommon.
- Abdominal exam often reveals distention, tenderness, prior surgical scars, or hernias. Rebound tenderness suggests more advanced disease.
- Bowel sounds are characterized by high-pitched tinkles and peristaltic rushes. Later in the disease, peristalsis may disappear.

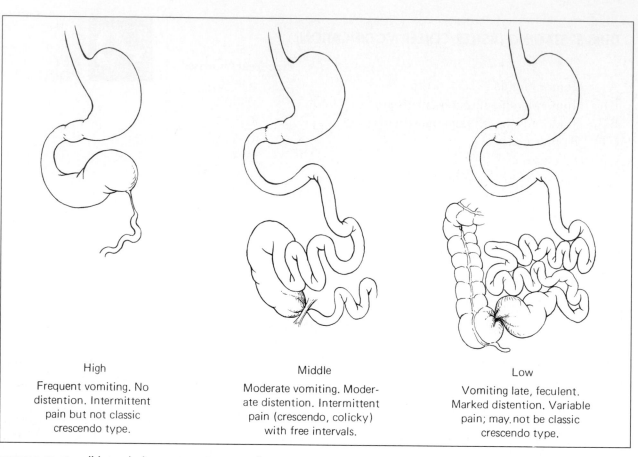

High	Middle	Low
Frequent vomiting. No distention. Intermittent pain but not classic crescendo type.	Moderate vomiting. Moderate distention. Intermittent pain (crescendo, colicky) with free intervals.	Vomiting late, feculent. Marked distention. Variable pain; may not be classic crescendo type.

FIGURE 8.10. Small bowel obstruction. Signs and symptoms vary with the level of blockage. (Reprinted, with permission, from Way L, Doherty G. *Current Surgical Diagnosis & Treatment,* 11th ed. New York: McGraw-Hill, 2003.)

Differential. The differential includes the following:

- **Adynamic ileus:** Postoperative ileus after abdominal surgery, hypokalemia, or medications.
- **Large bowel obstruction:** Colorectal cancer, diverticulitis, and sigmoid volvulus.
- Acute appendicitis (this should *always* be near the top of your differential for an acute abdomen).
- Inflammatory bowel disease.
- Mesenteric ischemia.
- Renal colic/pyelonephritis.

Workup

- **CBC:** Leukocytosis = strangulation.
- **chem-7:** Electrolytes often reflect dehydration (decreased K^+ and Na^+) and metabolic alkalosis due to vomiting.
- **Abdominal films:** A stepladder pattern of dilated small-bowel loops and air-fluid levels is seen (see Figure 8.11). It is possible to see an absent colon gas pattern. The presence of radiopaque material at the cecum is suggestive of gallstone ileus.

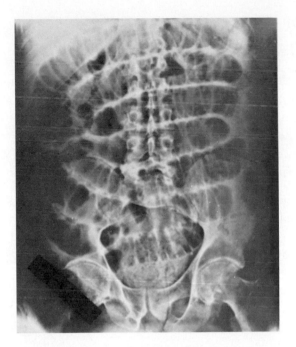

FIGURE 8.11. Small bowel obstruction of supine abdominal x-ray. Note dilated loops of small bowel in a ladderlike pattern. Air-fluid levels may be seen if upright x-ray is done. (Reprinted, with permission, from Way L, Doherty G. *Current Surgical Diagnosis & Treatment,* 11th ed. New York: McGraw-Hill, 2003.)

Treatment

- **Medical management:** Supportive care may be sufficient to treat partial SBO and may include NPO, NG suction to decompress the GI tract, IV hydration, correction of electrolyte abnormalities, and Foley catheterization to monitor fluid status.
- **Surgical management:** Surgery is required in cases of complete SBO, vascular compromise, or cases of more than three days' duration without resolution. Exploratory laparotomy may be performed with lysis of adhesions and resection of necrotic bowel as well as a bowel run (inspection of the entire length of bowel) with evaluation for stricture, IBD, and hernias.

Never let the sun rise or set on a complete small bowel obstruction.

STRANGULATED VERSUS NONSTRANGULATED SBO

Nonstrangulated SBO carries a total mortality of approximately 2%, while the risk of death from strangulated SBO increases in proportion to time from diagnosis to operative therapy, with a peak of roughly 25%. A second-look laparotomy or laparoscopy may be performed 18 to 36 hours after initial surgical treatment to reevaluate bowel viability.

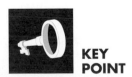

KEY POINT

DISEASES OF THE PANCREAS

Acute Pancreatitis

Acute pancreatitis is an acute pancreatic inflammation characterized by severe abdominal pain, nausea and vomiting, electrolyte and acid-base abnormalities, and, in some cases, hemorrhage, sepsis, and respiratory failure. Recurrent alcoholic pancreatitis often proceeds to chronic pancreatitis and subsequent pancreatic exocrine insufficiency (leading to malabsorption) and endocrine insufficiency (leading to diabetes).

Etiology. The most common etiologies for pancreatitis are gallstones and alcohol abuse. Gallstones account for 40% of cases; they cause pancreatitis by obstructing the pancreatic ductal system (see Figure 8.12). Alcohol abuse accounts for an additional 40% of cases; possible mechanisms include increased pancreatic ductal pressure or ethanol-induced increased ductal permeability. These and other etiologies can be remembered using the mnemonic "BAD HITS."

Signs and Symptoms

- **Abdominal pain:** Patients report acute, severe, "boring" epigastric pain, often radiating to the back (present in 90% of cases).
- Patients may present with nausea, vomiting, and fever.
- **Dehydration:** Severe hypovolemia is seen along with tachycardia, hypotension, and shock.
- Abdominal tenderness and/or an epigastric mass may be seen (suggestive of a pseudocyst, abscess, or phlegmon).
- Dullness over the left lower lung suggests a pleural effusion or pseudocyst.
- **Grey Turner's sign:** Ecchymotic discoloration of the flank from pancreatic hemorrhage is seen in 1–2% of cases.
- **Cullen's sign:** Ecchymosis of the periumbilical area from pancreatic hemorrhage is seen in 1–3% of cases.

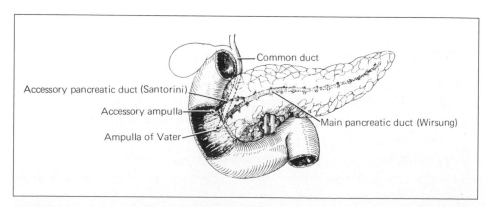

FIGURE 8.12. Anatomy of the pancreatic ductal system. (Reprinted, with permission, from Way L, Doherty G. *Current Surgical Diagnosis & Treatment,* 11th ed. New York: McGraw-Hill, 2003.)

Differential. Ruptured AAA, perforated peptic ulcer, acute appendicitis, acute cholecystitis, MI, mesenteric ischemia, SBO, nephrolithiasis, pyelonephritis, and hepatitis should be considered.

Workup. Workup includes the following:

- Amylase (increased in > 90% of cases), lipase (often increased but is less sensitive), CBC (moderate leukocytosis), chem-7, Ca^{2+} (decreased if severe), LFTs, and PT/PTT.
- **CXR:** May show basilar atelectasis indicative of a pleural effusion.
- **Three-way abdominal x-rays:** These may reveal "sentinel loop" or "colon cutoff" signs suggestive of peripancreatic inflammation; ileus may be present; and pancreatic calcifications may also be seen in cases of chronic pancreatitis.
- **Abdominal CT:** Not often used in initial management, but indicated in suspected cases of pancreatitis in which there is no clinical improvement. Abdominal CT can demonstrate pancreatic edema, necrosis, phlegmon, pancreatic calcifications, and pseudocysts (see Figure 8.13).

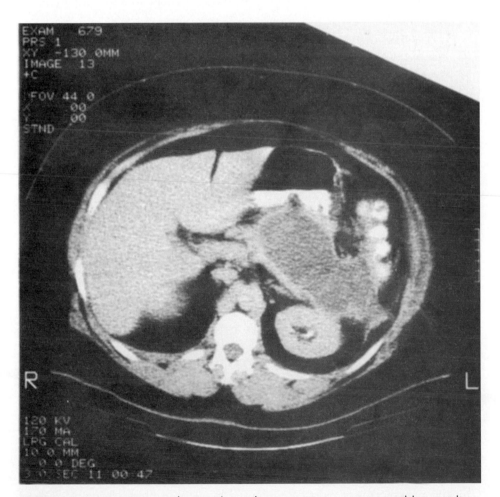

FIGURE 8.13. Pancreatic pseudocyst, shown here on CT scan, is a possible complication of acute pancreatitis. (Reprinted, with permission, from Way L, Doherty G. *Current Surgical Diagnosis & Treatment,* 11th ed. New York: McGraw-Hill, 2003.)

The false negative rate for abdominal CT in cases of pancreatitis is 15%.

Treatment. The treatment of acute pancreatitis can be operative or nonoperative depending on the severity of the disease and the presence of operable complications such as hemorrhage, pancreatic necrosis, or pseudocyst formation.

- **Nonoperative management** should proceed as follows:
  - NPO; consider NG intubation in cases with emesis.
  - Aggressive fluid and electrolyte repletion (consider patients with acute pancreatitis similar to burn victims in terms of severity of dehydration).
  - **Pain control:** Use meperidine (Demerol) rather than morphine in order to minimize spasm of the sphincter of Oddi.
  - Respiratory monitoring and support as necessary.
  - **Nutrition:** Patients may require TPN if they are to be NPO for more than several days.
  - Alcohol withdrawal prophylaxis should be initiated.
  - There is no benefit to using antibiotics except in cases of pancreatic sepsis/abscess.
- **Operative management** includes:
  - Surgical debridement of pancreatic necrosis.
  - Operative drainage of noninfected pseudocysts via cystogastrostomy, cystojejunostomy, or cystoduodenostomy (not usually performed in the acute setting). Infected pseudocysts must be drained externally.
  - Operative hemostasis in cases of pancreatic hemorrhage.
  - Diagnostic laparotomy in cases of uncertain diagnosis or deteriorating clinical status.
  - ERCP and sphincterotomy with stone extraction, then interval cholecystectomy for gallstone pancreatitis (usually done after pancreatitis has resolved).

Complications. The mortality rate for acute pancreatitis is 10–15%. The prognosis worsens with a higher Ranson's score or coexistent hemorrhage, respiratory failure, or severe persistent hypocalcemia. Pseudocysts develop in roughly 2–4% of cases and are initially managed nonoperatively, since 40% resolve spontaneously. Pseudocysts that are drained surgically have a roughly 10% recurrence rate. More dangerous complications include disseminated intravascular coagulation (DIC) and hemorrhage, sepsis, acute respiratory distress syndrome (ARDS), renal failure, and pleural effusion.

Chronic Pancreatitis

This disorder is characterized by chronic inflammation of the pancreas with damage to the parenchyma and resulting endocrine and exocrine dysfunction. Chronic pancreatitis is most often caused by alcohol abuse (roughly 70% of cases) but seems to be idiopathic in another 15% of cases. Other causes include hypercalcemia, hyperlipidemia, familial factors, trauma, and gallstones.

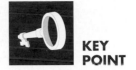

RANSON'S CRITERIA

Risk of mortality is 20% with three to four signs, 40% with five to six signs, and 100% with seven or more signs.

On Admission	Developing During Initial 24 to 48 Hours
Age > 55 years	Hematocrit fall > 10%
WBC > 16,000/mL	BUN rise > 5 mg/dL
SGOT (AST) > 250 IU/dL	Serum Ca^{2+} < 8 mg/dL
Serum LDH > 350 IU/L	Arterial P_{O_2} < 60 mmHg
Blood glucose > 200 mg/dL	Estimated fluid sequestration > 6 L
Base excess > 4 mEq/L	

Symptoms include recurrent epigastric pain that often radiates to the back as well as weight loss. In advanced disease, destruction of the exocrine pancreas leads to lipase insufficiency and resulting steatorrhea (fat malabsorption leading to stools that float in water). Damage to the endocrine pancreas leads to diabetes from a lack of insulin. Diagnosis is generally made with CT, although KUB reveals calcifications and ERCP shows ductal dilatation and strictures (the "chain of lakes" pattern). Treatment consists of alcohol cessation, insulin and pancreatic enzyme replacement, and pain control. Severe, prolonged cases may be treated with surgery (pancreaticojejunostomy or liver transplant).

Pancreatic Cancer

This disease is most often characterized by adenocarcinoma arising from the duct cells. It is more common in men and typically strikes those over 65. Risk factors include smoking, diabetes, alcohol abuse, and toxin exposure. Signs and symptoms include jaundice, anorexia, weight loss, abdominal and back pain, Courvoisier's sign (a nontender, distended gallbladder), and depression. Tumors are more often found in the head of the pancreas and are treated by a Whipple procedure. The prognosis for these patients is very poor, with only a 10% one-year survival rate.

Breast

BREAST CANCER

Approximately 10% of American women will be diagnosed with breast cancer during their lifetimes. Although women are most commonly affected, a small number of men get breast cancer as well. Major risk factors include female gender, age, prior breast cancer, a family history of breast cancer, ductal carcinoma in situ (DCIS), and lobular carcinoma in situ (LCIS). Minor risk factors include early menarche (before age 12), late menopause (after age 50), ovarian/

endometrial cancer, obesity, nulliparity, first pregnancy occurring after age 35, and OCP use. There is a higher incidence of breast cancer in women who carry the BRCAI/II genes.

Signs and Symptoms. Breast cancer often presents with a breast mass that does not change in size with menstrual cycle along with tenderness, nipple discharge or retraction, and/or changes in breast appearance/contour/symmetry. Malignant tumors will demonstrate spiculation, asymmetry, and/or microcalcifications on mammography.

Differential. The differential should include the following:

- **Benign mass:** Well circumscribed, mobile, tender, and changes in size with cycle.
  - **Fibrocystic change (most frequent breast lesion):** Painful (increased before menses), fluctuation in size, often multiple/bilateral. It is associated with increased breast cancer risk only in the presence of ductal/atypical hyperplasia.
  - **Fibroadenoma:** Firm, round, mobile, and nontender (most common breast mass in women under 30).
  - **Intraductal papilloma:** The most common cause of bloody nipple discharge.
  - Lipoma, breast abscess, fat necrosis, mastitis.
- **Malignant mass:** Hard, irregular, fixed, nipple retraction, dimpling of skin, edema, and lymphadenopathy (see Figure 8.14).
  - **Ductal carcinoma:** Most common breast malignancy (80% of cases).
  - **Lobar carcinoma:** 8–10% of cases.
  - **Paget's carcinoma:** Infiltrating ductal carcinoma in the nipple. Symptoms include itching/burning of the nipple with superficial ulceration or erosion.

Reinforce the importance of the breast self-exam to the patient.

DCIS increases the risk of breast cancer in the ipsilateral breast; LCIS increases the risk in either breast.

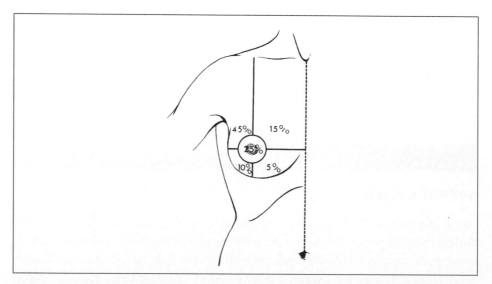

FIGURE 8.14. Frequency of breast cancer at various anatomic sites. (Reprinted, with permission, from Way L, Doherty G. *Current Surgical Diagnosis & Treatment,* 11th ed. New York: McGraw-Hill, 2003.)

- **Inflammatory carcinoma:** The most aggressive lesion; poorly differentiated and rapidly lethal. Symptoms include diffuse induration, warmth, erythema, edema, and axillary lymphadenopathy.

Workup. Workup consists of the following:

- Mammogram or ultrasound (in women over age 30)
- Fine-needle aspiration (FNA) of a palpable lump
- Core needle biopsy for nondiagnostic FNA
- Needle aspiration of a palpable cystic lesion (with or without ultrasound guidance)
- Open excisional biopsy (with or without needle wire localization) is definitive but the most invasive
- Ductography and cytology are often performed for nipple discharge

Treatment. Treatment options are as follows:

- **Modified radical mastectomy:** Removal of the breast and nipple with axillary node dissection (spares the chest wall muscles).
- **Wide local excision (lumpectomy) plus radiation of remaining breast tissue:** Complete excision of the tumor with margins and axillary node dissection, followed by radiotherapy.
- **Radical mastectomy:** Removal of the breast, nipple, axillary nodes, and chest wall muscles. This procedure is no longer commonly used to treat breast cancer.
- **Simple mastectomy:** Removal of the breast and nipple only. Simple mastectomy can be used as prophylaxis but does not represent adequate treatment of breast cancer.
- **Adjuvant therapy** is carried out to eliminate micrometastases responsible for late recurrence.
  - **Estrogen-receptor status:** Use tamoxifen for estrogen-sensitive tumors and combination chemotherapy for non-estrogen-receptive tumors.
  - **Nodal involvement:** If there is evidence of positive nodes, use combination chemotherapy.

Breast cancer is by far the most common type of cancer in women.

Vascular Surgery

ABDOMINAL AORTIC ANEURYSM

Abdominal aortic aneurysm is an abnormal dilation of the abdominal aorta that develops from weakness or a defect in the wall of the vessel; there is a strong association with atherosclerosis in the majority of cases. Risk factors include atherosclerosis, hypertension, smoking, and advanced age. AAAs are more common in men, are most often infrarenal, and frequently occur with aneurysms in other sites (e.g., popliteal). Symptoms are often absent, and AAAs can be discovered on routine abdominal exams. Elective surgical repair is indicated for cases in which the AAA is > 5 cm. AAAs < 5 cm have < 1% risk of rupture. Signs of rupture, however, include abdominal pain, the presence of a pulsatile abdominal mass, and hypotension. The differential includes acute pancreatitis, aortic dissection, MI, perforated viscus, and diverticulosis. Ruptured AAAs are a surgical emergency; treatment is emergent and often consists of a prosthetic graft placement. Repair is often undertaken when aneurysms reach a certain size in order to prevent catastrophic rupture. Operative mortality for cases of nonruptured AAA is < 5%, whereas mortality for cases of ruptured AAA is > 50%.

PERIPHERAL VASCULAR DISEASE

Peripheral vascular disease (PVD) is caused by occlusive atherosclerosis in the lower extremities. The most commonly involved artery is the superficial femoral artery (SFA) in Hunter's canal. Common symptoms include intermittent claudication (reproducible leg pain produced by walking a certain distance, with relief of the pain upon resting), pain at rest, impotence, and impaired sensation. Rest pain typically presents with pain over the distal metatarsals, often awakens the patient at night, and is relieved by hanging the feet over the edge of the bed or standing. The complication of limb loss (amputation) is only 5% at five years in patients with claudication but rises to over 50% of patients with rest pain. Signs of PVD include absent pulses, bruits, muscular atrophy, decreased hair growth, thickened toenails, and tissue infection. The severity of PVD is classified by means of the ankle-to-brachial index (ABI), which measures the ratio of systolic blood pressure at the ankle to that of the arm. Although claudication is often treated conservatively with exercise, smoking cessation, diet, hypertension treatment, and/or pentoxifylline (Trental), surgery is indicated in the presence of rest pain, tissue necrosis, infection, or severe effects on quality of life. Surgery is routinely carried out using an autologous vein graft or a prosthetic graft to bypass the area of arterial occlusion.

ACUTE ARTERIAL OCCLUSION

Acute arterial occlusion is generally embolic in nature, although other causes include acute thrombosis of an atherosclerotic lesion and vascular trauma. Signs and symptoms include the "six Ps:" **P**ain, **P**aralysis, **P**allor, **P**aresthesia, **P**olar (or **P**oikilothermia), and **P**ulselessness. The history will be significant for acute onset, and the most common site of occlusion is the common femoral artery. The workup consists of an arteriogram, ECG, and echocardiogram, and treatment consists of anticoagulation with IV heparin, surgical embolectomy, and Fogarty balloon placement.

GASTROENTEROLOGY

Appendicitis

Hardin DM Jr. Acute appendicitis: review and update. *Am Fam Physician* 1999;60:2027–2034. A good review of the pathogenesis, diagnostic evaluation, and treatment of acute appendicitis.

Jones PF. Suspected acute appendicitis: trends in management over 30 years. *Br J Surg* 2001;88:1570–1577. A comprehensive review of the treatment of appendicitis since 1970, with a specific focus on the "active observing" of patients with acute appendicitis.

Biliary Disease

Kalloo AN, Kantsevoy SV. Gallstones and biliary disease. *Prim Care* 2001;28:591–606. A thorough review of the definition, epidemiology, and pathophysiology of gallstones, acute cholecystitis, choledocholithiasis, and gallstone pancreatitis.

Moscati RM. Cholelithiasis, cholecystitis, and pancreatitis. *Emerg Med Clin North Am* 1996;14:719–737. A complete review of the pathophysiology of gallstones, their clinical presentation, and their treatment.

Upper GI Bleeding

Peter DJ, Dougherty JM. Evaluation of the patient with gastrointestinal bleeding: an evidence-based approach. *Emerg Med Clin North Am* 1999;17: 239–261. A comprehensive review of the diagnostic evaluation and treatment of upper and lower GI bleeding in an emergency setting.

Pianka JD, Affronti J. Management principles of gastrointestinal bleeding. *Prim Care* 2001;28:557–575. A good review of the management of UGIB along with a list of answers to commonly encountered clinical questions.

Lower GI Bleeding

Zuckerman GR, Prakash C. Acute lower intestinal bleeding: part I. Clinical presentation and diagnosis. *Gastrointest Endosc* 1998;48:606–617. The first of a two-part series reviewing the epidemiology, clinical course, and diagnosis of lower GI tract bleeding.

Zuckerman GR, Prakash C. Acute lower intestinal bleeding: part II. Etiology, therapy, and outcomes. *Gastrointest Endosc* 1999;49:228–238. A thorough review of the etiology, risk factors, therapy, and outcomes associated with lower GI tract bleeding.

Hernias

Bax T, Sheppard BC, Crass RA. Surgical options in the management of groin hernias. *Am Fam Physician* 1999;59:893–906. A good discussion of the anatomy and classification of groin hernias and the surgical techniques commonly used to treat these conditions.

Rutkows IM, Robbins AW. Classification systems and groin hernias. *Surg Clin North Am* 1998;78(6):1117–1127. Comprehensive review of the classification of groin hernias.

Inflammatory Bowel Disease

Andres PG, Friedman LS. Epidemiology and the natural course of inflammatory bowel disease. *Gastroenterol Clin North Am* 1999;28:255–281. A review of the epidemiology of IBD, risk factors for development, and the natural history of this disorder.

Chutkan RK. Inflammatory bowel disease. *Prim Care* 2001;28:539–556. A comprehensive comparative review of the clinical presentation of IBD, its pathology (including images), and medical and surgical therapy.

Stotland BR, Stein RB, Lichtenstein GR. Advances in inflammatory bowel disease. *Med Clin North Am* 2000;84:1107–1124. A thorough review of recent advances in diagnostics and therapies for IBD, along with an extensive bibliography.

Diverticular Disease

Farrell RJ, Farrell JJ, Morrin MM. Diverticular disease in the elderly. *Gastroenterol Clin North Am* 2001;30:475–496. A review of the epidemiology, pathogenesis, diagnosis, and management of diverticulosis and diverticulitis, including a thorough discussion of the complications of diverticular disease.

Stollman NH, Raskin JB. Diverticular disease of the colon. *J Clin Gastroenterol* 1999;29:241–252.

Colon Cancer

Blumberg D, Ramanathan RK. Treatment of colon and rectal cancer. *Clin Gastroenterol* 2002;34:15–26. A comprehensive review of existing surgical, radiologic, and chemotherapeutic treatment options for colon and rectal cancer.

Ponz de Leon M. Pathogenesis of colorectal cancer. *Dig Liver Dis* 2000;32:807–821. A useful review of the genetics and pathophysiology of colorectal cancer.

Small Bowel Obstruction

Wilson MS et al. A review of the management of small bowel obstruction. *Ann R Coll Surg Engl* 1999;81:320–328. A literature review of the diagnosis, evaluation, and management of SBO.

Pancreatitis

Cooperman AM. Surgery and chronic pancreatitis. *Surg Clin North Am* 2001;81:431–455. A comprehensive discussion of the evaluation and surgical management of chronic pancreatitis.

Moscati RM. Cholelithiasis, cholecystitis, and pancreatitis. *Emerg Med Clin North Am* 1996;14:719–737. A thorough review of the pathophysiology, clinical presentation, and management of acute and chronic pancreatitis.

Vlodov J, Tenner SM. Acute and chronic pancreatitis. *Prim Care* 2001;28: 607–628

BREAST

Breast Cancer

Apantaku LM. Breast cancer diagnosis and screening. *Am Fam Physician* 2000;62:596–602,605–606. A complete review of the epidemiology, symptomatology, and diagnosis of breast cancer.

Jatoi I. The natural history of breast cancer. *Surg Clin North Am* 1999;79: 949–960. An article addressing the history of breast cancer screening, diagnosis, and management.

VASCULAR SURGERY

Abdominal Aortic Aneurysm

Sternbergh WC et al. Abdominal and thoracoabdominal aortic aneurysm. *Surg Clin North Am* 1998;78: 827–843. A good review of the pathogenesis and operative management of AAAs.

Peripheral Vascular Disease

Newman AB. Peripheral arterial disease: insights from population studies of older adults. *J Am Geriatr Soc* 2000;48:1157–1162. A review of the epidemiology, symptomatology, natural history, and management of PVD.

HANDBOOK/POCKETBOOK

Handbook/Pocketbook

 Mont Reid Surgical Handbook $34.95

Berry

Mosby, 1997, 4th edition, 920 pages, ISBN 0815110073

A great pocketbook designed for interns and junior surgical residents but useful for motivated medical students as well. Rapid reading with quick, easily memorized facts for last-minute cramming before pimping sessions or entering OR. Outline format doesn't always provide adequate explanation of disease processes or operative procedures. Limited amount of pictures, tables, and figures. Latest edition includes chapters on gynecologic acute abdomens, laparoscopic procedures, and transplant medicine.

 Current Clinical Strategies: Surgery $12.95

Chan

Current Clinical Strategies, 2002 edition, 110 pages, ISBN 1929622066

A compact, quick-reference pocketbook that addresses common surgical problems in outline format. Includes sample admission orders and operative notes. Also offers good, high-yield descriptions of etiology, pathophysiology, clinical features, diagnostic procedures, and treatment. Contains few tables and no pictures to demonstrate anatomy or surgical techniques. Good overall value for its size and price.

 Pocket Companion to Sabiston Textbook of Surgery $39.95

Townsend

W. B. Saunders, 2002, 16th edition, 899 pages, ISBN 0721692796

A condensed version of its parent book written in bulleted, outline format, allowing for easy access to information. Would benefit from more illustrations, but a better quick reference than Schwartz's *Companion Handbook*. Size is an issue, however, as the book is a tight fit for the coat pocket. Consider carrying in backpack instead.

 Washington Manual of Surgery $39.95

Doherty

Lippincott Williams & Wilkins, 1999, 2nd edition, 698 pages, ISBN 0781716403

The counterpart to the *Washington Manual of Medical Therapeutics*, this text offers good coverage of basic general surgery as well as common problems in the surgical subspecialties. Practical chapters on day-to-day care of the surgical patient are also included. More appropriate for residents and subinterns, as there is little description of etiology, pathophysiology, and clinical features. Third edition not yet reviewed.

B The Cleveland Clinic Guide to Surgical Patient Management $34.95
Ponsky

Mosby, 2002, 1st edition, 441 pages, ISBN 0323017096

A comprehensive pocket guide that addresses common surgical problems with emphasis on surgical operations. Disease pathophysiology, typical presentation, clinical findings, and therapy are described in detail along with sample preoperative, postoperative, and discharge orders. The absence of illustrations makes it difficult to picture anatomy and procedures. Geared more toward intern- and resident-level education.

B On Call Surgery $29.95
Adams

W. B. Saunders, 2001, 2nd edition, 519 pages, ISBN 0721693512

A compact guide with a format similar to that of *Surgery On Call,* addressing common problems of surgeons on call. Not comprehensive enough for study, the pocketbook instead guides your clinical thinking and approach to emergent issues in a well-explained manner. Geared more toward residents on call than toward medical students.

B Pocket Surgery $22.95
Wrightson

Blackwell Science, 2001, 1st edition, 291 pages, ISBN 0632046155

A concise quick reference designed for students on their surgical clerkship. Bulleted text highlights key points of each disease with a brief discussion of etiology, epidemiology, clinical findings, workup, and management. Fact boxes provide useful clinical pearls. Not enough to provide a basis for study, but could be useful for rapid review before rounds. Bedside procedures and surgical medication sections in the back offer little detail or explanation.

B Principles of Surgery: Companion Handbook $39.95
Schwartz

McGraw-Hill, 1999, 7th edition, 1118 pages, ISBN 0070580855

A highly detailed handbook whose essay format lends itself more to in-depth review than to quick reference while on the wards. Includes discussions of basic anatomy and physiology. Paucity of tables and illustrations makes it difficult to understand anatomy and surgical procedures. A good supplement to the parent *Principles of Surgery* textbook. Too thick for coat pocket.

B⁻ Manual of Surgical Therapeutics $35.95
Condon

Little Brown and Company, 1996, 9th edition, 439 pages, ISBN 0316154024

Similar to the *Washington Manual of Surgery* although not as user-friendly or comprehensive, this book is written more at the intern and resident level. Index could be more complete and organized.

Surgical Intern Pocket Survival Guide $7.50

Chamberlain

International Medical Publishing, 1993, 1st edition, 74 pages, ISBN 0963406353

A practical pocketbook detailing the basic logistics of day-to-day surgical life. Written for the intern, but can serve as a guide for subinterns. Outlines the approach to the medical management of surgical patients, including sample orders and notes. Some parts may be too specific for beginning students, but most sections can be useful. Some therapeutic measures are out of date. Sparse on topics other than common problems, but small, compact, and inexpensive.

 Surgery On Call $29.95

Lefor

McGraw-Hill, 2001, 3rd edition, 577 pages, ISBN 0838588174

A practical handbook allowing for quick reference of common problems encountered by the physician on call. Provides guidelines for initial evaluation, differential, diagnostic workup, and management. Little discussion of pathophysiology is offered, and sections are divided by patient complaint, making it less useful for review. More useful for the subintern and resident than for the junior medical student.

 Handbook of Surgery $48.00

Schrock

Mosby, 1994, 10th edition, 1013 pages, ISBN 0801676371

A lengthy pocketbook with comprehensive coverage of surgical topics. Its full-paragraph form makes text difficult for quick reading on the wards. Often lacking in discussion of pathophysiology and differentials. Few tables, illustrations, and diagrams. *Principles of Surgery: Companion Handbook* is a more comprehensive source.

Surgical Recall $29.95

Blackbourne

Lippincott Williams & Wilkins, 1998, 2nd edition, 751 pages, ISBN 0683301020

A practical and useful adjunct to a reference text, presented in the typical question-and-answer format of the *Recall* series. Excellent for ward pimping preparation and great to use in spare moments, especially before entering the OR. Covers a wide breadth of topics and includes many surgical pearls. Quick, easy reading, although it covers most topics superficially and is insufficient for the shelf and USMLE Step 2 exams. Could also be better organized. Recommended for junior students looking to survive the common pimp questions of a difficult rotation.

Cope's Early Diagnosis of the Acute Abdomen $32.95

Silen

Oxford University Press, 2000, 20th edition, 296 pages, ISBN 0195136799

A classic, brief surgical textbook that every serious student of surgery should read. Offering an excellent exposition on differential diagnosis and physical exam, it helps students focus on the clinical skills necessary to diagnose an acute abdomen using a readable, personable approach. Ideally, should be read before the surgical rotation.

Introduction to Surgery $37.00

Levien

W. B. Saunders, 1999, 3rd edition, 303 pages, ISBN 0721676529

A clinically oriented, quick-review book written at a level appropriate for medical students. Each section begins with a clinical vignette followed by a well-written discussion of disease pathophysiology and management. Also offers helpful black-and-white illustrations of anatomy and surgical procedures. An excellent book to help guide one's transition into clinical thinking, especially for students interested in surgery.

Sabiston Essentials of Surgery $49.95

Sabiston

W. B. Saunders, 1994, 2nd edition, 774 pages, ISBN 0721650198

A thorough textbook condensed from the *Textbook of Surgery* with the primary goal of providing medical students with a full presentation of surgery, including major historical points, clinical features, and basic science aspects. Too long and detailed for end-of-rotation exam review, but an interesting read and a good foundation for serious surgical students. Includes a section on the surgical subspecialties.

Abernathy's Surgical Secrets $39.95

Harken

Hanley & Belfus, 2000, 4th edition, 344 pages, ISBN 1560533633

A text written in question-and-answer format with current references after each section. Comparable to *Surgical Recall* in that it is excellent preparation for pimping either on the wards or in the OR. A quick source for well-explained answers to the most commonly asked questions, but incomplete and somewhat limited in its discussion of treatment and management. Can be esoteric at times.

TOP-RATED BOOKS

Review/Mini-Reference

Essentials of General Surgery   **$42.95**

Lawrence

Lippincott Williams & Wilkins, 2000, 3rd edition, 650 pages, ISBN 0683301330

A basic introductory text to surgery that is written at the junior medical student level. Definitely an easy read, making it possible to cover the entire text within this busy rotation. Offers good pictorial and text reviews of pertinent anatomy and physiology, but lacks detail and depth in many areas. Weaker in its discussion of treatment and management, and does not cover subspecialties. Good questions and oral exam preparation are included at the end of each section. Appropriate as an introductory text for general surgery and for those not considering surgery as a career.

 NMS Surgery   **$42.95**

Jarrell

Lippincott Williams & Wilkins, 2000, 4th edition, 699 pages, ISBN 0683306154

An overview of surgery presented in outline format that falls between a true reference and a handbook in its detail. Offers ample coverage of common diseases, but needs more illustrations and anatomy. Includes questions following each chapter and a comprehensive exam at the end. Large review for shelf exam and USMLE Step 2 preparation for the highly motivated student, but not useful as a primary resource.

 Underground Clinical Vignettes: Surgery   **$24.95**

Bhushan

Blackwell Science, 2002, 2nd edition, 52 pages, ISBN 0632045752

A well-organized review of clinical vignettes commonly encountered on NBME shelf and USMLE Step 2 exams. Includes a focused, high-yield discussion of pathogenesis, epidemiology, management, and complications. Black-and-white images are included where relevant. Also contains several "mini-cases" in which only key facts related to each disease are presented. An entertaining, easy-to-use supplement for studying during your clinical rotation. May benefit from increased coverage of surgical subspecialties, including ophthalmology, anesthesiology, and pediatric surgery. The color atlas supplement comes with purchase of the full set of *Underground Clinical Vignettes*.

B **Blueprints in Surgery**   **$26.95**

Karp

Blackwell Science, 2001, 2nd edition, 160 pages, ISBN 063204487X

A well-organized, short text review of general surgery with good, clear tables and diagrams. Easy to read with a strong focus on high-yield topics. A brief question-and-answer section is included at the end of the text. Because it is geared toward study for shelf exam and USMLE Step 2, some of the information presented is over simplified, especially with relation to surgical operations and procedures. Excellent for the basics, but you will need a more detailed reference for the rotation. Some students feel it is one of the weaker review books of the *Blueprints* series.

B Colour Guide to Surgical Signs $21.95

Campbell

Churchill Livingstone, 1999, 2nd edition, 146 pages, ISBN 0443061459

Concise text descriptions with associated radiographs and color photographs of manifestations of surgical disease. Good illustrations but not complete, limiting its usefulness on the wards.

B General Surgical Anatomy and Examination $24.95

Thompson

Churchill Livingstone, 2002, 1st edition, 91 pages, ISBN 0443063761

An illustrative text that integrates knowledge of normal anatomy with the physical examination of the surgical patient. Line drawings overlaid on color photographs highlight abnormal areas in a clear manner. Short, but generally accomplishes its goals. Not a long-term investment for the wards, but may be good to review as pre- or early-rotation preparation.

B⁻ Most Commons in Surgery $26.95

Goljan

W. B. Saunders, 2001, 1st edition, 658 pages, ISBN 0721692915

A small reference book written in tabular format that describes the most common causes, manifestations, sites, signs or symptoms, complications, and management of all major surgical diseases. Includes sections on subspecialties. Format is not particularly useful or well organized for either study or review. Explanations to answers are minimal.

B⁻ Surgery Cue Cards $32.95

Hwang

F. A. Davis, 2000, 1st edition, 184 pages, ISBN 0803605420

Nonlaminated note cards for quick review of surgical disease written in outline and table form to highlight key points. Each card is a list of information without questions, making it not as useful for self-quizzing. Includes good black-and-white illustrations of anatomy and surgical procedures. Cards are flimsy and easy to lose or mix up. Would be a better reference if it were a complete book.

TOP-RATED BOOKS

Review/Mini-Reference

Principles of Surgery

$129.00

Schwartz

McGraw-Hill, 1998, 7th edition, 2176 pages, ISBN 0070542562

A reference textbook for the serious surgery student, and probably the most widely used of the surgical textbooks. Well organized and comprehensive, with a good discussion of surgical disease processes and in-depth, complex explanations of the diagnosis and treatment of surgical problems. Expensive and requires considerable reading time, but a great investment for those considering a surgical career. A valuable reference for presentations and in-depth study.

Sabiston Textbook of Surgery

$129.00

Townsend

W. B. Saunders, 2000, 16th edition, 2175 pages, ISBN 0721682693

An excellent reference book and a good read for medical students entering a surgical career. Places greater emphasis on basic science than does *Principles of Surgery*, with more discussion of normal anatomy and physiology. Well organized with good coverage of surgical disease. Not quite as readable.

Surgery: Scientific Principles and Practice

$149.00

Greenfield

Lippincott Williams & Wilkins, 2001, 3rd edition, 2381 pages, ISBN 0781722543

Similar to the *Sabiston Textbook of Surgery*, this is another excellent reference with a heavy emphasis on integrating the principles of basic science with its discussion of surgical disease. Good photos and diagrams.

Current Surgical Diagnosis and Treatment

$54.95

Way

McGraw-Hill, 1994, 10th edition, 1426 pages, ISBN 0838514391

A clinically practical reference book that is geared toward residents but should be useful for students considering surgery. Offers well-written explanations of the major diagnostic approaches toward and treatment options of surgical problems, but little information is given on operative procedures. Would also benefit from more illustrations. Includes chapters on most subspecialties of surgery. New edition not yet reviewed.

Current Surgical Therapy

$149.00

Cameron

Mosby, 2001, 7th edition, 1440 pages, ISBN 0323014283

A highly detailed and technical surgical textbook designed for the practicing surgeon with emphasis on evidence-based medicine. Too much for even the dedicated surgical student, although those going into surgery may consider buying this later in their career.

Abbreviations

Abbreviation	Meaning	Abbreviation	Meaning
A&O × 3	alert and oriented to person, place, and date	BUN	blood urea nitrogen
		BW	body weight
A&O × 4	alert and oriented to person, place, time, and date	c̄	with
		C&S	culture and sensitivity
AAA	abdominal aortic aneurysm	Ca	calcium
Ab	antibody	CA	cancer
ABCs	airway, breathing, circulation	CABG	coronary artery bypass grafting
ABD	abdomen	CAD	coronary artery disease
ABG	arterial blood gases	cal	calorie
ABX	antibiotics	CBC	complete blood count
ACE	angiotensin-converting enzyme	CBD	common bile duct
ACLS	advanced cardiac life support	CBT	cognitive behavioral therapy
ADA	American Diabetic Association	cc	cubic centimeter
ADH	antidiuretic hormone	CC	chief complaint
ADHD	attention-deficit hyperactivity disorder	C/C/E	clubbing, cyanosis, edema
AF	atrial fibrillation	C/D/I	clean, dry, intact
AFB	acid-fast bacillus	CEA	carcinoembryonic antigen
AIDS	acquired immune deficiency syndrome	CFTR	cystic fibrosis transmembrane regulation
Alk phos	alkaline phosphatase	chem 7	lab tests for sodium, potassium, chloride, carbon dioxide, bicarbonate, blood urea nitrogen, and glucose
ALS	amyotrophic lateral sclerosis		
ALT	alanine transaminase		
AMS	altered mental status	CHF	congestive heart failure
ANA	antinuclear antibody	CJD	Creutzfeldt-Jakob disease
ANCA	anti neutrophil cytoplasmic antibody	CK	creatine phosphokinase
AOM	acute otitis media	CK-MB	creatine phosphokinase, MB isoenzyme
AP	anterior/posterior	CL	contralateral
A/P	assessment and plan	CMT	cervical motion tenderness
ARBs	angiotensin receptor blockers	CMV	cytomegalovirus
ARDS	acute respiratory distress syndrome	CN	cranial nerve
ARF	acute rheumatic fever	CNS	central nervous system
ASDs	atrial septal defects	c/o	complains of
AST	aspartate transaminase	CO	cardiac output, carbon monoxide
AT	atraumatic	CO_2	carbon dioxide
ATS	American Thoracic Society	COPD	chronic obstructive pulmonary disease
AV	atrioventricular	CPR	cardiopulmonary resuscitation
AVM	arteriovenous malformation	Cr	creatinine
AXR	abdominal x-ray	CRNA	certified registered nurse anesthetist
AZT	azidothymidine	CRP	C-reactive protein
β-HCG	β-human chorionic gonadotropin	CSF	cerebrospinal fluid
BAEPs	brain stem auditory evoked potentials	CT	computed tomography
BBB	bundle branch block	CTA	clear to auscultation
BP	blood pressure	CTAB	clear to auscultation bilaterally
bpm	beats per minute	CTD	connective tissue disease
BPPV	benign paroxysmal positional vertigo	CV	cardiovascular
BR	bathroom	CVA	costovertebral angle/cardiovascular accidents
BRBPR	bright red blood per rectum		
BS	breath sounds, bowel sounds	CVP	central venous pressure

Abbreviation	Meaning		Abbreviation	Meaning
CVS	chorionic villi sampling		FFP	fresh frozen plasma
CW	compared with		FH	family history
CX	culture		FHT	fetal heart tone
CXR	chest x-ray		FLAIR	fluid attenuation inversion recovery
D&C	dilation and curettage		FM	fetal movement
D5	dextrose 5%		FNA	fine needle aspiration
DBP	diastolic blood pressure		FSH	follicle-stimulating hormone
DC	direct current		FTA/ABS	fluorescent treponemal antibody
DCIS	ductal carcinoma in situ			absorption (test)
D/C	discontinue		FTN	finger to nose
DEF	drugs/fluids, EKG, fibrillation		FTT	failure to thrive
DES	diethylstilbestrol		FUO	fever of unknown origin
DIC	disseminated intravascular coagulation		FVC	forced vital capacity
Dispo	disposition		G-tube	gastrostomy tube
DKA	diabetic ketoacidosis		GABA	gamma-aminobutyric acid
dL	deciliter		GAF	Global Assessment of Functioning
DLCO	diffusion capacity for carbon monoxide		GB	gallbladder
DM	diabetes mellitus		GBM	glioblastoma multiforme
DNR	do not resuscitate		GBS	Guillain-Barré syndrome
DOE	dyspnea on exertion		GCS	Glasgow Coma Scale
DPL	direct peritoneal lavage		GE	gastroesophageal
DRE	digital rectal exam		GEN	general
DSM	*Diagnostic and Statistical Manual*		GERD	gastroesophageal reflux disease
DT	delirium tremens		GFR	glomerular filtration rate
DTP	diphtheria, tetanus toxoids, pertussis		GGT	gamma-glutamyl-transferase
	(vaccine)		GI	gastrointestinal
DTR	deep tendon reflex		Glu	glucose
DU	duodenal ulcers		GNR	gram-negative rod
DUB	dysfunctional uterine bleeding		GnRH	gonadotropin-releasing hormone
DVT	deep venous thrombosis		GU	gastric ulcers/genitourinary
DWI	diffusion-weighted imaging		GUSTO	Global Utilization of Streptokinase and
dx	diagnosis			Tissue Plasminogen Activator for
EBL	estimated blood loss			Occluded Arteries
ECG	electrocardiogram		H&P	history and physical
ECT	electroconvulsive therapy		HA	headache
EDC	estimated date of confinement		HAART	highly active antiretroviral therapy
EDD	estimated date of delivery		HACEK	Haemophilus, Actinobacillus,
EEG	electroencephalogram			Cardiobacterium, Eikenella, Kingella
EF	ejection fraction		Hb	hemoglobin
EFW	estimated fetal weight		HBV	hepatitis B virus
EGD	esophagogastroduodenoscopy		HCT	hematocrit
EKG	electrocardiogram		HCV	hepatitis C virus
ELISA	enzyme-linked immunosorbent assay		HD	hospital day/Huntington Disease
EMG	electromyogram		HEENT	head, eyes, ears, nose, and throat
ENG	electronystagmogram		HELLP	hemolysis, elevated liver (enzymes), low
EOM	extraocular movement			platelets
EOMI	extraocular movements intact		hep	heparin
EPS	extrapyramidal symptoms		Hgb	hemoglobin
ER	emergency room		HHNK	hyperosmolar hyperglycemia nonketotic
ERCP	endoscopic retrograde			coma
	cholangiopancreatography		HIB	*Haemophilus influenzae* type B (vaccine)
ERRLA	equal, round, responsive to light and		HIDA	hepato-iminodiacetic acid
	accommodation		HIS	hospital information system
ESR	erythrocyte sedimentation rate		HITT	heparin-induced thrombocytopenia
ESWL	extracorporeal shock wave lithotripsy		HIV	human immunodeficiency virus
EtOH	ethanol		HLA	human leukocyte antigen
exp lap	exploratory laparotomy		HMO	health maintenance organization
EXT	extremities		HOCM	hypertrophic obstructive
FB	finger breadth			cardiomyopathy
F/C/S	fever, chills, sweating		h/o	history of
FEF$_{25-75}$	forced expiratory flow, mid-expiratory		HP	human papillomavirus
	phase		HPF	high-power field
FE$_{Na}$	excreted fraction of filtered sodium		HPI	history of present illness
FEV$_1$	forced expiratory volume in 1 second		HR	heart rate
FFM	fast finger movements			

Abbreviation	Meaning
HRT	hormone replacement therapy
HSM	hepatosplenomegaly
HSV	herpes simplex virus
HTN	hypertension
HTS	heel to shin
HVA	homovanillic acid
I&D	incision and drainage
IBD	inflammatory bowel disease
ICA	internal carotid artery
ICP	intracranial pressure
ICU	intensive care unit
ID	identification
IDDM	insulin-dependent diabetes mellitus
IE	infective endocarditis
IgA	immunoglobulin A
IHSS	idiopathic hypertrophic subaortic stenosis
IM	intramuscular
INH	isoniazid
INR	International Normalized Ratio
I/O	intake/output
IOC	intraoperative cholangiogram
ITP	idiopathic thrombocytopenic purpura
IUD	intrauterine device
IUGR	intrauterine growth retardation
IU/L	International Units per liter
IV	intravenous
IVC	inferior vena cava
IVDU	intravenous drug use
J	joules
J-tube	jejunostomy tube
JP	Jackson-Pratt
JPS	joint position sense
JRA	juvenile rheumatoid arthritis
JVD	jugular venous distention
JVP	jugular venous pressure
K	potassium
KCl	potassium chloride
KOH	potassium hydroxide
KUB	kidney, ureter, bladder
KVO	keep vein open
L&D	labor and delivery
L4–5	fourth and fifth lumbar vertebrae
LAR	low anterior resection
LCIS	lobular carcinoma in situ
LDH	lactate dehydrogenase
LEEP	loop electrosurgical excision procedure
LES	lower esophageal sphincter
LFT	liver function test
LGI	lower gastrointestinal
LGIB	lower gastrointestinal bleeding
LH	luteinizing hormone
Li	lithium
LLE	left lower extremity
LLQ	left lower quadrant
LMN	lower motor neuron
LMP	last menstrual period
LMWH	low-molecular weight heparin
LOC	laxative of choice, loss of consciousness
LP	lumbar puncture
LR	Ringer's lactate
LT	light touch
LUE	left upper extremity
LUQ	left upper quadrant

Abbreviation	Meaning
LV	left ventricle, left ventricular
LVEF	left ventricular ejection fraction
MAE	moves all extremities
MAI	*Mycobacterium avium-intracellulare*
MAO	monoamine oxidase
MAOI	monoamine oxidase inhibitor
MAT	multifocal atrial tachycardia
MCA	middle cerebral artery
MCV	mean corpuscular volume
MCTD	mixed connective tissue disorder
MDE	major depressive episode
MDI	metered dose inhaler
mEq/L	milliequivalents per liter
mg	milligram
Mg	magnesium
MG	myasthenia gravis
MHA-TP	microhemagglutination assay— *Treponema pallidum*
MI	myocardial infarction
mmHG	millimeter of mercury
MMR	measles, mumps, rubella (vaccine)
MPH	master's in public health
M/R/G	murmurs, rubs, gallops
MR	mitral regurgitation
MRI	magnetic resonance imaging
MS	multiple sclerosis/muscoskeletal
MS-I, II, etc	medical student (and year)
MSE	mental status examination
MRSA	methicillin-resistant staphylococcus aureus
MVP	mitral valve prolapse
Na	sodium
NABS	normal active bowel sounds
NASCET	North American Symptomatic Carotid Endarterectomy Trial
NC	nasal cannula, normocephalic
NCV	nerve conduction velocity
ND	nondistended
NDDG	National Diabetes Data Group
NEURO	neurologic
NFT	neurofibrillary tangles
NG	nasogastric
NICU	neonatal intensive care unit
NIDDM	non-insulin-dependent diabetes mellitus
NKDA	no known drug allergies
nl	normal
NMS	neuroleptic malignant syndrome
NP	nurse practitioner
NPH	normal pressure hydrocephalus
NPO	nil per os (nothing by mouth)
NQWMI	non-Q-wave myocardial infarction
NS	normal saline
NSAID	nonsteroidal anti-inflammatory drugs
NSCLC	non small cell lung carcinoma
NSVD	normal spontaneous vaginal delivery
NT	nontender
N/V	nausea, vomiting
NVE	native valve endocarditis
NYHA	New York Heart Association
O₂ sat	oxygen saturation
OB/GYN	obstetrics and gynecology
OCD	obsessive compulsive disorder
OCP	oral contraceptive pill
OGTT	oral glucose tolerance test

Abbreviation	Meaning		Abbreviation	Meaning
OI	opportunistic infection		qhs	every night
OOB	out of bed		qod	every other day
O/P	oropharynx		R	respiration
OR	operating room		RA	room air, rheumatoid arthritis
OTC	over the counter		RAAS	renin-angiotensin-aldosterone system
O/W	otherwise		RBC	red blood cell
P	pulse		RDS	respiratory distress syndrome
PA	posteroanterior		REM	random eye movement
PACs	paroxysmal atrial contractions		RF	rheumatoid factor
PaCO$_2$	partial pressure of carbon dioxide in arterial blood		Rh	Rhesus (factor)
			RHM	rapid hand movements
PCA	posterior cerebral artery, patient-controlled analgesia		RIND	reversible ischemic neurologic deficit
			RLQ	right lower quadrant
PCO	polycystic ovary		ROM	rupture of membranes
pCO$_2$	partial pressure of carbon dioxide		ROS	review of symptoms
PCOS	polycystic ovarian syndrome		RPGN	rapidly progressive glomerulonephritis
PCP	phencyclidine ("angel dust"), *Pneumocystis carinii* pneumonia		RPR	rapid plasma reagin (test)
			RR	rate regular, respiratory rate
P$_{Cr}$	plasma creatinine		RSV	respiratory syncytial virus
PD	Parkinson Disease		RT	recreation therapy, recreational therapist
PDA	patient ductus arteriosus/personal digital assistant		RUL	right upper lobe
			RUQ	right upper quadrant
PDR	*Physician's Desk Reference*		RV	residual volume, right ventricle, right ventricular
PDS	polydioxanone sutures			
PE	physical examination, pulmonary embolism		SA	sinoatrial
			SAB	spontaneous abortion
PEFR	peak expiratory flow rate		SAH	subarachnoid hemorrhage
PERRL	pupils equal, round, responsive to light		SBO	small bowel obstruction
			SBP	systolic blood pressure
PFT	pulmonary function test		SCLC	small cell lung carcinoma
PGY	postgraduate year		SCM	sternocleidomastoid
PID	pelvic inflammatory disease		SFA	superficial femoral artery
PIH	pregnancy-induced hypertension		SGOT	serum glutamic oxaloacetic transaminase
Plts	platelets			
PMH	past medical history		SH	social history
PMN	polymorphonuclear (leukocytes)		sl	slightly
PND	paroxysmal nocturnal dyspnea		SLE	systemic lupus erythematosus
PN	progress note		SMX	sulfamethoxazole
PNL	prenatal labs		SOAP	subjective (data), objective (data), assessment, and plan
P$_{Na}$	plasma sodium			
pO$_2$	partial pressure of oxygen		SOB	shortness of breath
POD	postoperative day		s/p	status post(operatively)
PP	pin prick		SPEP	serum protein electrophoresis
ppd	pack per day		SQ	subcutaneous
PPD	purified protein derivative (of tuberculin)		SSI	insulin sliding scale
			SSRIs	selective serotonin reuptake inhibitors
PPIs	proton pump inhibitors		STD	sexually transmitted disease
PR	per rectum		SVE	sterile vaginal exam
PRBC	packed red blood cells		SVR	systemic vascular resistance
prn	pro re nata (as required)		T	temperature
Pt	patient		T. bili	total bilirubin
PT	prothrombin time		T&P	tongue and palate
PTC	percutaneous transhepatic cholangiography		TAB	therapeutic abortion
			TB	tuberculosis
PTCA	percutaneous transluminal coronary angioplasty		TBW	total body water
			Tc	technetium
PTT	partial thromboplastin time		T$_c$	current temperature
PTSD	post-traumatic stress disorder		TCA	trichloroacetic acid/tricyclic antidepressant
PTX	Pneumothorax			
PUD	peptic ulcer disease		TD	tardive dyskinesia
PVCs	paroxysmal ventricular contractions		TEE	trans-esophageal echocardiography
PVD	peripheral vascular disease		TFT	thyroid function test
PVE	prostethic valve endocarditis		TIAs	transient ischemic attacks
q4h	every four hours		TID	three times a day
qd	every day		TIPS	transjugular intrahepatic portosystemic shunt

Abbreviation	Meaning	Abbreviation	Meaning
TLC	total lung capacity	URI	upper respiratory infection
TM	tympanic membrane	U/S	ultrasound
T_M	maximum temperature	USMLE	United States Medical Licensing Examination
TMP	trimethoprim		
TPAL	term, pre-term, abortion, living	UTI	urinary tract infection
TOA	tubo-ovarian abscess	VA	Veterans Administration
ToRCHeS	toxoplasmosis, rubella, cytomegalovirus, herpes simplex, syphilis	VB	vaginal bleeding
		VC	vital capacity
tPA	tissue-type plasminogen activator	VCUG	voiding cystourethrogram
TPN	total parenteral nutrition	VDRL	Venereal Disease Research Laboratory (test)
TSH	thyroid-stimulating hormone		
TTE	transthoracic echocardiography	VF	ventricular fibrillation
TTN	transient tachypnea of the newborn	VFFTC	visual fields full to confrontation
TTP	thrombotic thrombocytopenic purpura	V-fib	ventricular fibrillation
TyCo	Tylenol and codeine	VMA	vanillylmandelic acid
UA	urinalysis	V-Q	ventilation-perfusion
U_{Cr}	urinary concentration of creatinine	VS	vital signs
UGI	upper gastrointestinal	VSDs	ventricular septal defects
UGIB	upper gastrointestinal bleeding	V-tach	ventricular tachycardia
UMN	upper motor neuron	VT	ventricular tachycardia
U_{Na}	urinary concentration of sodium	VZV	varicella zoster virus
UO	urine output	WBC	white blood cell, white blood (cell) count
UP	universal precautions		
UPEP	urine protein electrophoresis	WHO	World Health Organization

Index

500

504

N

Nafcillin, 105
Nails
    anemia, 140
    menopause, 278
    peripheral vascular disease, 476
Naltrexone, 408
Naprosyn test, 146
Narcolepsy, 36
Nardil, 385
Nasal congestion, 329
Nasal flaring
    asthma, 344
    bronchiolitis, 348
    pneumonia, 331
    respiratory distress syndrome, 339
Nasal wash/swab, 331
Nasogastric (NG) tubes
    acute abdomen, 447
    acute appendicitis, 450
    acute pancreatitis, 472
    lower GI bleeding, 457
    overview, 438
    small bowel obstruction, 469
    upper GI bleeding, 455
National Center for Health Statistics, 355
National Diabetes Data Group
        (NDDG), 143–144
National Institute of Neurological Disor-
        ders and Stroke tPA Stroke
        Study Group, 228
Native Americans, 451
Native valve endocarditis (NVE), 105
Nausea
    acute abdomen, 445
    acute appendicitis, 448
    acute cholecystitis, 452
    acute myocardial infarction, 98
    acute pancreatitis, 470
    acute renal failure, 123
    alcohol withdrawal, 406
    angina pectoris, 93
    cholelithiasis and biliary colic, 451
    delirium, 192
    diverticulitis, 463
    ectopic pregnancy, 252
    gastritis, 135
    hepatitis, 133
    hyponatremia, 127
    nephrolithiasis, 129
    peptic ulcer disease, 137
    subarachnoid hemorrhage, 201
    tension headaches, 199
    urinary tract infections, 334
    Wilms' tumor, 320
Navane, 393
Neck
    epiglottitis, 351
    febrile seizures, 340
    pneumothorax, 120

Needle decompression, 120
Needlesticks, 33
Nefazodone, 386
Neisseria gonorrhoeae, 279
Neomycin, 132
Neonatology
    Apgar score, 335–336
    congenital infections, 336–338
    hyperbilirubinemia, 336, 338–339
    references, high-yield, 359
    respiratory distress syndrome, 339–340
    See also Congenital abnormalities
Neostigmine, 224
Nephritic syndrome, 125, 127
Nephritis, 123, 153
Nephrolithiasis
    acute renal failure, 123
    age, 128
    differential, 129
    signs and symptoms, 128–129
    treatment, 129
    urinary tract infections, 333
    workup, 129
Nephrolithotomy, 129
Nephrology
    acute renal failure
        causes, 123
        nephritic syndrome, 125
        nonspecific clinical manifestations,
            122
        signs and symptoms, 123, 124
        treatment, 124
        workup, 123–125
    glomerular disease
        acute renal failure, 123
        nephritic syndrome, 125, 127
        nephrotic syndrome, 125, 126
    hyponatremia
        causes, 127
        cirrhosis, 131
        signs and symptoms, 127–128
        treatment, 128
        workup, 128
    nephrolithiasis
        acute renal failure, 123
        age, 128
        differential, 129
        signs and symptoms, 128–129
        treatment, 129
        urinary tract infections, 333
        workup, 129
Nephrotic syndrome
    acute renal failure, 123
    causes, 125
    cirrhosis, 131
    pleural effusion, 116
    renal amyloidosis, 126
    treatment, 125
Nerve conduction velocity (NCV)
    carpal tunnel syndrome, 223
    Guillain-Barré syndrome, 224

myasthenia gravis, 224
weakness, 222
Nervous system. *See* Neurology
Neuroblastoma
    differential, 321
    references, high-yield
        "Neuroblastoma," 357
    signs and symptoms, 320–321
    treatment, 321
    workup, 321
Neurogenic shock, 65
Neuroleptic malignant syndrome
        (NMS), 394
Neuroleptics
    autistic disorder, 411
    brief psychotic disorder, 395
    schizophrenia, 392
Neurology
    Alzheimer's disease
        risk factors, 194
        signs and symptoms, 194
        treatment, 195
        workup, 195
    aphasias
        Alzheimer's disease, 194
        Broca's, 186–188
        conduction, 188
        global, 189
        references, high-yield
            "Multifactorial Processes in Re-
            covery From Aphasia," 225
        summary of, 186, 187
        transcortical, 188
        Wernicke's, 187, 188
    books
        Care of the Medical Patient (Ferri),
            174
        Clinical Neurology, 174
        Clinician's Pocket Reference, 174
        handbook/pocketbook
            *Handbook of Symptom-Oriented
            Neurology* (Remmel), 230
            Little Black Book of Neurology
            (Lerner), 230
            Manual of Neurologic Therapeutics
            (Samuels), 230
            Neurologic Pearls (Devinsky), 230
            Neurology (Weiner), 230
        review/mini-reference
            Clinical Neurology (Greenberg),
            231
            Four-Minute Neurologic Exam
            (Goldberg), 232
            High-Yield Neuroanatomy (Fix),
            232
            *Introduction to the Neurologic Ex-
            amination* (Nolan), 233
            Lecture Notes on Neurology (Gins-
            berg), 232
            *Manter and Gantz's Essentials of
            Clinical Neuroanatomy and
            Neurophysiology* (Gilman), 233

535

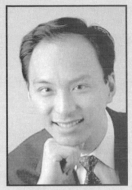
Tao Le, MD

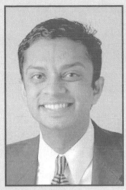
Vikas Bhushan, MD

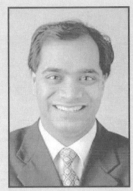
Chirag Amin, MD

Tao Le, MD   Dr. Le has led multiple medical education projects over the past seven years. As a medical student, he was editor-in-chief of the University of California, San Francisco Synapse, a university newspaper with a weekly circulation of 9,000. Subsequently, he authored *First Aid for the Wards* and *First Aid for the Match* and led the most recent revision of *First Aid for the USMLE Step 2*. At Yale, he was a regular guest lecturer on the USMLE review courses and an adviser to the Yale University School of Medicine curriculum committee. Dr. Le earned his medical degree from the University of California, San Francisco in 1996 and completed his residency training and board certification in internal medicine at Yale-New Haven Hospital. He subsequently went on to co-found Medsn and served as its Chief Medical Officer. Dr. Le is currently a fellow in allergy and clinical immunology at the Johns Hopkins Asthma and Allergy Center in Baltimore.

Vikas Bhushan, MD   Dr. Bhushan is a world-renowned author, publisher, entrepreneur, and board-certified diagnostic radiologist who resides in Los Angeles, California. Dr. Bhushan conceived and authored the original *First Aid for the USMLE Step 1* in 1992, which, after eleven consecutive editions, has become the most popular medical review book in the world. Following this, he co-authored three additional *First Aid* books as well as developed the highly acclaimed 17-title *Underground Clinical Vignettes* series. He completed his training in diagnostic radiology at the University of California, Los Angeles. Dr. Bhushan has more than 13 years of entrepreneurial experience and started two successful software and publishing companies prior to co-founding Medsn. He has worked directly with dozens of medical school faculty, colleagues, and consultants and corresponded with thousands of medical students from around the world. Dr. Bhushan earned his bachelor's degree in biochemistry from the University of California, Berkeley, and his MD with thesis from the University of California, San Francisco.

Chirag Amin, MD   Dr. Amin has extensive experience in the field of medical education and has served as a co-author with Drs. Bhushan and Le on the entire *First Aid* series. He also led the completion of *The Insider's Guide to the MCAT,* published by Lippincott Williams & Wilkins. Dr. Amin has an extensive background in Internet-related enterprises; he actively follows a number of development-stage Internet companies. Dr. Amin earned his BS in biology at the University of Illinois in 1992. He then went on to get his MD with Research Distinction from the University of Miami School of Medicine in 1996 and completed three years of residency training in orthopedic surgery at Orlando Regional Medical Center.

About the Authors

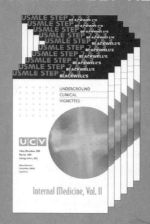
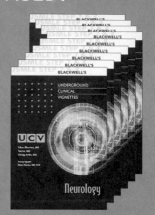
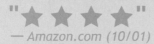